KU-158-922

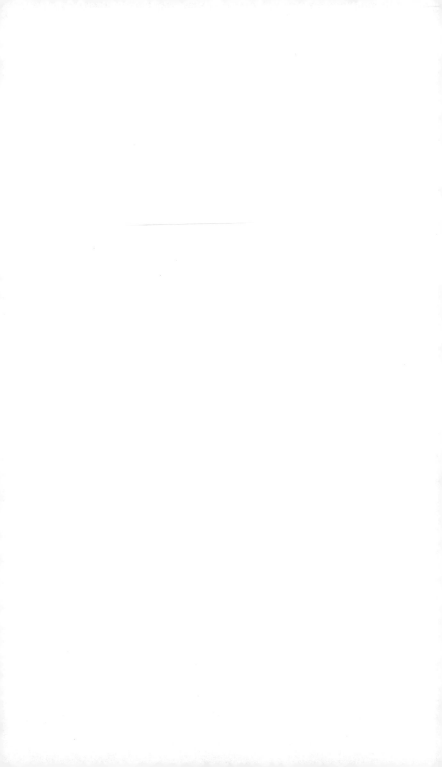

Social welfare with indigenous peoples

In many of the inhabited areas of the world, there has been an earlier population group (indigenous population) which has been subjugated or conquered by a more recent population group. In *Social Welfare with Indigenous Peoples* the editors and contributors have examined the treatment of many indigenous populations from five continental areas: Africa (Sierra Leone, Zimbabwe); Australasia (Australia, New Zealand); Central and South America (Mexico, Brazil); Europe (Nordic countries, Spain) and North America (Canada and the United States).

In investigating such questions as 'What are the social services that indigenous peoples receive?' and 'Are these services appropriate to their needs?', they found that, regardless of whether the newer immigrants became the majority population, as in North America, or the minority population, such as in Africa, there were many similarities in how the indigenous populations were treated and in their current situations. This treatment is examined from many perspectives – political subjugation; negligence; shifting focus of social policy; social and legal discrimination; provision of social services; and ethnic, cultural and political rejuvenation – to provide a complete picture of the treatment of indigenous peoples in comparison with other populations.

Social Welfare with Indigenous Peoples will be of particular value to undergraduates, researchers and lecturers in social anthropology, social policy and social administration.

Comparative Social Welfare Series
Edited by John Dixon

Social welfare in Asia
Edited by John Dixon and Hyung Shik Kim

Social welfare in the Middle East
Edited by John Dixon

Social welfare in Africa
Edited by John Dixon

Social welfare in Developed Market Countries
Edited by John Dixon and Robert P. Scheurell

Social welfare in Latin America
Edited by John Dixon and Robert P. Scheurell

Social welfare in Socialist Countries
Edited by John Dixon and David Macarou

Social welfare with indigenous peoples

Edited by
John Dixon and Robert P. Scheurell

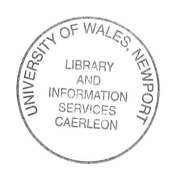

UNIVERSITY OF WALES, NEWPORT
LIBRARY
AND
INFORMATION
SERVICES
CAERLEON

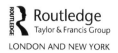

Routledge
Taylor & Francis Group

LONDON AND NEW YORK

First published in 1995
by Routledge
2 Park Square, Milton Park, Abingdon, Oxon, OX14 4RN

Transferred to Digital Printing 2005

Simultaneously published in the USA and Canada
by Routledge
270 Madison Ave, New York NY 10016

© 1995 John Dixon and Robert P. Scheurell, selection and editorial matter;
individual chapters, the contributors

Typeset in Times by
J&L Composition Ltd, Filey, North Yorkshire

All rights reserved. No part of this book may be reprinted or
reproduced or utilised in any form or by any electronic,
mechanical, or other means, now known or hereafter
invented, including photocopying and recording, or in any
information storage or retrieval system, without permission in
writing from the publishers.

British Library Cataloguing in Publication Data
A catalogue record for this book is available from the British Library

Library of Congress Cataloging in Publication Data
A catalogue record for this book has been requested

ISBN 0–415–05564–4

Printed and bound by Antony Rowe Ltd, Eastbourne

Contents

Contributors

J. C. Altman is the Director of the Centre for Aboriginal Economic Policy Research, Australian National University, Canberra, Australia.

Carmen Carriga is Vice-Directora of the Escola Universitaria de Treball Social, Barcelona, Spain.

Ian Culpitt is Senior Lecturer in Social Policy in the Department of Sociology and Social Work, Victoria University of Wellington, Wellington, New Zealand.

Alfred A. Jarrett is a Professor in the Graduate School of Social Work at the University of Texas at Arlington, Texas, USA.

Saliwe M. Kawewe is an Assistant Professor of Social Work in the Department of Social Work at Wichita State University, Kansas, USA.

Joyce M. Kramer is a Professor in the Department of Social Work at the University of Minnesota, Duluth, USA.

Celso Barroso Leite is in the Centro de Estudios de Providencia Social, Rio de Janeiro, Brazil.

Dave Lewis is an instructor at the International Graduate School, Stockholm University and is currently conducting research on Sami culture and welfare at the Department of Sociology, Stockholm University.

Sven E. Olsson is the Director of Graduate Studies in the Department of Sociology, Stockholm University.

Sandra Luz Navarro Pulgarin is a cross-cultural social worker in Durango, Mexico.

W. Sanders is a National Research Fellow in the Urban Research Programme in the Research School of Social Sciences, Australian National University, Canberra, Australia.

Hugh Shewell is a National Welfare Fellow and PhD candidate in the Faculty of Social Work, University of Toronto, Canada.

Annabella Spagnut is a practising social worker in Vancouver, Canada.

Preface

In all of the inhabited areas of the world there has been an earlier population group (indigenous population) which has been subjugated or conquered by a more recent population group. This volume in comparative social welfare policy consists of representative articles from five continental areas: Africa (Sierra Leone, Zimbabwe); Australia/Pacific (Australia, New Zealand); Central and South America (Mexico, Brazil); Europe (Nordic countries, Spain) and North America (Canada and the United States).

Regardless of whether the newer immigrants become the majority population, such as in North America, or the minority population, such as in Africa, there are many similarities in how the indigenous populations were treated and in their current situation. The treatment of indigenous populations can be viewed from the perspective of political subjugation; negligence; shifting focus of social policy; social and legal discrimination; provision of social services; and ethnic, cultural and political rejuvenation.

POLITICAL SUBJUGATION

In all of the countries represented there has been political subjugation of the indigenous population either through military action or economic/cultural encroachment. In all countries except two (Sierra Leone and Zimbabwe) there was initial subjugation, isolation and segregation of the indigenous populations, followed by a period of attempts at assimilation (an attempt to change and subvert the indigenous culture), followed again by periods of protection of the indigenous population up to the current demands for self-government, limited autonomy and legal rights.

In Africa (Sierra Leone and Zimbabwe) the circumstances were somewhat different since the indigenous population was the majority population. The tribes were allowed to maintain part of their old political and cultural traditions. The result was not assimilation as the goal, but coexistence. In both cases the majority indigenous population ultimately obtained their political independence from the conqueror. Sierra Leone gained its independence in 1961 and Zimbabwe in 1980.

In some countries there were attempts to enslave the population which were unsuccessful (United States) and successful for a time (Brazil).

In most of the countries the indigenous population have a special legal status. Only recently, however, have they been enfranchised and granted protected lands known as reservations, reserves, grazing land and so on.

NEGLIGENCE

In all of the countries represented there has been a tendency to neglect the social, educational and health needs of the indigenous population. In all of them there was a neglect of physical and health needs and educational opportunity, and housing and financial support was inadequate. Subsequently, the indigenous population relied on mutual aid (self-help) and traditional means of coping with problems. Initially, church or religious groups were predominant in working with the indigenous population group in all countries represented. The anticipation was to convert the indigenous population to a specific religion, mainly some branch of Christianity.

One of the reasons for the neglect of the indigenous population was the attempt to assimilate them, but this was generally unsuccessful, and special legislation was enacted, which created a separate or isolated population. In some cases, the neglect is partly attributed to the resistance of the indigenous population to assimilation (Mexico, the United States, Canada, the Nordic countries), which further created a sense of isolation.

SHIFTING FOCUS OF SOCIAL POLICY

In all countries, once subjugation was accomplished a general pattern emerged of separation (protective reserves, reservations, trust land, communal grazing land and so on); *assimilation* (special education, boarding schools, restriction on the practice of religion or of the use of language), *cultural protection* (recognition and preservation of cultural differences), and, more recently, *political and cultural rejuvenation* (claiming treaty rights, recognition of the maintenance of the culture).

The time sequence for this shifting pattern of the focal concern of social policy varies from indigenous groups, such as the Gypsies in Spain, the Sami in Nordic countries, the Temne in Sierra Leone and, more recently, the Canadian and American Indians. The overall time span of these changes in social policy covers 400 years (1500–1900), except for the Gypsies, where it was even earlier. It is noteworthy that in all cases there are currently demands (since 1960–70) for the fulfilment of treaty rights and some degree of autonomy, and in the cases of Sierra Leone and Zimbabwe the indigenous population (the majority) have assumed political control of the country.

SOCIAL AND LEGAL DISCRIMINATION

In all the countries represented there has been social and legal discrimination directed towards the indigenous population group. All of the countries have (or have had) special laws restricting the indigenous population to second-class status. The extent of this social and legal discrimination varied, from barring from citizenship (Brazil) to dual citizenship (United States). The previous attempt at assimilation through special schools is an example of this, such as in Mexico, United States and Canada, where individuals were not allowed to speak their own language or practise their own religion.

Currently, in all countries there has been great political and economic concern about social and legal discrimination, and attempts are being made to rectify the situation.

PROVISION OF SOCIAL WELFARE SERVICES

All of the countries represented have social-welfare services which are available to the indigenous populations, and they consist of housing, education, employment and social services (family and individual). The adequacy of these services is highly variable; for example, from inadequate (Brazil, Mexico) to minimally adequate (Australia, New Zealand and the United States).

In some countries there is a dual provision of services through organizations accessible to all citizens and those that focus on the indigenous population (for example, in the Nordic countries and the United States). In other countries the services provided to the indigenous population are no different from those offered to any citizen (for example, Sierra Leone and Zimbabwe). In other countries there are specialized programmes only; for example, Brazil. There is no clear pattern overall for the delivery of social welfare programmes.

ETHNIC, CULTURAL AND POLITICAL REJUVENATION

In all countries represented, since 1960 there has been a political, cultural, legal and economic rejuvenation. There is now a growing acceptance of the need for indigenous peoples to maintain their cultural identity. This has generated a growing demand that a society recognizes and tolerates the resultant cultural differences and that it acknowledges and deals with the serious social problems confronting indigenous peoples – in particular, problems of alcohol, suicide, cultural diffusion and changing family patterns.

OVERALL PERSPECTIVE

Similar patterns were found amongst all of the countries represented, with periods of subjugation, isolation/separation, assimilation, protection and ethnic/cultural and political rejuvenation. Differences were found in the role of the family and church as mutual aid elements, in maintaining the indigenous population, in the degree of separation – in Brazil and the Nordic countries – and in the provision of social services – in the United States and Zimbabwe.

Acknowledgements

We would like to thank all the contributors for their enthusiastic support of this volume.

To Mrs Cheryl Leeton go our thanks for typing the manuscript in its various drafts and in its final form.

Publication of this book, indeed the entire comparative series, would not be possible without the support received from the International Fellowship for Social and Economic Development Inc. (IFSED).

To our wives, Tina and Sally, go our thanks for putting up with our idiosyncrasies throughout the preparation of this manuscript.

For any errors of fact and for all opinions and interpretations, the authors and the editors accept responsibility.

John Dixon and *Robert P. Scheurell*

1 The First Nations of Canada: social welfare and the quest for self-government

Hugh Shewell and Annabella Spagnut

There are three distinct groupings of native peoples in Canada: the Indians, the Inuit and the Metis (McMillan, 1988). Amongst them there are many differences in social organization, culture and demographics, and, in this chapter, it would be impossible to explain in any detail the genesis and impact of government social policies upon all of them. Our discussion, then, will focus on the Indian (First Nations) populations of Canada. We do this for two reasons. First, they are the only native group defined and governed by specific legislation of the dominant Canadian state; that is, the Indian Act (Canada, Revised Statutes of Canada, 1988). Second, the general group of peoples referred to as Indians have inhabited North America for the longest period. Their historical relationship with the western European cultures is especially symbolic of the intrinsic dilemmas facing all native nations in Canada today and, in particular, is embodied in their present relationship with the federal Department of Indian Affairs and Northern Development.

THE HISTORICAL CONTEXT OF FIRST NATIONS–EUROPEAN RELATIONS IN CANADA

The fur trade, dispossession and subjugation

The history of First Nations–European relations originates during the period of the fur trade beginning in the sixteenth century. The fur trade can be seen as a period in which First Nations were not only drawn inexorably into the history of western European capitalism and expansion but also, as a result, one in which their own cultures and national groupings experienced profound changes in population, economies, social organization and geographic distribution (Trigger, 1985; Wolf, 1982).

The colonial period from the late eighteenth to the mid-nineteenth centuries was characterized by a distinct change in the attitude of Europeans towards First Nations and in the accelerated dispossession of their lands. Fisher (1977: 73) observed:

> Indigenous society and behaviour is viewed through a cultural filter that distorts 'reality' into an image that is more consistent with European preconceptions and purposes. The process is complete when the image . . . becomes the basis for policy and action.

The change in Europeans' attitude can be linked directly to their change in purpose from trade to settlement. Once the land became the object of European possession, Indians came to be seen as a hostile force, primitive savages who obstructed progress (Fisher, 1977: 94).

Following Canadian Confederation in 1867 the federal government, which had been given responsibility for Indian matters under the new constitution, continued the policy of 'civilization' and assimilation under laws carried forward from the colonial legislatures. Also, the government continued to make treaties with First Nations in western Ontario and the prairie territories as these areas became the object of rapid settlement and economic expansion (Frideres, 1988; McNaught, 1988). The post-Confederation period from 1867 until 1945 was a period best described as Indian subjugation, during which successive federal administrations attempted to make Indians completely subject to the will of the state. The federal government, in concert with provincial legislatures, continued to displace Indians from their lands and confined them to reserves for the purpose of civilizing them with white, European ways, and sought to create among them a menial, working-class population (Titley, 1986).

Beyond the world of Indian affairs Canada was changing. Rapid industrialization, the Great Depression of the 1930s and the Second World War had an enormous impact on social and economic thought in Canada. The inability of capitalism and free market principles to provide and distribute social and economic goods equitably and adequately, the sacrifice of life for the state in two world wars, and a state which was wanting in its constitutional functioning and responsiveness to economic crisis created a climate for significant domestic reforms in the post-Second World War period (Banting, 1987; Guest, 1985; Owram, 1986). By the end of the war Canada was a nation concerned about equality and the rights of citizenship: it was a nation set to embark on the path of the interventionist welfare state

(Guest, 1985; Owram, 1986). In the spirit of a new social consciousness, mainstream Canadians became more aware of the impoverishment of Indians and, with a certain collective shame, sought the amelioration of their condition in Canada (Miller, 1991).

The era of citizenship

Following the recommendations of the 1944 Parliamentary Committee on Post-war Reconstruction, and in response to public pressure, the federal government, in 1946, appointed a Joint House of Commons and Senate Committee on Indian Affairs. Its mandate was to enquire into the policies of the Indian Affairs Branch of the Department of Mines and Resources as well as into the general conditions of Indians living on reserves, with special emphasis on their status as citizens of Canada (Tobias, 1976; Canada, Special Joint Committee, Session No. 1, 1946, pp. iii–iv). The Committee reported to Parliament periodically over the course of its mandate, and these reports consistently centred on the necessity of advancing Indians to full citizenship. The fundamental assumption that Indians were to be assimilated was not questioned, but the tone of the assumption changed. It was no longer a question of subjugating Indians and of degrading their cultures, but of extending to them their rightful opportunities to be full and equal citizens of Canada. This required the state to become more active in their development and welfare. The state, through the Indian Affairs Branch, was to assume a positive mantle and become the advocate of Indian interests and the agent of their democratic equality.

The recommendations of the Special Joint Committee in 1948 set the policy agenda of Indian Affairs for the next 35 years. In 1949, in a symbolic move, Indian Affairs was made a branch of the Department of Citizenship and Immigration. This was followed in 1951 by the enactment of a new Indian Act which, while eliminating the worst features of the original Act, continued to mandate the Department to accomplish its same 'civilizing' aims (Tobias, 1976: 25–6). Throughout the 1950s and into the 1960s the Department emphasized the integration of Indians into mainstream society. Three areas were stressed: the education and social integration of Indian children; the provision of public works programmes on reserves to create the illusion of economic integration; and, the extension of provincial laws and services on to reserves so that Indians might be treated exactly like other Canadians (Miller, 1991; Shewell, 1991a; Weaver, 1981).

Persistent and endemic Indian poverty and unemployment gave rise to a further Joint Parliamentary Committee review of the Department's policies and progress beginning in 1959. One important outcome of this committee was the unconditional extension of the federal franchise to adult Indians in 1960. However, the work of the Indian Affairs Branch posed a more difficult problem. Citizenship and Indian integration had become yet another paternalistic mission of the government. In their own testimony before the Committee, Branch officials maintained that progress was slow partly because of varying degrees of Indian readiness to enter 'modern' Canadian life and partly because of the reluctance of the provinces to extend their services – especially welfare services – on to the reserves (Canada, Joint Committee of the Senate and of the House of Commons on Indian Affairs, *Minutes of Proceedings and Evidence*, 1959–61). The Committee ended by endorsing the objectives of Indian Affairs and called for more federal–provincial co-operation in their achievement.

In early 1963 influential pressure was again brought to bear on the federal government to find ways to alleviate Indian poverty and to develop programmes that would bring Indians into the mainstream of Canadian life (Weaver, 1981: 20–1). This pressure resulted in a commissioned, independent study of the Indian Affairs Branch, *A Survey of the Contemporary Indians of Canada*, known as the Hawthorn Report (Hawthorn, 1966; Weaver, 1981: 20–1). Central to the Report was a powerful theme supporting the integration of Indians into Canadian society through the full extension of social, political and civil rights coupled with the protection of their historically special status. Indians, the Report argued, should be regarded as 'citizens plus'. The Report, while critical of the Indian Affairs Branch, recommended its thorough reorganization (not its abolition, as some had hoped) and reiterated the necessity of the Branch being an advocate of Indian interests and a co-operative partner with them in future policy development (Weaver, 1981: 23–4).

Finally, the Hawthorn Report was especially critical of the provinces which, it opined, were at best indifferent to the plight of the First Nations. As the other key players to integration, the provinces were decidedly resistant to involvement in Indian matters (Hawthorn, 1966, in Getty and Lussier, 1983). Constitutionally, the provinces continued to insist that Indians were the sole responsibility of the federal government despite considerable opinion to the contrary (Shewell, 1991a; Weaver, 1981: 27). This created a *de facto* situation where Indian Affairs, in order to continue to promote integration, increasingly began to provide the services and infrastructure akin to provincial and municipal government at the band level.

We now come to a watershed period in the history of First Nations–Canada relations. The Hawthorn Report, while never fully endorsed by the federal government, did inspire considerable reform within Indian Affairs. But it was its theme of equal citizenship which carried forward into the federal government's next and boldest attempt to resolve the 'Indian problem'. Beginning in the late 1960s, the federal, Liberal administration of Pierre Elliott Trudeau entered into on-going consultation with First Nations' leadership to determine the future of Indian policy and of the Indian Act (Weaver, 1981; Miller, 1991: 223–9). In June 1969 it tabled in Parliament the *Statement of the Government of Canada on Indian Policy*, known as the White Paper. The White Paper proposed fundamental changes in the status of Indian peoples in the social structure of Canada. It recommended: the repeal of the Indian Act and its replacement by an Indian Lands Act; the end of the distinct status for Indians and the speedy assurance of full citizenship with attendant services and opportunities; and finally, the dissolution of Indian Affairs (Weaver, 1981: 166–7). The White Paper was seen by many to be a progressive document of the 1960s, in tune with social reform and civil rights. It proposed to end not only discrimination but also the insular colonialism of Indian Affairs, something the Hawthorn Report had failed to do (Weaver, 1981: 24). Yet its objectives were troubling. Upon analysis it was the continuation of a familiar theme: civilization and assimilation. But this time it was to be civilization without protection, citizen status without the 'plus'. Existing historical and treaty rights were to be ended and any outstanding grievances resolved through the proposed Indian Lands Act. Indians were to shed their Indian status forever, get on with being full and equal citizens, and forget about historical might-have-beens (Weaver, 1981: 55; Gibbins and Ponting, 1986; Tobias, 1976: 26).

Indian leaders condemned the government proposals. So intense was their opposition that the federal government withdrew the White Paper in 1971 and declared an end to assimilation policy (Weaver, 1981: 187). Some analysts (Gibbins and Ponting, 1986) assert that Indian policy has since been thrown into purgatory and never reformulated. We take a somewhat different view. Although the federal government dropped the legislative proposals of the White Paper the programme objectives remained in place. This meant that throughout the 1970s Indian bands were increasingly developed as modified forms of municipal governments. The federal government infused large amounts of funds into the provision of administrative and service infrastructures, as well as creating employment both in the on-reserve management of band affairs, the delivery of services and in community and public works (Driben and Trudeau, 1983). What could not be accomplished through legislation could still be done through the relentless expansion of federal and quasi-provincial programmes.

The quest for self-government

After 1971 the landscape against which the Department of Indian Affairs conducted its business changed rapidly. Up to 1971 the Department had administered its policy and programmes relatively unchallenged; now the entire Indian agenda of the Canadian government was under scrutiny not only by the Indian First Nations and their allied organizations but also by public policy groups and interested academics. The White Paper rejuvenated Indian politicization. Although Indians had always resisted government policies that resistance now entered a confrontational phase. Until 1969 Indians had sought economic and social justice through a co-operative strategy and had complied somewhat with the goals of citizenship providing they could maintain their unique status in Canada. The First Nations wanted to share in Canada without having to compromise their heritage and inherent rights. When, in 1969, it became apparent that the government still intended that they be assimilated, Indian strategy became proactive. Although Indian Affairs continued to expand and enrich its programmes, the political relationship with First Nations changed. Beset by government programmes which they were increasingly required to administer, but faced with continued economic and social deprivation, a politically articulate Indian leadership began to demand the right to self-government (Frideres, 1988; Miller, 1991).

In 1980, in an effort to allay Quebec separatism, Prime Minister Trudeau decided the country was ready to establish a renewed federalism through the repatriation of the constitution together with a charter of entrenched rights and freedoms. The task of repatriation was politically and legally difficult. Not only did the provinces have to agree to repatriation and an amending formula, but also to the principles and contents of the proposed charter (McNaught, 1988). The proposed charter attracted intense lobbying from various groups anxious to ensure that their rights were recognized and entrenched.

Significant among these groups were aboriginal peoples. At first, the provincial premiers refused to entrench the basic rights of aboriginals. But continued lobbying by their national organizations finally resulted in existing aboriginal rights being affirmed in principle, together with a specified, time-limited constitutional process during which those rights would be defined (Greene, 1989: 58–9, 234). All the provinces – with the critical exception of Quebec – agreed to the new accord, and the Constitution Act, including the Charter of Rights and Freedoms, became law in 1982.

Although federal government programmes continued to foster integration and 'mainstream normalization', there was a growing public understanding of the unique historical status of First Nations and of their demand for self-government. This was remarkably demonstrated in the 1983 *Report of the Special Committee on Indian Self-Government in Canada* (or the *Penner Report*) which repudiated assimilation policy and called on the federal government to entrench Indian self-government in the constitution. Moreover, the report urged the federal government to repeal the Indian Act and to replace it with legislation to maximize self-government until such time as it was entrenched. The Report did not specify the level of government Indians should have, but the recommended scope of powers, combined with fiscal transfer arrangements, implied a level akin to provincial jurisdiction (Canada, House of Commons, 1983: 63–4). Additionally, the federal government was to phase out the Department of Indian Affairs while also creating a Ministry of State for Indian First Nations Relations to protect and advocate Indian rights and interests (Canada, House of Commons, 1983: 122–5).

The *Penner Report* was not fully endorsed by the federal government but it did form the basis for much of the federal government's position during the follow-up constitutional task to define existing aboriginal rights. Unfortunately, the talks, chaired first by Prime Minister Trudeau and then, in 1984, by the new Prime Minister, Brian Mulroney, failed to achieve the necessary consensus, and aboriginal rights remained undefined. Ominously, however, self-government became a programme mission of the Department of Indian Affairs. It is important to observe that, as a programme, it ran – and continues to run – the danger of being absorbed into overall government policy (Boldt and Long, 1988) and – as Weaver (1981: xii) has warned – into the fabric of liberal ideology.

Quebec's failure to ratify the Constitution Act 1982 resulted in a new initiative by the Progressive Conservative government of Brian Mulroney. In 1987, Mulroney and the ten provincial premiers reached a secretive agreement known as the Meech Lake Accord. The Accord recognized Quebec as a 'distinct society' and, in so doing, in the opinion of many observers considerably weakened the powers of the federal government to the advantage of the provinces, not just Quebec (Behiels, 1989; Forsey, 1990; Granatstein and McNaught, 1991; Trudeau, 1988). Aboriginal peoples were particularly angered by the Accord. It again failed to acknowledge their distinct status in Canada and left them without a voice at the constitutional table. The impression was left that, in the nation-building process, the First Nations were politically irrelevant and, in the liberal, pluralistic state, were nothing more than another interest group (Miller, 1991). The provinces had three years in which to ratify the Accord, and the failure of even one to do so would result in its demise. As the 1990 deadline neared it was increasingly obvious that the Accord was in trouble. In Manitoba, through both a quirk in the debate procedure and a lack of will on the part of the governing party, the sole Indian member of the legislature, Elijah Harper, brought about the Accord's defeat (Miller, 1991).

The process of constitutional renewal, however, did not die. Through a complicated and complex array of subsequent government hearings and reports the beginnings of a new agreement took shape. Importantly, as this new agreement reached a stage when the elected provincial representatives were ready to finalize its substantive content, the aboriginal leaders – at their and Ontario's insistence – were included at the constitutional table. On 28 August 1992 the Prime Minister of Canada, the ten provincial premiers, the leaders of the two territorial governments and of the aboriginal peoples reached a new constitutional agreement. Critical to the agreement, termed the Charlottetown Accord, was the recognition and entrenchment of the inherent right of aboriginal self-government as well as re-defined powers for Quebec and the other provinces (*Globe and Mail*, 29 August 1992). The new accord, at the time we write, while representing a breakthrough for the First Nations of Canada, faces many hurdles. The first is a national referendum on its acceptance scheduled for 26 October 1992. Although Canadians would seem to support the provisions for aboriginal self-government, there is emerging discontent in English Canada for often divergent reasons over various aspects of the Accord as well as strong separatist opposition in Quebec (*Globe and Mail*, 14 September 1992).

CULTURAL AND DEMOGRAPHIC CHARACTERISTICS

Cultural characteristics

Within First Nations there are ten major cultural and linguistic groups, made up of 58 dialects living within five main regions of Canada. The groupings are outlined in Tables 1.1 and 1.2 and shown in Map 1.1. These groupings are by no means static but have changed, and will continue to change over time as people move and circumstances change (McMillan, 1988: 6). Today these groupings are located on about 2,241 reserves and divided among 592 different bands. Like the cultural groupings, the number of bands and reserves also varies over time according to government policy (Frideres, 1988: 150). Indian First Nations in Canada are as culturally diverse from one another as they are from the mainstream Canadian population. This means that it is possible only to identify certain common characteristics which might be said to differentiate them from other Canadians. We have selected two which we believe highlight this difference.

Perhaps the most important cultural characteristic of the First Nations is embodied in their attachment to and relationship with the land. This relationship is best reflected in the following statement:

> For thousands of years, we have lived with the land, we have taken care of the land, and the land has taken care of us. . . . We have been satisfied to see our wealth as ourselves and the land we live with. It is our greatest wish to be able to pass on this land to succeeding generations on the same condition that our fathers have

Table 1.1 First Nations: cultural and linguistic groupings by region

Linguistic group	Region
1 Algonquian	Eastern woodlands, Plains Subarctic
2 Athapaskan	Subarctic Plateau, Plains
3 Siouan	Plateau, Plains
4 Wakashan	Northwest coast
5 Salishan	Plateau, Northwest coast
6 Iroquoian	Eastern woodlands
7 Tsimshian	Northwest coast
8 Haida	Northwest coast
9 Tlingit	Northwest coast
10 Kutenai	Plateau

Source: McMillan (1988: 3–6)

Table 1.2 Distribution of status Indian population by provinces and territories, 1990

	Population	
Province	*Total*	*On-reserve*
1 Atlantic (Newfoundland, Nova Scotia, New Brunswick, Prince Edward Island)	19,319	12,968
2 Quebec	48,551	33,802
3 Ontario	112,826	58,702
4 Manitoba	72,238	46,708
5 Saskatchewan	75,441	39,336
6 Alberta	60,303	37,873
7 British Columbia	83,894	44,064
8 Northwest Territories	11,379	194
9 Yukon	6,227	345

Source: Canada, Indian and Northern Affairs, *Indian Register Population by Sex and Residence*, 1990: xi

> given it to us. We did not try to improve the land and we did not try
> to destroy it. That is not our way.
>
> (Blake, 1975, cited in: Watkins, 1977: 8)

This concept of the land, and its association with identity and culture, are inherent in the definition of Indians and their rights. It is a concept which non-Indians have difficulty in understanding. The land possesses and nourishes the Indian: in return, the Indian cares for and celebrates the land. Land is not a commodity: it is the gift of life, and it is the way of life. From this idea of the land flows the meaning of Indian spirituality, community, self-government and sovereignty.

The second, significant, common attribute of First Nations' cultures is their understanding of the individual. In the dominant culture's view the individual is the fundamental unit of society and is thought of as self-reliant, competitive and acquisitive. Society, or the community, is considered to be merely a collection of individuals each looking after their own interests and needs. The sense of community is derived from the role of the state as a regulator and arbitrator of competition so that each individual's freedom to pursue their interests is protected. In summary, the dominant culture views the individual as primarily sovereign, a state unto themselves. It is the fundamental premise of liberal society, the premise of possessive individualism (Macpherson, 1962).

In First Nations' cultures there is a fundamental respect for the individual. However, this respect should not be confused with the possessive individuals of the dominant culture; rather, respect for the individual is intrinsically tied to the equal value accorded to the community collective. The unique value of individuals is determined through their contribution to the well-being of the collectivity, not through their personal achievements or 'successes'. The community – the interconnectedness of individuals, families, kinship systems and the land – is the source of the individual's complete being. Thus, the individual's existence, material and spiritual, derives its entire meaning from the community: the two are inseparable (Ontario, 1992: 6–7).

Demographic characteristics

Status Indians (those persons registered under the Indian Act) are the fastest growing population group in Canada. Their total population on and off reserve has increased by 45.5 per cent in the nine-year period 1981–90 from 336,900 to 490,178. By 1991, the total status population was projected to be 521,500, a further 6.4 per cent increase. In 1991, status Indians represented about 2 per cent of the total Canadian population. A breakdown of the 1990 population by the provinces and territories of Canada is shown in Table 1.2.

The Indian on-reserve population in 1990 was 273,992 or 56 per cent of the total status population (Canada, Department of Indian Affairs and Northern Development, *Highlights of Indian Register Population by Sex and Residence*, 1990: xi; *Aboriginal Conditions, 1981–2001*, Part I: 4). Of this number, 133,697 (49 per cent) were female and 140,295 (51 per cent) were male. Of all male and female status Indians, 59 and 53 per cent respectively lived on-reserve. Finally, status Indians on-reserve are a young population with a median age in 1991 of 22 years. Table 1.3 shows on-reserve age distribution from 1981 projected to 2001.

Occupation and sources of income

There are few current data on occupational distribution among Canada's First Nations. The most recent data from 1989 (Table 1.4) provide a basic distribution of the experienced labour force by occupation type, and reflect a significant trend away from primary to tertiary (service) occupations. Siggner (1986: 72–4) already noted this trend in occupational distribution of occupations and sex. Siggner found that, of the women in the labour force living on-reserve, about

Table 1.3 On-reserve age distribution (percentages) 1981–2001

Ages	1981 (%)	1991 (%)	2001 (%)
0–14	40	37	34
15–64	55	59	62
65 +	5	4.37	5

Source: Canada, Indian and Northern Affairs, *Highlights of Aboriginal Conditions 1981–2001*, Part I, 'Demographic trends': 11 & 26

Table 1.4 Distribution of experienced Indian labour force (percentages)

Group	Occupation type Primary (%)	Secondary (%)	Tertiary (%)
Total Status Indians	12.9	8.9	68.6
Indians on-reserve	15.5	6.7	67.6

Source: Canada, Indian and Northern Affairs, *Highlights of Aboriginal Conditions 1981–2001*, Part III, 'Economic conditions': 34.

30 per cent were engaged in managerial or professional occupations, compared to about 14 per cent of the men. Similarly, women compared to men on-reserve were both numerically and proportionately higher in all the tertiary occupations, such as clerical (23.3 to 2.8 per cent) and services (24.7 to 8.8 per cent). He concluded that it 'would appear that the majority of the experienced Indian labour force as of the 1980s is now engaged in tertiary occupations and that Indian women lead the way in terms of occupying the managerial/ professional/technical category' (1986: 74).

In the 1986 Canadian mid-census, the on-reserve labour-force participation rate for persons over the age of 15 years was about 43 per cent. Among Indian males the participation rate was 53.3 per cent, and among females, 32.3 per cent. Of the on-reserve Indian population over the age of 15 years, 57 per cent did not participate in the labour force, while, of those participating in the labour force, the employment rate was 28 per cent. Not only do less than half of those eligible to participate in the labour force report that they do so, but only slightly more than a quarter of those report employment. In comparable non-aboriginal populations living near reserves the employment rate was almost 52 per cent, and the labour force participation rate 59.6 per cent (Canada (1989) *1986 Census*

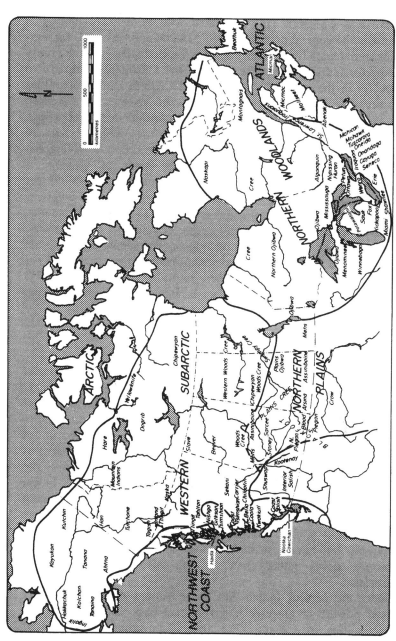

Map 1.1 The First Nations of Canada
Source: Miller, 1991: xii

Highlights on Registered Indians: 20–1; Canada, *Basic Departmental Data*, 1990: 74–9).

In 1985 the average individual income of registered Indians on-reserve was C\$9,300. This compared with an average individual income in the general population of C\$18,200 and C\$14,700 for non-Indian individuals living near reserves. Similarly, the average family income for Indians on-reserve in 1985 was C\$20,900, compared to C\$38,700 in the general population and C\$29,800 in communities near reserves. These comparisons are useful because, in a market, cash economy, Indians on-reserve are at a considerable disadvantage with respect to their earning and purchasing power. Although data are not available, it is generally conceded that the cost of living on-reserve, especially in rural and remote areas of Canada, is considerably higher than elsewhere. Additionally, almost 50 per cent of on-reserve Indians rely on government transfer payments (social assistance, old age pensions and so on) as a source of income, compared to 28 per cent of comparable populations near reserves. Finally, of those Indians living on-reserve who reported income, 48 per cent stated that it derived from employment compared to 63 per cent in non-Indian communities near reserves (Canada (1989) *1986 Census Highlights*: 20–1, 24–7; Canada, Indian and Northern Affairs (1989) *Highlights of Aboriginal Conditions*, Part III: 15, 38).

Legal and political status

Registered Indians, on- and off-reserve, are Canadian citizens and enjoy the rights and most benefits of Canadian citizenship. A main exception to benefits is that most provincial governments do not extend their social services on to reserves. This is an issue related to the constitutional division of powers and will be discussed in the following section. Indians are eligible to vote in provincial elections within the province of their residence and in all federal elections. The meaning of citizenship is historically problematic to Canada's Indian peoples. Until 1960 citizenship was equated with enfranchisement and the loss of legal Indian status. Since that year, when Indians were unconditionally granted the franchise, they have enjoyed the rights of citizenship but have also had to fight continually to protect their collective rights rather than be subsumed into the pluralist mainstream.

Under the present Indian Act, First Nations communities have limited powers of on-reserve government akin to but lesser than municipalities in Canada. The federal government has always envisaged municipal status as the preferred level of government for First Nations communities, and one community, the Sechelt Indian Band of British Columbia, has chosen this level for itself (Cassidy and Bish, 1989). Despite the entrenchment of the inherent right of aboriginal self-government in the Charlottetown Accord, the Accord has yet to be approved; thus the scope of self-government remains to be negotiated.

THE SYSTEM OF SERVICES

The constitutional division of powers and the Indian Act: the system in context

Canada is a Confederation made up of ten provinces and two territories. The division of powers between the federal state and the provinces is articulated principally under Sections 91 and 92 of the Constitution Act 1867. These sections are referred to as the enumerated powers: Section 91 defines the federal powers; Section 92, the provincial (Irving, 1987: 327). Importantly, Section 91 (24) gives the federal government exclusive responsibility for matters related to 'Indians and lands reserved for Indians'. Through this power the federal government derives its authority to legislate and administer the Indian Act.

Of importance to social policy in Canada are subsections 91(1a) and 91(3), which, over time, have come to be interpreted as the general spending power of the federal government (Irving, 1987: 327–8). The spending power provides the federal government with the means by which to provide direct 'payments to individuals, institutions, or other governments for purposes on which Parliament does not necessarily have the power to regulate' (Banting, 1987: 52). Through this power and through constitutional amendment the federal government has been able to provide universal welfare benefits, such as the Family Allowance and the Old Age Pension, simply on the basis of citizenship and *without encroaching on provincial jurisdiction*. After the Second World War, and in line with its Indian policy, the federal government used the general spending power to foster Indian citizenship and to set an example to the provinces. Today, Indian persons continue to benefit directly from these universal programmes like all other citizens of Canada.

Under Section 92 of the Constitution Act the provinces were given the responsibility for social welfare matters, including health and education. Pursuant to this section the provinces have the sole responsibility to legislate and make regulations for health and welfare services. Accordingly, only the provinces legislate, regulate and provide a broad range of personal social services, child and family services, basic social assistance and adult institutional care. Provinces also legislate and provide public health, hospital and medical services as well as housing and all matters related to education (Armitage, 1988; Banting, 1987; Manzer, 1985).

An unresolved question in Canadian constitutional law continues to be whether or not federal responsibility for Indians under Section 91 (24) includes Indian social welfare. There are various complicated arguments related to this question. Some centre on the relationship between the enumerated federal and provincial powers (federal powers superseded provincial powers) and the unique status of Indians; while others focus on the extent, if any, to which Section 88 of the Indian Act – a section which declares that all laws of general applicability in a province apply to Indians in the province – includes provincial social welfare legislation. At this time, with the principal exception of Ontario, the only provincial welfare service extended on-reserve is statutory child protection. This jurisdictional impasse affects other areas in the general scope of welfare, such as education, housing and health. The federal government assumes, without prejudice, responsibility for assuring the general health and welfare of First Nations but it will not legislate specifically in these areas (DIAND, 1984).

Beyond questions of jurisdiction between Ottawa and the provinces is the fundamental issue of Indian self-government. It can be seen from the preceding description that jurisdiction has been a bilateral issue between the federal and provincial governments. Since their rejection of the 1969 White Paper, the First Nations have been openly hostile to agreements made between Ottawa and the provinces, the federal government and themselves, especially in child welfare and education services. But it became evident that, even with such agreements, ultimate statutory authority still lay with the provincial governments. Indians, as interested third parties, established only the right to administer programmes according to provincial policies and federal-provincial funding formulas while the issue of control remained unresolved (DIAND, 1984: 68; DIAND, 1991).

A more recent strategy was a First Nations demand for federal legislation in these service areas. In their view federal legislation would further the fiduciary trust relationship implicit in the Royal Proclamation and required of the federal government. Furthermore, it would symbolize a more equal relationship between federal and First

Nations' governments in that it would evoke the historic principles of partnership and coexistence. First Nations argue, and rightly so, that they treated with the federal government and its predecessors, not with the provinces. Federal legislation would therefore emphasize and confirm the unique status of First Nations within Canada and their special relationship with the government of Canada. This strategy continues to some extent.

The latest jurisdictional strategy of the First Nations was the entrenchment of their inherent right to self-government in the Canadian constitution. This right, as we have noted, was recently incorporated in the Charlottetown Accord, but the scope of jurisdiction has yet to be determined. Undoubtedly, First Nations will contend that the powers of self-government must include jurisdiction over such matters as health, justice, education, housing, social security, child welfare and social services. It is within this context of constitutional reform, therefore, that the ensuing description of the present system of services occurs.

The current service delivery system

Because of the various federal–provincial issues affecting the nature of service provision on Indian reserves it is impossible to describe one uniform system throughout the country. However, some common characteristics do apply. The federal government derives authority from the Constitution Act 1867 to administer matters of concern to Indian peoples and the Department of Indian Affairs and Northern Development (DIAND) through the powers of the Indian Act (Revised Statutes of Canada, 1988) is the federal agency responsible for its administration. Because Canada is a parliamentary democracy the Department is accountable through the Minister of Indian Affairs and Northern Development to Cabinet and thus to Parliament in Ottawa. Today, the Department is a large, complex bureaucracy centralized in its corporate policy and programme structure but decentralized in its programme and service delivery (see Figures 1.1 and 1.2).

During the 1970s the Department placed special emphasis on community development and Indian band management training with the expectation that Indians themselves would eventually assume the responsibility of administering the Department's programmes on the reserves (Shewell, 1991b: 63; Weaver, 1981). Throughout the 1980s this theme continued, but with added emphasis placed on self-government in the wake of the Penner Report. In effect, DIAND contrived its own interpretation of Indian self-government as an enriched version of its on-going ideas on self-government from as early as the late 1950s: absolute devolution of programme administration to the Indian band level. Devolution, together with the idea of self-government as a form of municipal administration, resulted in the restructuring of the Department depicted in Figure 1.1.

In the field there are nine Regional offices, each headed by a Regional Director General (see starred boxes, Figure 1.1), and each reflecting key components of the central administration. The Regional offices relate directly with Ottawa and, with their District offices (see Regional Office example, Figure 1.2). The District Offices are responsible for the operation of the Indian bands within defined geographic areas. In recent years the cost-cutting measures of the Progressive Conservative government and a certain desire to reduce direct bureaucratic interference in Indian communities has entailed the considerable reduction of personnel and the restructuring and refinement of the functions of the central and regional operations. However, the essential policy–programme relationships between headquarters and the regions remain the same.

The on-going, daily service functions are subsumed under the Intergovernmental Relations sector. In Ottawa, this sector develops the broad guidelines, standards and funding levels for the various services in consultation with both the Policy and Financial sectors. At the Regional level (see, for example, Figure 1.2, page 20) programme services are part of Operational Policy. While Operational Policy is responsible for the functional direction of these programmes, Funding Services, together with Finance, controls annual programme planning and fiscal allocations, and Intergovernmental Affairs provides the developmental, substantive context of self-government as well as liaison with provincial administrations where this is necessary. At the Regional level there is a certain amount of autonomy in Operational Policy. Although Ottawa provides overall functional direction and support, the Regions have considerable flexibility in adapting programmes to their own requirements in response to the uniqueness of their constituent Indian bands and of the provinces in which they are situated.

Entry into the service system is at the band level. There are few bands which do not administer at least some of the Department's programmes. Over the past twenty years, First Nations communities have developed significant planning and administrative bureaucracies with which both to negotiate and deliver these programmes. The size and capacity of the band administrations vary depending upon the

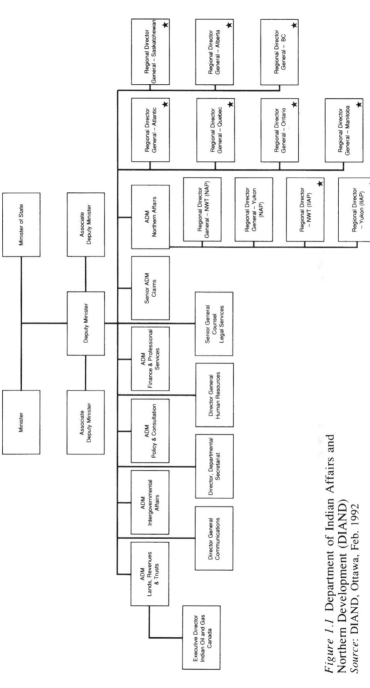

Figure 1.1 Department of Indian Affairs and
Northern Development (DIAND)
Source: DIAND, Ottawa, Feb. 1992

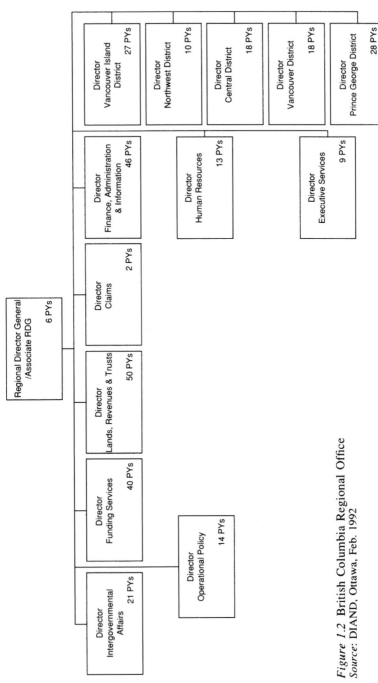

Figure 1.2 British Columbia Regional Office
Source: DIAND, Ottawa, Feb. 1992

populations of the communities and their own perceived expertise in providing any or all of the direct services. Small bands, for example, will often ally with other bands from their tribal grouping to form a tribal council. Such a council serves as a master planning and funding conduit for all the member bands as well as providing professional advice, consultation and training. Also, a larger band will occasionally administer programmes on behalf of a smaller band, For our purposes, however, it is best to describe the service delivery system as delivered through a single band administration.

Although administrations vary depending upon the size of a band, its wealth, geographic location, needs and so on, they share many attributes. Typically, a band replicates liberal forms of democratic government: there is an elected chief and council pursuant to the Indian Act and a separate band administration accountable to the council. Bands are empowered to enact and administer by-laws in functional areas specified under Section 81 of the Indian Act but in fact their jurisdictions out of necessity exceed their defined authorities. This is generally because the Department itself offers programmes which are outside its own authority to do so (Frideres, 1988: 242). Band administrations tend to be organized around the Departmental programmes they deliver. Most have a core staff consisting of a band manager, secretary, bookkeeper, and maintenance person. In addition, there are frequently some or all of the following staff functions: finance and accounting, economic development, education, social work, drug and alcohol counselling, community health band membership, land use, recreation, housing, employment, community planning, community maintenance and engineering, and so on. Occasionally two or three functions might be performed by one person. In small bands it is not uncommon, for example, for the band manager to perform other functions like social work or housing.

In the past these programme functions were performed by departmental personnel. Now they are performed by band employees whose line accountability is to the chief and council but who receive constant advice, consultation and policy directives from the Department. This bifurcation is – or can be – a constant source of conflict between bands and the Department. We will return to this issue later in the chapter. In a very real sense, however, band administrations have simply replaced Departmental line staff as the entry point for services. They follow Departmental policies and procedures and access funds using Departmental formulas and fiscal planning instruments. Thus they, like many other quasi-governmental organizations, enjoy administrative independence but in fact represent an extension of the government itself. Nevertheless, an Indian individual no longer depends upon DIAND officials for services but can go to the local band office and receive services or gain access to them directly. This is an improvement over past practices, but it is a long way from Indian autonomy and control over their own programmes.

THE SOCIAL DEVELOPMENT PROGRAMME: THREE SERVICES PROVIDED

Background

We turn now to a description of the principal social services provided by the Department of Indian Affairs through its Social Development Programme. The Social Development Programme is comprised of three main elements: Child Welfare, Individual and Family Care; Adult Care; and Social (Income) Assistance. Today, the programme accounts for at least one-quarter of the annual C$2.25 billion budget for Indian Affairs (Canada, DIAND, *Indian Education*, 1989). Until after the Second World War the only welfare expenditure of any significance was for basic relief. As early as the immediate post-Confederation period the Department authorized the issue of 'relief assistance' in the form of rations to destitute Indians. It was provided to the sick, the elderly, and to widowed women and their children, but able-bodied adults were assisted only in unusual circumstances. In most cases relief was in response to widespread starvation or extreme hardship and was limited to essential staples, blankets, clothing and ammunition. Relief was granted on authority of the Department by the church missions, by the Hudson's Bay Company trading posts and, as the agency system expanded, by the Indian Agents. Funds expended for relief were charged against a band's trust account or, where a band did not have sufficient funds to meets its own needs, were approved specially by Parliament. There was no statutory provision for welfare expenditure, and the Department, in keeping with the *laissez-faire* attitudes of the period, generally held to the idea that Indians, like all individuals, were responsible for their own well-being.

Only after the Second World War, and following the recommendations of the 1946–48 Parliamentary Committee, did a more articulate policy begin to develop on welfare matters. Because it was now held that welfare services were integral to the rights of citizenship, the extension of welfare services on to the reserves would constitute an important gesture on the part of the provinces in bringing Indians into the Canadian fold. But the continuing refusal of all the provinces – with the important exception of Ontario – to provide services led the federal government to develop a comprehensive policy for social assistance. Throughout the 1950s Indian welfare expenditures rose dramatically, necessitating a more rationalized method for its administration. This resulted in the introduction of a needs test, a nationally standardized scale of benefits, and the introduction of individualized cheque payments to welfare recipients (Shewell, 1991a). But the Department did not give up its overall objective to have the provinces provide services.

In July 1964, the Department received permission from the Treasury Board to allow each region to adopt local municipal or provincial rates and administrative standards in the provision of social assistance. It also received further permission from the Treasury Board to relieve bands of the financial responsibility for social assistance. Funds were now directly budgeted by the federal government. These changes were partly due to the Department's fear that its own benefit scale was contributing to a shamefully high Indian mortality rate. But they also fit a wider strategy to provide provincially comparable services which would facilitate their transfer to provincial jurisdiction (Shewell, 1991a). A federal–provincial conference in late 1964, however, failed to produce the agreement the federal government sought. Instead, there was a general agreement that provincial welfare services be extended on the basis of *separately* negotiated agreements with each province and then only to those First Nations communities which agreed to accept them. Ontario – which as early as 1955 had extended its Child Welfare and Social Assistance services on to reserves – was the only province to enter such an agreement with the federal government (Shewell, 1992). The 1965 'Canada-Ontario Indian Welfare Services Agreement' – which remains in effect – was, much as the Department's Welfare Division bureaucrats had originally envisaged, a blanket provincial agreement. Despite the success of the Ontario agreement as a funding mechanism, similar provisions under Part II of the Canada Assistance Plan 1966 – the federal welfare cost-sharing legislation – failed to induce the provinces to follow suit (Shewell, 1992).

Although the provinces have refused to extend their social assistance, family and personal services on to reserves, they have reached individual agreements with the federal government for the provision of child protection. This has meant, as we noted earlier, the exercise of mandatory child apprehension according to the terms outlined in each province's legislation. It is not entirely clear why the other provinces chose to isolate and provide this one service without similarly providing the support and preventive services associated with family and child welfare. Presumably the answer lies in the interpretation of Section 88 of the Indian Act and what has been perceived to be the sole aspect of jurisdictional applicability: the *action* of protecting a child due to parental *failure to comply* with community standards of acceptable care (Canada, DIAND, *Indian Child and Family Services in Canada – Final Report*, 1987: 4; Hawley, 1986).

Child welfare and individual and family care

The child welfare programme has three main parts: protection, foster care (including treatment and adoption) and support services. Child protection and foster-care services are provided by each province, while support services are provided by the Department.

Child protection and subsequent foster-care services are the sole domain of the provinces. Indian child welfare has thus been subject to the statutory terms and policies enunciated by provincial legislatures and their welfare departments. Although there is a strong liberal tradition in Canada to respect the privacy of the family, there is a degree of public consensus on the necessity of state intervention when a child is believed to be in need of protection. Commonly, situations requiring intervention are defined by community standards surrounding physical, sexual and emotional abuse as well as physical and emotional neglect. In the past, Indians have exercised little or no control or influence over these programmes and their mainly white, European, bourgeois origins.

Child welfare programmes had little impact on First Nations until the 1960s. This was due to the existence of residential schools, to the absence of children from the reserves, and to the relatively minimal presence of child welfare authorities in provinces prior to the expansionary influence of the Canada Assistance Plan. The late 1960s, however, produced what has been referred to as 'the sixties swoop' (Johnston, 1983). In the final years of that decade child welfare authorities apprehended Indian children from their homes on-reserve in unprecedented numbers and placed them in white foster homes, usually far away. In many instances these children were placed for adoption; most never to return to, or indeed never to know

Table 1.5 On-reserve children in care, registered Indian population, Canada, selected years 1966/67–1990/91

Fiscal year	Children in care	Children aged 16 and under	Percentage
1966/67	3,201	93,101	3.4
1971/72	5,336	94,777	5.6
1976/77	6,247	96,417	6.5
1978/79	6,177	94,866	6.5
1981/82	5,144	94,608	5.4
1986/87	3,603	101,841	3.5
1990/91	4,352	109,165	4.0

Source: DIAND, Canada, *Basic Departmental Data*, 1991: 47

or remember their native background. The pattern worsened during the 1970s, and only the strengthening political voice of the First Nations created a gradual decline in the rate of Indian children in care. By the middle 1970s the 'swoop' had peaked at 6.5 per cent, but even by 1991 had not returned to the more 'moderate' levels of the early 1960s. In comparison, the mainstream rate of children in care was 1.2 per cent in 1981 and 0.8 per cent in 1987. Thus, Indian children in those years were 4.50 and 4.75 times as likely to be in care (Canada, DIAND, *Highlights of Aboriginal Conditions 1981–2001*, Part II, 1989: 17). Table 1.5 highlights the pattern and extent of the problem.

Several factors no doubt accounted for this phenomenon. The residential school system resulted in generations of children growing up knowing only institutional care. As these children became adults and parents, many lacked the skills to raise children and were often ignorant of their own cultures' indigenous nurturing patterns. At the same time the 1960s witnessed a significant expansion of the welfare state in Canada, including the growth of child welfare services and the concurrent employment of both trained and untrained social workers (Guest, 1985). The desire to ameliorate the plight of Canada's native peoples led to a misguided, culturally biased perception that the 'rescue' of Indian children from the dire poverty on the reserves and their placement in white foster homes would afford them the love and opportunity they required to be happy and successful adults in Canadian society. This was simply a new wrinkle on the integration theme, and has since been roundly condemned by First Nations' leaders as nothing less than cultural genocide (Johnston, 1983; Wharf, 1987: 9–10). Because child welfare was a provincial responsibility, and because 'the sixties swoop' abetted integration objectives by placing Indian children in white homes, the Department of Indian Affairs did not question the unfolding reality of Indian children permanently removed from their communities. Finally, child apprehension was a powerful procedure. Social workers exercised a professional judgement based on legal criteria to decide if a child should be removed from a home. Once they made the decision to apprehend, there was little a parent could do to stop its occurrence. Indeed, in difficult situations social workers would be accompanied by the police. When First Nations communities became a target for child welfare concerns they discovered themselves to be isolated and virtually powerless in trying to prevent the removal of their children. They were confronted by provincial systems which, in most other respects, ignored them, and by their own federal Department which did not consider child welfare any of its concern. Thus, unlike any other programme affecting their communities, the First Nations had no clear means by which to influence provincial child welfare policy.

Now, in the early 1990s, although the numbers of Indian children in care remain too high, there are indications that they will continue to decline. Underlying the decline is an increasing assertion by First Nations of control over their own child welfare. Before examining this issue, however, it is necessary to review briefly the child welfare programme as it continues to function – Ontario excepted – for about 50 per cent of First Nations communities.

- Under provincial child welfare legislation social workers investigate any report that a child may be in need of protection.
- Depending upon the circumstance a decision may be made to remove a child from her/his home or to provide support and remedial services to prevent such action. Until the early 1980s these alternatives to apprehension were not available to First Nation communities. Conditions were allowed to deteriorate until removal became necessary.
- Following provincial family court hearings children who remain in care are placed in foster homes, group homes, or treatment facilities if required. Services are then provided to the family in an attempt to enable the return of the child to home. Similarly, until the 1980s these services were not available to the First Nations. Children who were apprehended from reserves stood a far greater chance of remaining in care and of being placed for adoption.
- The federal government, through the Department of Indian Affairs,

assumes responsibility for the costs of care only; that is, once a child is apprehended and placed in care the federal government pays the province a negotiated per diem allowance. The per diem may vary depending upon the type of care and services provided *to the child*. Since 1982 however, increasing funds have been available to bands prepared and able to provide preventive and support services.

(DIAND, 1987)

Although Ontario has been an exception to this pattern, the services it has provided – as with mandatory child protection – have been culturally dissonant. Even though there has been a richer service delivery pattern in Ontario, the services have been largely seen as inappropriate (Interview, Director, Ontario Indian Social Services Council, 1991).

First Nations control of child welfare

The control of child welfare and its related services has become a dominant issue for First Nations and has paralleled the demand for self-government (Wharf, 1987). Indian concerns about child welfare and autonomy became apparent as early as 1969 when the Blackfoot Band of Alberta first began to develop and provide on-reserve services to prevent the apprehension of their children. This led in 1973 to the first tripartite agreement between a First Nation, the provincial and federal governments for the provision and funding of a range of family and children's services subject to provincial supervision (DIAND, *Indian Child and Family Services in Canada – Final Report* 1987: 17). Then, in 1980, a dramatic confrontation in British Columbia between the Spallumcheen Band and the provincial Welfare Minister, Grace McCarthy, resulted in her acquiescing to the band's demand for control of its child welfare programme. The band enacted a child welfare by-law under Section 81 of the Indian Act. Although the band by-law was outside the jurisdiction of the Indian Act, the federal Minister of Indian Affairs failed to veto it. Thus, it remains in effect (Johnston, 1983; Wharf, 1987).

Under the by-law the band enters into annual funding agreements with the federal government to provide a range of protective, support and prevention services. While the Spallumcheen model is technically illegal under current law, the band's actions at the time served to catalyse First Nations to pressure both provincial and federal levels of government to accord them greater involvement in child welfare matters (DIAND, *Indian Child and Family Services in Canada – Final Report*, 1987: Appendices 2, 4). Since then, and in response to Indian representations, both the federal and provincial governments have gradually moderated their positions with respect to jurisdiction, funding and control. Initial changes came mainly from the provinces, many of which introduced new or amended child welfare legislation which required First Nations representatives to be notified and involved in protection proceedings and in-care planning. In some instances legislation also permitted the province to enter into service agreements with First Nations representatives to deliver both statutory and non-statutory services. New policies also required social workers to account for social and cultural differences and to be more involved with band social workers in prevention and support (DIAND, 1987: 3–5).

The changes in provincial legislation and the strong Indian representation obliged the Department of Indian Affairs to revise its own policies and to develop a long-range strategy for increased Indian control over child welfare services. Central to the federal approach, however, was its insistence not to legislate in the area of Indian child welfare believing that such action would infringe on provincial jurisdiction. In May 1982, the Department issued a policy statement in which it endorsed the transfer of government-administered social services to First Nations communities as and when they were ready to assume control. This policy fostered an increase in the already established mechanisms of bipartite and tripartite agreements among the three levels of government. Nevertheless, by 1986 there was such a variety of agreements in place that the Department decided it was necessary to conduct a review of the national situation with a view to Cabinet approving a fully rationalized policy (DIAND, 1987: 1–5). A task force was appointed and, in 1987, it produced a report, *Indian Child and Family Services in Canada – Final Report*. The Report and its recommendations formed the basis for present federal Indian child welfare policy.

The Report found that in 1985/86 there were 292 service agreements in place, among which there were four distinct variants. Rather than stating a preference for one type of agreement over another, the Report simply analysed the features of each and examined the relative costs of service delivery in relation to the levels of transferred provincial authority and the patterns of services offered in different provincial jurisdictions. What the Report did note was that, as service delivery and transferred levels of authority became more complex, it was preferable that a band develop its own

Indian Child and Family Service Agency (ICFS) distinct from the band administration *per se* (DIAND, 1987). In 1989, Cabinet approved what might best be termed a developmental policy with respect to Indian child welfare:

> Cabinet did endorse several basic principles . . . the federal government will continue to fund and support the expansion of Indian child and family services on reserve as resources become available, in cooperation with Indian people and the provincial governments. This funding and support will be in accordance with provincial legislation and at a level comparable to the services provided off reserve in similar circumstances. . . . Cabinet also approved the basic objectives of a . . . management framework which would not only make life easier for Indian child welfare agencies by providing them with stable . . . funding, and more flexibility in their budgets, but would also improve agency management and accountability.
>
> (DIAND, *Indian Child and Family Services in Canada*, 1987
> Management regime discussion paper, 1989: 2.)

Under the new policy bands enter a process in which they progress to the highest level of transferred authority permitted under their provincial law. This can include the power to apprehend as well as to plan and provide appropriate preventive, remedial, support and in-care services. Adoption services may be included, but day care services – an area of great need on many reserves – may not. The Department further seeks to negotiate standardized tripartite agreements with each province with a funding formula applicable to each level of service that a band assumes, beginning with the provision of preventive services only up to the provision of a completely comprehensive family and child welfare programme. The negotiated funding formula applies both to the actual service and to its staffing. In addition to the negotiated agreement there must be a provincially approved statement by the band of its family and child welfare standards (DIAND, Programme Directive, ICFS Programme Directive, 1991; ICFS Management Regime Discussion Paper, 1989: 10).

There are, however, certain constraints on the policy. First, developmental and operational funding is limited on the basis of the availability of resources. Developmental costs are especially high because they include professional consultation and initial capitalization (see Tables 1.7 and 1.8). Thus, the number of bands able to enter the process in any one year is limited. This leads to further methods

Table 1.6 Child welfare and individual and family care, actual and projected expenditures, 1989/90–1991/92

	Actual 1989/90	Projected 1990/91	1991/92
Developmental funding	404,400	1,561,600	526,500
Operations	53,851,900	60,336,500	62,044,900
Maintenance	53,412,000	57,756,800	65,721,400
Total	107,668,300	119,654,900	128,292,900

Notes:
Development includes costs of pre-planning, start-up, development and negotiation of Indian standards and consultation.
Operations covers the costs of Indian social services, ICFS agencies, staffing, administration, etc.
Maintenance refers to the costs of children-in-care, including provincial and on-reserve care, group homes and institutions.
Source: Canada, DIAND, Social Development Directorate, 'SEAS national report, child welfare and individual and family care', Ottawa, 1990

Table 1.7 Total and per child-in-care expenditures, registered Indian children living on-reserve, 1965/66–1990/91

1 Fiscal year	2 Children in care	3 Total C$ exp	4 Per child C$ exp	5 Total C$ exp 1986 C$ exp
1965/66	2,889	2,464.0	853	n/a
1970/71	5,156	10,042.0	1,948	31,479.6
1975/76	6,078	16,076.0	2,645	36,371.0
1980/81	5,716	29,485.7	5,158	43,877.5
1981/82	5,144	34,740.7	6,754	46,014.2
1986/87	3,603	71,979.7	19,978	71,979.7
1989/90	4,178	102,797.6	24,605	90,173.3
1990/91	4,352	122,456.3	28,150	102,519.4

Note: C$ in columns 3 and 5 reported in millions rounded to nearest hundred; e.g. 1980/81: C$29,485.7 = C$29,485,700.00. All C$ are based on a constant dollar using the 1986 Consumer Price Index.
Source: Canada, DIAND, *Basic Departmental Data – 1991*, 1991: 49

of assessing and establishing priorities for band proposals. Second, proposals are preferred from bands or groups of bands with an on-reserve child population (0–18 years) of at least 1,000, although bands with less population will be considered. It is thought that small populations are neither cost-effective nor suitable for acceptable professional intervention given the greater likelihood of relatives

Table 1.8 Registered Indian adults from on-reserve in residential care, 1971/72–1990/91

Fiscal Year	Adults in care	Adult population over 17 years	Ratio per 1,000
1971/72	335	87,585	3.8
1975/76	318	102,282	3.1
1980/81	567	121,263	4.7
1986/87	459	153,947	3.0
1990/91	561	174,445	3.2

Source: DIAND, Canada, *Basic Departmental Data*, 1991: 51

having to deal with one another. Herein lies the source of the child welfare quagmire. Many bands simply don't have that number of children, nor are they close to other bands which do, nor would they necessarily wish to affiliate with them.

Because the federal government refuses to pass Indian child welfare legislation, First Nations are left with a model of family and child welfare which, regardless of the extent to which it is adapted, remains essentially alien to their own social systems. It is not a model of their choosing. Within provincial legislation and programmes are tacit assumptions about privacy, about families, their function, roles and responsibilities in liberal society, their appropriate caring patterns and their relationship with the wider community. The idea of professional intervention is thus defined by these assumptions. They are not in the least Indian. Although the federal policy appears progressive – and it is a clear improvement over past policy – ultimately it fails to consider the possibility of other models of child welfare natural to each First Nation. Thus, the extent to which First Nations can adapt the concept of child welfare and its services to their own cultures remains subject solely to provincial authority.

Not surprisingly, there is some ambivalence on the part of First Nations to embrace the federal policy wholeheartedly. Naturally, many are taking advantage of a policy which permits them, within their respective provincial jurisdictions, to acquire as much control as possible. Yet the real issue is jurisdiction. First Nations are generally opposed to provincial statutory authority, and most prefer the idea of federal legislation, which, they believe, would be more responsive to their cultural concerns. But ideally they desire, through recognition of the inherent right to self-government, the jurisdiction to conceive, legislate and administer their own family and child services completely within their own cultural and legal traditions (Wharf, 1987; Interview, Ontario Indian Social Services Council, 1991).

Adult care

Adult care is subdivided into two elements: In-home Care and Institutional Care.

In-home care

This programme provides basic homemaking services to the chronically ill and the elderly, and to physically or mentally disabled persons, with the objective of assisting them to remain at home within their own communities. Services provided under this programme include meal preparation, cleaning, laundry, essential shopping, and other chores related to housekeeping. The service is available on a comparable basis with the relevant provincial programme and is offered under the same terms and conditions. Thus, eligibility, needs testing, recipient contribution and the actual range of services provided vary from province to province.

Access to the service is through the band social worker. The assessment of need for the service may be made by a provincial public health nurse, and on-reserve community health nurse, or some other person recognized as having the skills to make an informed judgement. A needs test to determine if the programme will contribute to all or part of the cost of the service is conducted by the social worker. In most regions, a set number of hours per month is available for any one recipient, and recipients may therefore only receive financial assistance according to the number of hours of service they receive up to the set maximum. The service may be provided by a recognized off- or on-reserve agency (sometimes part of the band's social service administration) or by an individual. Funds for In-home Care are determined and allocated through the annual database exercise. They are based on the band's own projections, using the required number of hours multiplied by the approved hourly rates. Further analysis of band submissions by the region, headquarters and Treasury Board determines the final allocations (DIAND, BC Region, *Policy and Procedure Manual*, Vancouver, 1991).

Institutional care

Adult persons who require protected, supervised care due to chronic illness, age, physical or mental disability must often be institutionalized in a suitable facility. The Department, through the Institutional Care programme, pays for the costs of care of eligible registered Indians (*Policy and Procedures Manual*, 1991; DIAND, BC Region, *Basic Departmental Data*, 1990: 97; DIAND, Kovach, 1990: 31–5). Because many reserves lack a sufficient population base to build and support the operation of even a small facility, the likelihood is great that Institutional Care must be found off-reserve and purchased through provincial or proprietary operators. Institutional Care may be for limited or indefinite periods, and in most provinces falls under the jurisdiction of the department responsible for health, hospitals and medical treatment.

Many provinces refer to the entire system of Adult Care as long-term care, meaning that there is a continuity of care beginning with In-home Care and progressing, by levels of institutionalization, to extended care requiring constant nursing. Thus, Indian adults who receive In-home Care on-reserve are often already known to provincial authorities since they have 'entered the system'. Ideally, this ensures a regular reassessment of an individual's condition and the identification of future care requirements.

Access to Institutional Care, like In-home Care, is a dual process. The band social worker is responsible for assessing an individual's financial ability to pay for the care, and a provincial health authority usually assesses the level of care required. Funding is projected and allocated on an annual basis through the database exercise similar to and in conjunction with In-home Care. Approved per diem rates and total care days are used to determine the amounts required. In most regions the per diem rate for Institutional Care varies according to the level of care required and whether or not the institution is privately or publicly operated. Recipients of care who can do so must pay all or part of the applicable per diem charge. The band social worker's financial assessment, conducted according to provincial guidelines, determines what, if any, contribution a recipient is required to make. Recipients of full or partial subsidy may, depending upon prevailing provincial social assistance policy, receive an additional monthly 'comforts' allowance for personal and recreational needs and periodic clothing allowances.

Jurisdiction is an issue of particular importance in these cases. Depending upon the province, rules concerning residence and responsibility may apply. In some provinces, like British Columbia, the Department is responsible for the recipient's per diem contribution if the recipient lived on-reserve at the time of admission. Otherwise, the province accepts responsibility. In other provinces the Department is expected to pay for the costs of institutionalization whether or not the recipient of care lived on-reserve at the time of admission (DIAND, Kovach, 1990).

Although the numbers of Indian adults in Institutional Care are not many, the issues related to the provision of care are sensitive. Indians, like other Canadians in the twentieth century, have benefited from advances in medicine and health care. Many Indian health problems and a resultant shortened lifespan arose from disease introduced by Europeans, inadequate sanitation and housing, and poor diet caused by the severe disruption of traditional methods of food production and preparation. Life expectancy, while still below that of other Canadians, has continued to rise from an average 63 years in 1976 to 69 years in 1991 (DIAND, Canada, *Basic Departmental Data*, 1991: 22–3; Frideres, 1988: 144). Increased life expectancy has created a greater need for Adult Care institutions. But, like the removal of children from reserves, the necessity of placing adults – usually elders – in institutions off-reserve can be distressing not only for the adult but also for the family group and the community life and detrimental to the imparting of wisdom and spirituality to the youth and the leaders of the band. Thus, when disability or old age necessitates their extended care in institutions off-reserve it can be a confusing and lonely experience for them as well as a loss to the community.

There are no easy resolutions to this problem. Besides the lack of a large enough base population to warrant the development of facilities on most reserves, there is also a problem with respect to their licensing. Because Adult Care constitutionally falls under provincial jurisdiction, provinces have been reluctant to enter reserves and approve those facilities which do exist for fear that they appear to be accepting responsibility for Indians (DIAND, Kovach, 1990: 32). The absence of licensing, however, presents legal problems with respect to supervision, the quality of care received and responsibility for negligence or malpractice, fire, and so on. Nevertheless, a growing sentiment exists amongst First Nations that Adult Care institutions can and must be situated on-reserve and that alternative, innovative forms of providing such care can be developed. Part of the solution lies, then, in the ability to create culturally appropriate models of adult care on a scale which is compatible to their present and

Table 1.9 Total and per adult-in-care expenditures, registered Indian adults living on-reserve, 1971/72–1990/91

1 Fiscal year	2 Adults in care	3 Total C$ exp	4 Per adult C$ exp	5 Total C$ exp constant
1971/72	335	663.0	1,979	2,078.4
1975/76	318	1,330.0	4,182	3,009.1
1980/81	567	4,257.0	7,508	6,334.8
1986/87	459	8,916.3	19,425	8,916.3
1990/91	561	15,853.9	28,412	13,266.9

Note: C$ in columns 3 and 5 reported in millions rounded to nearest hundred; e.g. 1975/76: C$3,009.1 = C$3,009,100.00. All C$ are based on a constant dollar using the 1986 Consumer Price Index.
Source: DIAND, Canada, *Basic Departmental Data*, 1991: 53

relatively stable elderly population of about 5 per cent. Another problem lies in the current round of constitutional reform, and whether or not First Nations – within a recognized right to be self-governing – are able to negotiate jurisdiction over health as well as welfare matters.

Social assistance

Social Assistance is not only the largest single annual expenditure within the Social Development programme (DIAND, Canada, *Basic Departmental Data*, 1991) but it also symbolizes the overwhelmingly dependent condition in which First Nations' communities find themselves. We have already observed its importance to the issues of integration, constitutional jurisdiction and the extension of provincial services. We have also noted that in 1964 the Treasury Board authorized the Department to issue assistance according to local municipal or provincial rates and standards. Since 1964 – despite the defeat of the 1969 White Paper – and while other Departmental programmes have been modified in an attempt to reflect changing Indian realities, the Social Assistance programme continues to be governed by this same authority, a symbol of the aims of integration and citizenship (Cassidy, 1991: 8).

Of course, since 1964 the Social Assistance programme has increased in scope and complexity; but its fundamental aim – to offer to First Nations communities welfare services comparable to those available to mainstream Canadians – has remained unchanged. Because it adopts the essence of each provincial system it is not possible to describe one programme which applies universally. Still, the provincial systems, including Ontario's, are derived from a common model of social assistance which is categorical and residual in nature. It is characterized by the idea of individual self-reliance and the principle that assistance by the state to persons in need is a measure of last resort. Persons are categorized as either employable or unemployable, and this categorization generally determines both the level of benefit and the conditions attached to eligibility. Certain traditional, moral pejoratives are also publicly attached to all recipients of social assistance, but especially to the 'employable', who are seen to be less deserving and who must be constantly admonished to seek their welfare through the labour market (Guest, 1985; Ontario, *First Nations' Project Team Report* 1992: 6–10; Shewell, 1991b).

There are three main components of the Social Assistance programme: Basic Needs, Special Needs and Service Delivery (*Policy and Procedures Manual*, 1991; Canada, DIAND, 1984).

Basic Needs

The Basic Needs component of Social Assistance is the core benefit package of the programme. In departmental language it is referred to as 'mandatory, non-controllable', meaning that if eligibility is established for Basic Needs the benefits *must* be provided. Basic Needs is comprised of two allowances: support and shelter. The support allowance is intended to provide recipients sufficient monthly payment for the costs of food, clothing and personal necessities. Eligibility for Social Assistance immediately entitles a recipient to the support allowance, the amount of which is determined by a scale of benefits set by family size. However, employable status may reduce support entitlement, while age and/or disability will increase it. The shelter allowance is intended to cover the essential monthly shelter costs of eligible recipients. Depending upon the provincial system, essential shelter costs can include rent or mortgage payments, heating, electricity, telephone, fire insurance, water, garbage and sewage disposal costs. Shelter allowances are also set according to family size but may vary depending upon actual costs. Although shelter allowances parallel those of the provincial system, the Department contends that on-reserve shelter costs should be lower than off-reserve. The shelter costs should be lower because government contributions to the Indian housing and its maintenance supposedly minimize the need to charge rent. The reason for this is that most on-reserve housing stock is built by departmental funds and managed by the bands. Bands may charge a small rent to offset some costs, but it will never approach off-reserve, for-profit, market rent. This situation is gradually changing due to an increase in mortgageable housing through the on-reserve Social Housing programme sponsored by the federal Central Mortgage and Housing Corporation.

Four variants of Basic Needs bear mentioning:

1 The monthly 'comforts' and the occasional clothing allowances mentioned in the adult care section are a form of Basic Needs allowances. Adults in institutions who are eligible for subsidized care are therefore eligible for these additional benefits.

2 Children who require temporary care outside their own home due to the temporary absence or disability of the usual parent or custodian may receive a monthly allowance payable to the temporary caregiver. Sometimes referred to as Child Outside Parental Home (COPH) or Guardian Financial Assistance (GFA), this allowance is not intended to replace child welfare intervention. In reality, because of First Nations' resistance to provincial statutory intervention COPH/GFA is often used as a method of avoiding provincial authorities, sometimes with their knowledge and consent.

3 Room and board allowances are issued as Basic Needs, but in most provinces they are a variation of the combined support and shelter allowances. The actual costs of room and board may be paid up to a maximum based on family size. In some cases a 'comforts' portion is factored out for the personal needs of the recipient.

4 Increased Basic Needs to assist with extra costs associated with a permanent mental or physical disability are available to persons who meet provincial eligibility guidelines. Referred to as Handicapped or Disabled Person's Allowances, they are normally available to persons who (a) are eligible for Basic Needs; (b) have a medically certified condition or permanent disability; and (c) can demonstrate that the condition incurs additional monthly expenses.

Special needs

These are a range of supplementary allowances which may only be accessed if eligibility for Basic Needs has been established. Most of the allowances are one-time grants although some, such as special diet or natal allowances, may continue over a set period. Special Needs allowances are defined by the Department as 'mandatory, controllable', meaning that they must be paid but only if funds are available within the budget allocation. Each allowance usually has its own eligibility criteria patterned after the comparable provincial benefit. Special Needs usually includes a discretionary, crisis or emergency grant. Frequently it is used as a one-time supplement to the support allowance so that a recipient may purchase extra food or clothing. The governing criteria normally entail an appraisal of the hardship which might be suffered if the grant was denied.

Funding for Special Needs is problematic. The Department considers it a controllable expenditure and allocates set budgets to band administrations. Also, due to fiscal restraint its annual growth rate has been severely restricted. But Special Needs allowances often respond to situations which are unpredictable and for which provision *must* be made. Typical of these are funerals, house fires and extra food. Unexpected emergencies can decimate Special Needs, thus limiting the extent to which other projected needs can be met. Conversely, an unexpected emergency need near the end of a fiscal year may go unmet if the Special Needs budget has already been expended. The Department at both regional and national levels is attempting to devise a funding formula for Special Needs which might address this problem. However, in our opinion, until certain items like burials, December bonus, diet and natal allowances are charged to Basic Needs – as is the case in the provincial systems – the problem cannot be resolved.

Service delivery

The Social Assistance programme was one of the first departmental programmes to permit administrative devolution to the band level, and, since the middle 1960s, band social workers have become an important occupational group on-reserve. Before bands assume any responsibility for child welfare services they nearly always have a history of administering Social Assistance and Adult Care. Because of the complexity of the issues and programmes which they administer, and the skills they require to perform their jobs effectively, band social workers as a group have become a major factor in influencing universities and community colleges to develop social work education and training programmes unique to their needs and communities.

Through the Service Delivery component, the Department funds annual salary, benefits and travel costs of band social workers responsible for Social Assistance. The number of workers per band that the Department is willing to fund varies from region to region, depending upon the formula that each region has devised. Most formulas are based on on-reserve population, historical caseloads or a combination of both. Salary levels are determined by qualification and experience, and conform either to provincial or federal salary scales. Travel funds cover routine trips to reserve lands isolated from the main reserve or to regularly scheduled training and information meetings with other workers and departmental officials.

As the Service Delivery component implies, applicants for Social Assistance apply through the social worker at their band office. Band social workers take all applications, determine eligibility and authorize the issue of benefits. They also provide information, counselling and referral services. Benefits are issued at the band office or – in the case of larger bands – are mailed directly to the recipients. Applicants or recipients who feel aggrieved by a social worker's decision have the right to appeal, and this process also begins at the band level, although its final outcome may be determined at the regional office of the Department.

Band social workers and the band administration are responsible for maintaining monthly and annual statistical data for auditing and database funding purposes. Each region has its own variant on the database exercise. In Ontario, where the relationship with the federal government is purely administrative, the database tends to be conducted as a global exercise. But in British Columbia, for example, band social workers are required to project the size and demographic make-up of the Basic Needs caseloads, together with their average unit costs and known provincial rate adjustments. Similarly, they must project and justify their Special Needs and Service Delivery requirements. In every other respect the database exercise follows the same process as in Adult Care. Administrative costs for Service Delivery are funded through Indian Government Support, a separate Department programme.

Dependency, cultural compatibility and control

The most disturbing aspect of Social Assistance on-reserve is the high level of dependence upon it as a sole source of income and support. Tables 1.10 and 1.11 outline the Indian aggregate on- and off-reserve dependency rate and expenditures. Where data have been available, the on-reserve rate is consistently 1.5 times that of the aggregate. In comparison the aggregate rate is about 3.5 to 4 times greater than the national rate of 7.25 per cent (Canada, Department of Health and

Table 1.10 Average number of Social Assistance cases and total dependants per month, registered Indian population on- and off-reserve, 1981/82–1990/91

Fiscal year	Average no. of cases per month	Average no. of dependants per month	Dependency rate (%)
1981/92	39,146	88,079	27.2
1986/87	50,879	114,478	29.5
1987/88	54,170	121,882	29.3
1988/89	56,573	127,290	28.7
1989/90	59,680	134,280	28.8
1990/91	64,360	144,810*	29.6*

Note: The on-reserve figures were not separately available except for 1986/87 and 1989/90. In those years, the on-reserve dependency rate was 43.7 and 42.3% respectively. It is probably reasonable to assume that the on-reserve rate is consistently about 1.5 times the aggregate rate.
* The 1990/91 figures are estimates based on preliminary data.
Sources: Canada, DIAND, *Basic Departmental Data*, 1991: 5, 55; DIAND, Social Development, '1989–90 Average monthly Social Assistance recipients and dependency rate by Region', MYOP DISK 2, Ottawa: 25 Oct. 1990; Shewell, 1991b: 20

Table 1.11 Social Assistance expenditures, registered Indian population, Canada, 1976/77–1990/91

1 Fiscal year	2 Number of cases	3 Total C$ expenditure	4 C$ per case	5 Total expenditure
1976/77	n/a	78,660,000	n/a	165,600,600
1980/81	n/a	141,985,300	n/a	211,287,649
1981/82	39,146	165,030,100	4,216	218,582,914
1985/86	48,494	255,288,200	5,264	265,925,208
1986/87	50,879	278,070,900	5,465	278,070,900
1990/91	64,360	459,634,000	7,154	384,631,297

Source: DIAND, Canada, *Basic Departmental Data*, 1991: 57

Welfare, Telephone Information Services, 1990), whereas the on-reserve rate can be at least six times greater. The dependency rates are all the more disturbing when it is understood that Social Assistance is generally designed to be a temporary means of support, and that the benefits themselves are well below government defined poverty lines (Canada, *National Council of Welfare Incomes, 1991*, 1992). This means that in a liberal market economy where cash is critical to the acquisition of goods, First Nations' communities are significantly deprived.

The problem of Social Assistance on-reserve reaches far deeper than the dependence itself. It can be convincingly argued that Social Assistance, a programme which implicitly assumes a 'private trouble' to be resolved through individual self-reliance, is indeed very much a 'public issue' which can only be addressed through economically and politically empowering means. The issue of Social Assistance dependence in First Nations communities is intimately linked to the history of the fur trade, dispossession and the policies of assimilation and integration. Moreover, the idea that Indian poverty can be relieved and solutions found through Euro-Canadian welfare state measures was, and is, a profoundly, ethnocentrically misguided assumption (Asch, 1977: 50–6; Ontario, *First Nations' Project Team Report*, 1992: 5; Shewell, 1991b). Historically, like any independent and economically self-sufficient peoples, First Nations had their own ways of coping with times of scarcity and hardship. But the hegemony of the Canadian state and their reduction to wards of the federal Crown systematically denied First Nations their inherent capacities to develop solutions to their own problems (Ontario, *First Nations' Project Team Report*, 1992: 5).

The main impact of the Euro-Canadian Social Assistance programme has been its individualization of poverty and the undermining of the collective and traditional patterns of helping, sharing and co-operation centred on interconnected kinship systems (Asch, 1977: 55–6; Ontario, *First Nations' Project Team Report*, 1992: 8). There is an important reason for the individualization of poverty in a liberal society. Dependence on collective or state charity is perceived to be a burden on the collective since a basic principle of liberal society is the freedom of the individual to accrue wealth to herself or himself. Thus, to support others is understood to undermine the principle. But, as we noted in our discussion of cultural characteristics, the interdependence of the individual and the collective in First Nations' cultures is fundamental to their social organization. Thus, benefits directed solely at the individual or the nuclear family are detrimental to collective responses to scarcity and the distribution of wealth.

Not only is the organizing principle of categorical Social Assistance inappropriate to First Nations' cultures but it is also largely impractical. The desired solution to reliance on state support is that the recipient obtain employment in the wage economy. The securing of employment depends on the existence of a vibrant, accessible labour market. In Canada, nearly 63 per cent of the First Nations population live in rural or remote locations. This means that the majority of the First Nations live *at least* 50 kilometres from a centre where there is a labour market (DIAND, Canada, *Basic Departmental Data*, 1991: 14, 99). A recent report observes:

> First Nations experiencing . . . lower dependency rates are . . . in areas that have fairly ready access to the wage economy – there appears to be a . . . correlation between dependency rate and increasing remoteness from such areas. Clearly, a system designed to assist individuals . . . to make it through short term weakness in the wage economy is not and has not been an adequate response to the needs of communities that are . . . on the outside or on the periphery of this economy.
>
> (Ontario, 1992: 9)

Even where wage labour is more accessible, results have been mixed. On the whole, Indians are underemployed given their labour market participation rate, and this is largely due to employer discrimination and the loss of jobs to technological change (Frideres, 1988; Shewell, 1991b). Opinions differ about the harmfulness of wage labour on First Nations societies (Asch, 1977; 1984; Usher, 1985; 1993: 114–15), but one point is clear: the high dependency rate occasioned by the relationship between wage labour and Social Assistance can only be resolved if First Nations gain jurisdiction over their own social welfare policy and achieve significant control over the development of their own economies and their relationship with the outside labour market.

It is remarkable that the Social Assistance programme – the subject of considerable criticism by the First Nations and the symbol of such economic dispossession – has received so little attention from the Department. Social Assistance is a mark of powerlessness. Criticism of the programme is a double-edged sword because, whereas it may be valid, it is nevertheless necessary to have the infusion of money into the communities if only to ensure a baseline survival. This point was not lost in a cogent report (TAP Associates, 1979) on the programme's impact in Ontario, sardonically entitled, *A Starving Man Doesn't Argue*. The Department's chief response to welfare dependency has been the initiation of on-reserve employment creation programmes which utilize Social Assistance Basic Needs entitlements to make up part of a wage. These programmes, while producing limited community benefits, have largely failed in their overall objectives; that is, the creation of permanent employment on-reserve or the development of transferable skills to the outside labour market. In effect, Social Assistance transfer programmes have simply moved money around while temporarily masking the continuing dependency (Shewell, 1991b).

The Department is reluctant to look at how Social Assistance might be better conceived in First Nations communities for two reasons: first, at a basic level the Department remains committed to the principle of comparability to the provincial systems; and second, the 1964 Treasury Board authority – which binds the Department to that principle – is a secure and easily justified funding source. To abandon the 1964 authority might jeopardize what are now relatively assured budget levels. For their own part, First Nations have little leverage, with the exception of Ontario, in effecting change in the provincial systems. The federal government will not interfere in an area of provincial jurisdiction, nor, as in child welfare, will it legislate its own Social Assistance programme. But the fact that the federal government chooses to deliver Social Assistance according to provincial regulations is only of incidental interest to the provinces. Because First Nations are not direct recipients of provincial Social Assistance, whatever they might think of the provincial programmes is of little concern to the provinces. Consequently, First Nations have no choice but to pressure the federal government to change its policy or – as often happens now – simply to ignore or stretch regulations under a policy which they perceive to be inappropriate or counter-productive (Shewell, 1991b).

But what of Ontario, the exception? The province is presently undertaking substantial reform of its Social Assistance legislation as the result of an influential 1988 report, *Transitions,* in which considerable attention was devoted to the unique issues affecting First Nations. Because under current Ontario legislation First Nations are delegated considerable administrative powers, they are considered legitimate stakeholders in the reform process. A recent task force composed mainly of First Nations representatives recommended the inclusion in new provincial legislation of a specific First Nations clause. The special clause would permit First Nations a range of options from adherence to the mainstream programme to acquisition of almost complete jurisdiction and the capacity to develop their own models of social assistance (Ontario, 1992: 19, 26–35). Jurisdiction, as it is in all the Social Development programmes, is at the heart of the issue. Ideally, Ontario's First Nations desire the constitutional right to legislate their own Social Assistance programme. But in the absence of that right – and with questions of jurisdiction still to be negotiated even if the right to self-government is achieved – the proposed Ontario legislation is an important step forward. Should Ontario accept the recommended legislative approach – and there is reason to believe that it will – First Nations in other provinces will be hard-pressed to ignore its significance. It will represent the example they require to push the federal government to abandon the policy of comparability and to encourage the exploration of real alternatives.

CONCLUSION

Three distinct themes emerge from our discussion of the Social Development programme which can be said to apply to and reflect the history of the relationship between the Department of Indian Affairs and the First Nations. These are paternalism, programme devolution and the quest for self-government. Although the days of more overt forms of paternalism – where Indian Agents treated and referred to Indians as children – have passed, its vestige and the aims of assimilation policies remain in the concepts and conditions implicit not only in Social Development but in most of the Department's programmes as well. In a sense, it is a more insidious form of paternalism, couched in technocratic and bureaucratic language and appearing rational and benign.

This new form of paternalism began to take significant form as the period of subjugation passed and the Canadian perception of Indian issues changed from one where Indians *were* the problem to one where Indians, like all citizens, *had* problems. In response, the government increasingly introduced full welfare-state measures in an effort to create greater equality of citizenship and opportunity for the First Nations. But, for them, the welfare state has consisted of an onslaught of government programmes to achieve their social integration which have resulted in a situation of imposed and ghettoized dependency. Moreover, welfare-state measures for First Nations have not fostered equality with other Canadians either materially or socially. On the contrary, the welfare state has been but another chapter in the history of liberal capitalism bringing a peculiar notion of 'progress' and 'enlightenment' to peoples presumed to be underdeveloped and inferior. As long as First Nations are thought to be not ready developmentally and are subject to models of social policy assumed to be better, yet are alien to their societies and incongruent with their economies and politics, then paternalism will continue to flourish.

The administrative devolution of government programmes to the bands has had many implications for the First Nations. Positively, it has increased access to services and lessened the tension of interface between a dominant and subordinate culture. But it has also served to satisfy current neo-conservative agendas such as cost-cutting and government down-sizing in the name of First Nations self-government. A justifiable complaint of First Nations is that they have been asked to do the Department's dirty work but have not benefited directly or indirectly from positions lost to the Department. Thus, they are required to 'do more with less' (Interview, Assembly of First Nations, Media Relations Department, 13 Nov. 1991). Devolution has also tacitly compelled bands to adopt forms of organization distinct from their own and more congruent with departmental and, in some cases, provincial structures. In addition, band administrations answer to two lines of authority: as employees they are responsible to their chief and council, but their programme direction comes from the Department. This can create an internal conflict, where the elected council may direct an employee to administer a programme in a manner contrary to departmental regulations. But in the end, either by virtue of the Indian Act or by the terms of their administration agreements with the government, the Department's authority prevails. There is then the sense of a charade: the continuing management of Indians under the guise of Indian self-management (Cassidy, 1991: 9); AFN, Media Relations, 1991).

Related to devolution is the way in which First Nations have been drawn into competition for scarce resources. Scarcity is generated by the Department, which determines the fiscal amounts available for each programme area and sets the terms of the competition. It is, as some First Nation members have wryly observed, the old game of divide and conquer. Indeed, it is often too easy to be diverted from the fundamental issues when daily bread and butter are at stake. In this sense, according to AFN officials (Media Relations, 1991), devolution has been a headache and a hindrance to substantive change.

The most problematic issue of devolution is the cultural incompatibility of the programmes First Nations are asked to administer. In addition to the programmes' inherently alien administrative process, there is, in the genesis of the programme models, a basic conflict with Indian cultures. This is the incompatibility rooted in the differences of world-view, in the meaning of community and of individualism. Current departmental initiatives are designed to address some of these concerns, notably the Alternative Funding Arrangements Program (a form of limited block funding) and the Self-government Sector (an opportunity to opt out of the Indian Act and become a form of municipal-style government). But even these initiatives, although representing some improvement, are still constrained by standards and ideas about 'readiness' rooted in the perceptions of the dominant society (DIAND, Alternative Funding Arrangements, 'Entry assessment', 1990; interview, DIAND, National Director, Alternative Funding Arrangements Programme, Ottawa, 12 Nov. 1991. DIAND, 'Indian Self-government Negotiations Policy', 1990; interview, Self-government Negotiator, 13 Nov. 1991). Thus, the Social Development programmes we reviewed, despite their attempts to respond to First Nation concerns and to lend themselves to adaptation, inescapably continue to represent the historical trajectory of assimilation and integration. How can it be otherwise when they are programmes whose very origins and premises are located in twentieth-century liberalism and the problems and solutions of the liberal state?

No other theme has stood out so clearly in this chapter as jurisdiction. Whether it has been the history of their dispossession since the Royal Proclamation of 1763, the conflict between federal and provincial jurisdictions, or the endless struggle with a bureaucracy of programmes and conditions, the First Nations have emerged socially battered but spiritually intact. Their attachment to the land, their historical memory and their indomitable resistance to Canadian governments have first sustained and now rejuvenated them. The First Nations have survived as distinct peoples and that survival has restored the consciousness of independence and the unstoppable quest for self-government.

In order to achieve meaningful self-government, the current constitutional accord must be affirmed by the Canadian people. This means that the people of Canada acknowledge that First Nations never surrendered their right to self-determination, and that they agreed to coexist and share the land with newcomers. For their part, the First Nations already agree that their inherent right to self-government exists within what is now Canada and that it is, therefore, a third order of government. First Nations, in our view, must define where exactly their 'comfort zone' exists in their relationship with Canada. This premise must guide how First Nations approach the issues raised in areas of social policy discussed in this chapter. Child welfare is an excellent example. Responsibility for developing programme models, services and practice must lie with the First Nations and must not be surreptitiously couched in the policy expectations of an outside body. The legitimization of new models need only come from within their own communities.

It is true that the development of new models, of new policy and practices may not come easily. This problem and its resolution were discussed with us by an Indian band councillor from the Six Nations reserve in southern Ontario (Six Nations Band Councillor, Interview, 8 Nov. 1991). He observed that government programmes are foreign to many people on his reserve despite its proximity to Canada's largest concentrations of population. 'They are used to living on the reserve,' he said.

> The outside work, its infrastructure are just not comfortable for them. It is not their system. In order to make changes . . . the federal and provincial governments should let us identify our own needs and design programmes to meet those needs. We are the ones who live in the community and know what the problems are. We experience them and see them every day. Yet we do not have the power and the authority to do that.

But new approaches will not materialize easily. The councillor used the present Social Assistance programme in Ontario as an example of how pervasive non-Indian thinking has been amongst First Nations and how difficult it is to create new programmes based on traditional cultures.

> With our assemblies, most of the time is spent on changes in required policy, programmes and planning. They are not looking at issues like developing a new system, there is no discussion around that. What you have is discussion about how the system is now, changes that can be made, where we can offer services; all within the existing regulations. . . . Some of us get brainwashed into the provincial system. A lot of people have to get it out of their heads. They see change as radical, [yet they] are not happy with the system.
>
> (Six Nations Band Councillor, Interview, 8 Nov. 1991)

The councillor, however, did not see this as an insurmountable issue, nor as a 'There, I told you so!' indictment of First Nations' aspirations. Rather, he had a clear vision of new programmes, and of a new relationship with Ottawa.

> The federal government would have to work out a process of yearly allocations based on money owed to us for the resources we once owned. It would be like them paying us rent for the land they

occupy. We would exist on that money, one block, that's all. And, if we go under, we go under. We would be accountable to our own people. All the government would need to be concerned about is that they would be paying rent. And, when you pay your rent you do not tell the landlord how to spend it.

(Six Nations Band Councillor, Interview, 8 Nov. 1991)

This solution is a nutshell summary of the 1983 Penner Report. More importantly, it speaks plainly and simply to the principles of jurisdiction, of self-government and for the future: the right of First Nations to conduct their own affairs in ways appropriate to themselves and to their own needs and priorities, without fear of external judgement and with the realization that mistakes will be made but that their resolutions will be found from within.

In conclusion, social welfare programming is inextricably linked to the entire future of First Nations in Canada. It goes to the heart of how all societies maintain and nourish themselves, of how they cope with the present and plan for the future. In short, it symbolizes the sense of control all societies must have over the destiny of their cultures. The Assembly of First Nations (Interview, Assembly of First Nations, Media Relations, 1991) realizes that self-government will not occur immediately. Besides the further negotiation required to determine the scope of jurisdiction, there is the pressing reality of economic deprivation and the need for fiscal resourcing and self-sufficiency which must support and sustain self-government. But, as a priority, the transfer of jurisdiction to the First Nations of the broad areas of social welfare, such as social security, family and child welfare, health, education and housing, will be a decisive and necessary step towards their self-determination.

ACKNOWLEDGEMENT

The extract on p. 42 is reproduced with the kind permission of the publisher. © The Queen's Printer for Ontario, 1994.

REFERENCES AND FURTHER READING

Books and articles

Armitage, A. (1988) *Social Welfare in Canada: Ideals, Realities, and Future Paths*, 2nd edn, Toronto: McClelland & Stewart.
Asch, M. (1977) 'The Dene Economy', In Mel Watkins (ed.) *Dene Nation:*

The Colony Within, for the University League for Social Reform, Toronto: University of Toronto Press, pp. 47–61.

—— (1984) *Home and Native Land: Aboriginal Rights and the Canadian Constitution*. Agincourt, Ont.: Methuen Publications.

Banting, K. G. (1987) *The Welfare State and Canadian Federalism*, 2nd edn, Kingston, Ont.: McGill-Queen's University Press.

Behiels, M. D. (ed.) (1989) *The Meech Lake Primer: Conflicting Views of the 1987 Constitutional Accord*, Ottawa: University of Ottawa Press.

Blake, P. (1975) Statement to the Mackenzie Valley Pipeline Inquiry, in Mel Watkins (ed.) *Dene Nation: The Colony Within*, for the University League for Social Reform, Toronto: University of Toronto Press, 1977, pp. 5–9.

Boldt, M. and Long, A. J. (1988) 'Native Indian Self-Government: Instrument of Autonomy or Assimilation?', in Anthony J. Long and Menno Boldt (eds) *Governments in Conflict? Provinces and Indian Nations in Canada*, Toronto: University of Toronto Press, pp. 38–56.

Cassidy, Frank (1991) 'Approaches to Welfare Reform in Indian Communities', in Frank Cassidy and Shirley Seward (eds) *Alternatives to Social Assistance in Indian Communities*, Halifax: The Institute for Research on Public Policy, pp. 1–14.

Cassidy, Frank and Bish, Robert L. (1989) *Indian Government: Its Meaning in Practice*, Lantzville, BC, and Halifax: Oolichan Books with the Institute for Research on Public Policy.

Cumming, Peter A. and Mickenberg, Neil H. (eds) (1972) *Native Rights in Canada*, 2nd edn, Toronto: The Indian-Eskimo Association of Canada and General Publishing.

Driben, Paul and Trudeau, Robert S. (1983) *When Freedom is Lost: The Dark Side of the Relationship between Government and the Fort Hope Band*, Toronto: University of Toronto Press.

Fisher, Robin (1977) *Contact and Conflict: Indian–European Relations in British Columbia, 1774–1890*, Vancouver: University of British Columbia.

Forsey, E. (1990) *A Life on the Fringe: The Memoirs of Eugene Forsey*, Toronto: Oxford University Press.

Frideres, J. S. (1988) *Native Peoples in Canada: Contemporary Conflicts*, 3rd edn, Scarborough, Ont.: Prentice-Hall Canada.

Getty, I. A. L. and Lussier, A. S. (eds) (1983) *As Long as the Sun Shines and Water Flows: A Reader in Canadian Native Studies*, Nakoda Institute Occasional Paper No. 1, Vancouver: University of British Columbia Press.

Gibbins, Roger and Ponting, J. Rick (1986) 'Historical Overview and Background', in J. Rick Ponting (ed.) *Arduous Journey: Canadian Indians and Decolonization*, Toronto: McClelland & Stewart, pp. 18–56.

Granatstein, J. L. and McNaught, K. (eds) (1991) *'English Canada' Speaks Out*, Toronto: Doubleday, Canada.

Greene, Ian (1989) *The Charter of Rights*, 'Foreword' by Peter H. Russell, Toronto: James Lorimer & Co.

Guest, Dennis (1985) *The Emergence of Social Security in Canada*, 2nd edn, rev., Vancouver: University of British Columbia Press.

Hawley, D. L. (1986) *The Indian Act Annotated*, 2nd edn, Toronto: The Carswell Co.

Hawthorn, Harry B. (ed.) (1966) 'The politics of Indian Affairs', in Ian A. L. Getty and Antoine S. Lussier (eds) *As Long as the Sun Shines and Water*

Flows: a Reader in Canadian Native Studies, Nakoda Institute Occasional Paper No. 1. Vancouver: University of British Columbia Press, 1983, pp. 164–87. Abridged from *A Survey of Contemporary Indians of Canada*, Part 1, chap. 17, Ottawa: The Queen's Printer, 1966.

Irving, Allan (1987) 'Federal–Provincial Issues in Social Policy', in Shankar A. Yelaja (ed.) *Canadian Social Policy*, 2nd edn, Waterloo, Ont.: Wilfrid Laurier University Press, pp. 326–49.

Johnston, Patrick (1983) *Native Children and the Child Welfare System*, Ottawa: Canadian Council on Social Development.

McMillan, Alan D. (1988) *Native Peoples and Cultures of Canada*, Vancouver: Douglas & McIntyre.

McNaught, Kenneth (1988) *The Penguin History of Canada*, new, rev. edn, London: Penguin Books. First published as *The Pelican History of Canada*, London: Penguin Books, 1969.

Macpherson, C. B. (1962) *The Political Theory of Possessive Individualism: Hobbes to Locke*, Oxford: Oxford University Press.

Manzer, Ronald (1985) *Public Policies and Political Development in Canada*, Toronto: University of Toronto Press.

Miller, J. R. (1991) *Skyscrapers Hide the Heavens: a History of Indian White Relations in Canada*, rev., paperback edn, Toronto: University of Toronto Press.

Owram, Doug (1986) *The Government Generation: Canadian Intellectuals and the State 1900–1945*, Toronto: University of Toronto Press.

Shewell, H. (1991a) Social Policy and the Liberal State: A Case Study of the Authority to Provide Social Assistance on Indian Reserves in Canada', Comprehensive paper in partial fulfilment of PhD, University of Toronto.

—— (1991b) 'The Use of Social Assistance for Employment Creation on Indian Reserves: An Appraisal', in Frank Cassidy and Shirley B. Seward (eds) *Alternatives to Social Assistance in Indian Communities*, Halifax: The Institute for Research on Public Policy, pp. 17–81.

—— (1992) 'The Impact of the Constitution and Federal–Provincial Issues on Social Policy and Canada's First Nations', unpublished paper.

Siggner, Andrew J. (1986) 'The Socio-Demographic Conditions of Registered Indians', in J. Rick Ponting (ed.) *Arduous Journey: Canadian Indians and Decolonization*, Toronto: McClelland and Stewart, pp. 57–83.

The Globe and Mail (Toronto) 29 Aug.–14 Sept. 1992.

Titley, E. Brian (1986) *A Narrow Vision: Duncan Campbell Scott and the Administration of Indian Affairs in Canada*, Vancouver: University of British Columbia Press.

Tobias, John L. (1976) 'Protection, Civilization, Assimilation: An Outline History of Canada's Indian Policy', *The Western Canadian Journal of Anthropology* VI (2): 13–30.

Trigger, Bruce G. (1985) *Natives and Newcomers: Canada's 'Heroic Age' Reconsidered*, Montreal: McGill-Queen's University Press.

Trudeau, P. E. (1988) *With a Bang, not a Whimper: Pierre Trudeau Speaks Out*, ed. and with an introduction by D. Johnston, Toronto: Stoddart.

Usher, Peter J. (1985) 'An Hypothesis on the Effects of Wage Employment on Subsistence Harvesting in the Canadian Western Arctic', Panel on Modern Hunting and Fishing Adaptations in Northern North America,

Meetings of the American Anthropological Association, Washington, DC, 7 Dec. 1985. Photocopied.

—— (1993) 'Northern Development, Impact Assessment, and Social Change', in Noel Dyck and J. B. Waldron (eds) *Anthropology, Public Policy, and Native Peoples in Canada*. Montreal: McGill-Queen's University Press.

Watkins, M. (ed.) (1977) *Dene Nation: The Colony Within*, University League for Social Reform, Toronto: University of Toronto Press.

Weaver, S. M. (1981) *Making Canadian Indian Policy: The Hidden Agenda 1968–1970*, Studies in the Structure of Power: Decision-Making in Canada, Jack Grove (ed.) No. 9, Toronto: University of Toronto Press.

Wharf, B. (1987) *Toward First Nation Control of Child Welfare: A Review of Emerging Developments in BC*, Victoria: University of Victoria.

Wolf, Eric R. (1982) *Europe and the People without History*, Berkeley: University of California Press.

Government documents, publications and reports

Canada Alternative Funding Arrangements Programme (1990) 'Alternative Funding Entry assessment: a management development approach for interested bands', Ottawa; Alternative Funding Arrangements, Standard Agreement, Ottawa.

—— Department of Citizenship and Immigration, Indian Affairs Branch, (1966, 1969) *A Survey of the Contemporary Indians of Canada: Economic, Political, and Educational Needs and Policies*, Harry B. Hawthorn (ed.) Ottawa: The Queen's Printer, 2 vols.

—— Department of Indian Affairs and Northern Development (DIAND), Indian and Inuit Affairs (1984) Social Development Programme, 'Interpretation of the Legal Mandate and Responsibilities of Federal, Provincial, Municipal and Indian Band Governments for Social Services to Indian People with Special Reference to the Canada-Ontario Welfare Services Agreement of 1965', Draft Discussion Paper, Ottawa.

—— Education Branch (1989), *Indian Education*, Ottawa.

—— (1991) Social Development Programme, 'Indian Child and Family Services', Programme directive, chap. 5, Social Development, 'Indian Child and Family Services,' (Draft). Ottawa, 22 March.

—— (1990) 'Registration, Revenues and Band Governance', *Indian Register Population by Sex and Residence*, Ottawa.

—— (1990) Social Development Directorate, 'SEAS National Report, Child Welfare and Individual and Family Care', Ottawa.

—— Self-government Sector, (1990) 'Indian Social Services within a Self-Government Framework: Issues to Consider', Prepared by Margaret Kovach, Ottawa.

—— Social Development Programme (1989). Indian Child and Family Services, 'Management regime discussion paper', Ottawa.

—— Department of National Health and Welfare Canada, (1990) Canada Assistance Plan Division, Telephone Information Services, Ottawa.

—— House of Commons (1983). Report of the Special Committee on

Indian Self-government in Canada, Keith Penner, Chairman, Ottawa: The Queen's Printer.

―――― House of Commons (1988) Indian Act, Revised Statutes of Canada, Ottawa.

―――― DIAND, (1987) Child and Family Services Task Force, *Indian Child and Family Services in Canada*, Final Report, Ottawa.

―――― DIAND, Communications Branch. Indian Services Sector (1989). Ottawa.

―――― DIAND, (1989) Finance and Professional Services, *Highlights of Aboriginal Conditions 1981–2001*, Part I, 'Demographic Trends'; Part II, 'Social Conditions'; Part III, 'Economic Conditions', prepared by N. Janet Hagey, Gilles Larocque and Catherine McBride, Ottawa.

―――― Finance and Professional Services (1989), *1986 Census Highlights on Registered Indians: Annotated Tables*, prepared by Gilles Y. Larocque and R. Pierre Gauvin, Ottawa: Supply and Services Canada.

―――― DIAND, (1989) Self-government Sector, Indian self-government community negotiations, questions and answers; process, Ottawa.

―――― Finance and Professional Services (1991). *Basic Departmental Data*, Ottawa: Supply and Services Canada.

―――― (1989) 'Indian Self-Government Community Negotiations – Process', Ottawa.

―――― Self-government Sector. (1990) 'Indian Self-government Community Negotiations – Policy', Ottawa.

―――― DIAND, BC Region. (1991) *Policy and Procedures Manual: Social Development Program*, Vancouver, BC.

―――― (1959–61) Joint Committee of the Senate and the House of Commons on Indian Affairs, *Minutes of Proceedings and Evidence*, Ottawa: The Queen's Printer.

―――― National Council of Welfare. (1992) *Welfare Incomes, 1991*, Ottawa: Supply and Services Canada.

―――― Special Joint Committee of the Senate and the House of Commons, Appointed to Examine and Consider the Indian Act. (1946–48) *Minutes of Proceedings and Evidence*, Ottawa: Edmond Cloutier, Printer to the King's Most Excellent Majesty.

Ontario Ministry of Community and Social Services. (1979) *A Starving Man Doesn't Argue*, Report prepared by TAP Associates Ltd for the Tripartite Social Services Review Committee, Toronto.

―――― Social Assistance Legislation Review. (1992) *First Nations' Project Team Report*, Toronto: The Queen's Printer.

―――― (1988) *Transitions*, Report of the Social Assistance Review Committee, Toronto: The Queen's Printer.

Public Archives of Canada, Government Records Division. (1944–46) Record Group 10, CR Series, Vol. 8585, File 1/1–2–17, Special Committee on Postwar Reconstruction and Re-establishment of Indian Population, Ottawa.

―――― Record Group 10, Red Series, Vol. 2071, File 10589, Rev. E. Langevin on the extreme poverty of the Indians on the Coast from Nabaskowan to Bonne Esperance and asking that aid may be sent to them this fall, 1878. Vol. 1903, File 2162, North Shore River St Lawrence

Superintendency – Mingan Reserve – Reports Concerning the death by starvation of several Indians in the winter, 1873.

Interviews

Assembly of First Nations, Media Relations Department, Ottawa, 13 Nov. 1991.

Department of Indian Affairs and Northern Development (DIAND), Indian and Inuit Affairs, National Director, Alternative Funding Arrangements Programme, Ottawa-Hull, 12 Nov. 1991.

—— Self-government Sector, Self-government Negotiator, Ottawa-Hull, 13 Nov. 1991.

Ontario Indian Social Services Council, Director of Social Services, Toronto, 8 Nov. 1991.

Six Nations Band Council, Councillor, Toronto, 8 Nov. 1991.

2 Social welfare of the indigenous peoples within the United States of America

Joyce M. Kramer

The earliest written history of the indigenous people of the Americas is obtained from Christopher Columbus's 1492 chronicle of the first day of his fleet's arrival on the continent's shores.

> No sooner had we concluded the formalities of taking possession of the island than people began to come to the beach, all as naked as their mothers bore them. . . . They are well-built people, with handsome bodies and very fine faces. . . . Their eyes are large and very pretty, and their skin is the colour of Canary Islanders or of sunburned peasants. . . . These are tall people and their legs, with no exceptions, are quite straight, and none of them has a paunch. They are, in fact well proportioned.
>
> (Fuson, 1987)

In a later entry, Columbus describes the population as the 'best and gentlest people in the world' (Fuson, 1987). Throughout his journal, Columbus repeatedly marvels about the good health and general well-being of the indigenous people and the pristine beauty of the land. One must remember that Columbus was coming from a Europe which was still exhibiting the scars of repeated bouts with the plague and which was endemically disease-ridden as a result of social and economic inequities and the unwholesomeness of urban living during the mercantile era.

Ironically, the condition of America's indigenous people has changed drastically subsequent to this early contact with Europe. Within a couple of centuries, the indigenous population was reduced to less than half due to famine, exposure, disease and violence (Denevan, 1976). Many of the deaths can be attributed to the blatantly genocidal policies and practices of the European powers and their successors in the hemisphere. Now, 500 years later, on-going economic exploitation, misguided welfare policies, as well as insensitive neglect by federal and State authorities continue to contribute to unacceptably high morbidity and mortality rates amongst America's indigenous people. Nevertheless, a reformation is occurring as indigenous Americans reclaim control over what is left of their natural resources, administratively take over the human service systems affecting their lives, and promote a renaissance of their cultural heritages.

Before proceeding, a note about the terminology used in this text is in order. It is difficult to write about the indigenous people within the United States because there is a marked lack of consensus regarding appropriate terminology. In fact, words commonly used to describe the people and their social organizations, such as 'American Indian', 'Native American', 'Alaska Native', 'tribe' and 'chief', are inventions arising out of the colonial and neo-colonial experience. They are 'loaded' terms which are often stereotypic and/or grossly misrepresent the social reality (Berkhoffer, 1978). Consequently, except when other sources are quoted in the text or when the terms used have precise legal meaning, an attempt is made to utilize generic terminology throughout the text. For example, given the overlapping usages in the literature of the terms 'nation', 'tribe' and 'band', and the more generic term 'society', the latter is used in this text as referring to the basic inter-familial community which confers an individual's identity and membership at birth.

Five hundred years ago, prior to the arrival of Columbus, there are estimated to have been more than 150 distinct aboriginal cultures in what is currently the lower 48 states (Ubelaker, 1976). Each of these peoples referred to themselves in their own languages as 'We, the People', while members of the other societies were typically referenced by some distinctive characteristic such as 'They, the Blackfoot; . . . the Nez Percés (Pierced Noses); . . . the Ojibwe (Puckered Moccasins)'. Prior to colonization, the indigenous inhabitants of North America did not call themselves by a single term nor perceive of themselves as a single collectivity, and to this day, it is generally considered more appropriate to identify an individual by his or her culture than to refer to them simply by 'race'.

In general, throughout the text, the term 'indigenous' is used to refer to all the people who trace their ancestry to the aboriginal inhabitants of what is currently the continental United States. Apologies are in order, in this regard, to indigenous Hawaiians who, like other indigenous Americans, have experienced many problems as a consequence of encroachments by colonial and neo-colonial forces. However, indigenous Hawaiians' history and current conditions are somewhat unique in that their legal status with respect to the federal government is different from that of 'American Indians and Alaska Natives'. Therefore, although indigenous Hawaiians definitely deserve scholarly attention, it is not within the scope of this chapter to include Hawaii.

'Indigenous Americans' are differentiated from 'European Americans', 'African Americans', 'Asian Americans', and 'Latino Americans', who trace their ancestry principally from Europe, Africa, Asia, or Latin America respectively. Whereas many Americans acknowledge genetically mixed ancestry, thereby confounding categorization, it is the people's primary identity which is of interest in this text. The primary identity of 'indigenous Americans' is with one or more of the aboriginal peoples in what is currently the United States. In other words, a sociological rather than biological definition of ethnic identity is utilized in this text.

ENVIRONMENT

Historical eras

As should be apparent in the following description of eras, the policies of the European colonists followed by those of the US government have historically been fraught with contradictions and inconsistencies regarding relationships with and responsibilities to the indigenous people of the United States. One way in which these contradictions have exhibited themselves is in pendulum-like shifts from (1) acknowledging the rights of indigenous people to govern themselves, to (2) denying these rights and attempting to force indigenous people to become 'acculturated' and 'assimilated' into the European-American life-ways.

Early contact and treaty-making

This begins with Leif Ericsson's journeys in the eleventh century, and continues to the late eighteenth century. European colonial forces brought missionaries, fur traders, armies and settlers who came armed with attractive merchandise and technologies as well as deadlier weapons than the indigenous societies had ever known. It was an overwhelming combination which was to affect the life-ways of the indigenous people profoundly.

Throughout the British colonies, patterns of purchasing lands from indigenous societies superseded formalized treaties. The first written land transactions appear to have taken place in 1633. Nation-to-nation treaties were used initially in order to seek the allegiance of indigenous societies in the wars between the European powers and later between the United States, Canada and Mexico in the scramble for territorial 'spheres of influence'. Also, the peace treaties facilitated lucrative trade with the indigenous societies and facilitated missionaries' endeavours to convert the people to Christianity.

Britain's Royal Proclamation of 1763 codified the treaty process for acquiring lands from the 'nations or tribes of Indians with whom we are connected, and who live under our protection', and it delineated the definition of 'Indian country' (Sanders, 1985). Under the proclamation, private transactions by individuals to acquire 'Indian country' were explicitly prohibited. The Proclamation set the precedent officially practised in the United States after the War of Independence (1776–83) (Sanders, 1985): that is, the federal government is constitutionally obliged to deal with indigenous societies as distinct political entities whose governments have sovereignty over internal affairs. Because of this special relationship codified by treaty and statute, many indigenous peoples have distinct rights which differ from those of the majority culture as well as of other racial and ethnic minorities in the United States.

After the War of Independence, the administration of indigenous affairs came under the Department of War, which was responsible for enforcing the Trade and Intercourse Acts passed by Congress between 1790 and 1834. These acts focused exclusively on external relations with indigenous societies and authorized the War Department to protect indigenous territories by removing unauthorized settlers (Sanders, 1985). Such federal prohibitions, however, were not well enforced, and unauthorized intrusions and settlement into 'Indian country' continued.

Conquest and removal

Beginning in the early eighteenth century, treaty-making continued with indigenous societies, but the purposes changed. As acquisitive European settlers and their descendants sought to gratify their lust for land and precious metals, the US government turned its armies from fighting its neighbours to the task of pacifying the indigenous societies. Under duress, indigenous governments agreed, through the treaty-making process, to give up rights to vast expanses of land, and indigenous people were confined to 'reservation' lands. In exchange, the US government promised to provide the material goods and services required to survive.

Given the enforced dependency of indigenous people upon the federal government, a legal 'trust' relationship was acknowledged whereby the federal government accepted fiduciary responsibilities for their indigenous wards' well-being. In 1824, the Bureau of Indian Affairs (BIA) was established under the War Department to enforce and administer federal policies on reservations 'in a government to government relationship' (Bureau of Indian Affairs, 1986). However, there was widespread corruption in the BIA, and in many places the promised food, supplies and services were never provided. Faced with starvation, some indigenous societies revolted but were ultimately defeated (Brown, 1971).

As early as 1817, treaties were used for moving indigenous peoples westwards, and removal reached a pinnacle after the 1830 passage by Congress of the Indian Removal Act. Considered a 'permanent solution' to the 'Indian problem', the Act facilitated the removal of indigenous societies from their homelands. Most were moved into the newly designated 'Indian country' – that is, to the relatively dry and infertile land in what is now Oklahoma. Affected societies include the Cherokee, Choctaw, Chickasaw, Chippewa, Creek, Delaware, Fox, Kaskasias, Kickapoo, Ottawa, Pawnee, Peoria, Piankashaw, Potawatomi, Quapaw, Sac, Seminole, Shawnee, Wea and Winnebago (Sanders, 1985). An estimated one-third of the people who were moved died. Thousands died in transit on the 'Trail of Tears' from exposure, starvation and exhaustion, and as many more died within a year of arrival due to insufficient food, clothing and shelter as well as to the social turmoil and emotional anguish of drastic upheaval.

By the middle of the nineteenth century, indigenous people no longer posed a military threat, at least in the more populated eastern and midwestern States. Because the War Department had demonstrated itself to be ill-equipped to administer the needs of its wards, in 1849 the Bureau of Indian Affairs was transferred to a newly created Department of the Interior (Bureau of Indian Affairs, 1986).

'Allotment' and 'acculturation' beginning in the late nineteenth century and lasting until the 1920s

During this era, the authority of the indigenous governments to represent their people and to be responsive to their people's needs was systematically undermined. At the same time, residential schools were used as instruments of 'acculturation'.

With the discovery of gold in the West and the mass movements of migrants of European heritage along the Oregon Trail, the federal government abandoned treaty-making and removal as viable policies, and allotment was substituted as a means of responding to the demands of European Americans for land. Initially, starting in 1854, treaties were utilized to disintegrate tribal lands into individually held allotments which could be sold. However, there was an inherent contradiction in this tactic in that treaty-making inherently acknowledges tribal sovereignty, and in 1871, the treaty period was officially terminated by a provision of the Appropriations Act.

Aptly referred to as the 'vanishing policy' (Hertzberg, 1971), the 'Dawes (General Allotment) Act' was passed in 1887. It was followed in 1898 and 1906 by Acts stripping indigenous governments of their powers. Under the 'Dawes Act', reservation lands were subdivided into 40- to 60-acre parcels, and title was given to indigenous individuals provided they were certified as 'competent' by a commission of the Bureau of Indian Affairs. Given the prejudices of commission members, applications were attributed greater credibility if the applicant claimed some European American ancestry. Such documentation has subsequently been detrimental to the descendants of allotment holders, because they sometimes have difficulty proving that they have sufficiently high 'blood quantum' to entitle them for enrolment on their reservation. In part, because of illegal taxation and other forms of deception, much of the allotted land was eventually sold to European Americans, and by 1934, when the distribution of allotments was finally halted, 140 million acres of reservation land had been reduced to under 50 million acres, and most reservations are a 'chequer-board' of land owned by indigenous people and their governments interspersed with land owned by European American interests. However, approximately 140 reservations (out of a total of about 300) managed to resist allotment and to maintain the integrity of their territory (Bureau of Indian Affairs, 1986). These reservations are often referred to as 'closed', and, unlike 'open' reservations, they are not subject to State laws.

The overall effects of the loss of land and reduction of indigenous governments' powers proved extremely detrimental to the health and welfare of most indigenous people (Meriam, 1928). Very few indigenous people became fully assimilated into European American society. Rather, most were forced because of economic necessity to adapt to living marginally at the bottom of the American economic hierarchy.

The federal government's assimilationist policies have been based, in part, on the ethnocentric beliefs of European American reformers that indigenous cultures have little if any redeeming features, and that the best thing that could happen to indigenous people would be for them to become fully acculturated and assimilated into European American culture. Such ethnocentrism on the part of federal policy-makers was particularly apparent in the establishment of residential schools for indigenous children. 'Kill the Indian and save the man', was the slogan coined by General Richard Henry Pratt, who in 1879 founded Carlisle, the first non-reservation boarding school for indigenous children in the United States (Hertzberg, 1971).

The basic intent, to repress the indigenous cultures, was a principal purpose of residential schools. Interestingly, the principle, sanctified by the First Amendment to the United States Constitution of 'separation of church and state' was not practised with respect to indigenous people, and the US government resorted to requiring indigenous children to attend missionary as well as government-run residential institutions called 'boarding schools'. The children were stripped of their traditional attire and punished if they spoke the language or practised the religion of their people.

Because of the partial effectiveness of these culturally genocidal practices, many indigenous people lost their original language and failed to learn the basic skills, such as hunting and parenting, needed to live effectively among their people. Many also internalized feelings of ambivalence regarding what they had been taught in boarding schools to be their 'savage' and 'heathen' heritage. Although 'Some adjusted fairly well either at home or off the reservation . . . [others] went utterly to pieces. An appallingly large number died prematurely' (Hertzberg, 1971). They suffered from identity problems, because they

> were cut off from tribal life or their relationship to it had changed. Many of them felt the need for a more generalized Indian identity within which a tribal identity might also function. They lived in two, or three worlds, and most of them were not quite comfortable in any.
>
> (Hertzberg, 1971)

A positive outcome of the boarding school experience was that indigenous children of many diverse cultures were mixed together and learned a common language with which to communicate. They learned about one another, and out of the shared experience they began to forge a shared identity. 'For many students . . . Pan Indian movements provided a psychological home, a place where they belonged' (Hertzberg, 1971).

Reorganization

The assault on indigenous governments during the preceding era resulted in extreme poverty and a malaise within indigenous communities. In lieu of effective indigenous governments, the people had become dependent for direct services upon the federal government. Basically unwilling and ill-equipped to address the problems, the 'pendulum' swung, and from the 1930s to the 1950s federal policies reverted to reorganization of indigenous governments in an attempt to shift some of the responsibility away from the federal government.

The Reorganization Policy was flawed in that the United States Congress created the new 'Tribal Governments' in its own image. That is, instead of acknowledging the legitimacy of traditional modes of government, the Bureau of Indian Affairs was mandated to oversee the subdivision of each reservation into electoral districts for the purpose of electing a 'Tribal Council'. In some places, the electoral process has gone smoothly and is generally accepted by the people. However, in others, problems have occurred because people preferred the traditional methods for selecting leadership. For example, among the Hopi, the vast majority of the population have boycotted elections in support of the Council of Elders, who have governed the Hopi since time immemorial. As a result, the 'Tribal Council', which is officially recognized by the federal government, continues to be composed of somewhat marginal 'upstarts' who lack legitimacy in the eyes of many of the Hopi people.

Also, most human services continued to be administered centrally 'from the top down' by federal bureaucracies. However, some progress was made by the new governments in regaining effective control of their land. For example, on the San Carlos Apache Reservation, land which had been leased to European American ranchers by the Bureau of Indian Affairs was returned to the San Carlos Apache Tribal Council, and a reservation-owned herd of cattle was established there. It is particularly significant that the principles of 'tribal sovereignty' and 'self-government' were reaffirmed during this era.

Termination and urbanization

Again the 'pendulum' swung and, beginning in the 1950s until the 1970s, federal policy was directed towards reducing the number of people who had treaty rights to goods and services. Monetary inducements were offered to lure indigenous people away from their reservations to urban centres where they were to receive job training and employment opportunities. Many of the people who moved were ill-equipped for city life. Those who did receive employment tended to work for very low pay in unskilled and semi-skilled positions. Many were chronically unemployed or underemployed. Their 'assimilation', if it can be correctly called that, was at the bottom of the US class structure. At the same time, monetary inducements were offered to entire societies to give up their treaty rights. Between 1953 and 1968, more than 100 tribes, bands and rancherias were terminated (affecting 12,000 individuals and 2.5 million acres of land). The effects were devastating in terms of general health and well-being. High indigenous death rates, continuing poverty, chronic unemployment, and escalating rates of alcohol abuse attested to the failure of the federal government's 'assimilationist' policies.

Self-determination

Mobilized by the disastrous policies of the federal government during the 1950s and 1960s, beginning in 1968, indigenous organizations throughout the United States protested and lobbied for change. The primary thrust of this widespread movement is for indigenous people to regain control over their own affairs and over the land and other natural resources to which they are entitled by treaty. Some of the societies which had been terminated, including the Menominee in Wisconsin and the Klamath in Oregon, who were the largest societies terminated, were reinstated.

The cornerstone of the new era has been the 1975 passage by the federal government of the 'Indian Self-determination and Educational Assistance Act' (Public Law 93–638). This law provides a procedure whereby indigenous governments can contract with the federal government to assume administrative control of all the services which federal agencies such as the Bureau of Indian Affairs and the Indian Health Service have been mandated to provide. Most State governments have followed the federal government's leadership and have enacted similar legislation of their own. Although many indigenous governments have opted to take over services formerly offered by the federal and State authorities, others are reluctant. Despite the fact that the 'Indian Self-determination Act' explicitly prohibits the federal government from diminishing the amount of budgetary resources allocated for contracted services, many indigenous people are distrustful of the government because of its long history of broken promises. They fear that once the federal government abdicates responsibility for administering services, budgetary support for those services will also eventually be withdrawn. 'Self-determination', they fear, may actually be 'self-termination' in disguise. Given subsequent attempts by the Reagan, Bush and Clinton administrations to reduce budgetary allocations for services to indigenous people, these fears are not unfounded. For the most part, Congress has successfully resisted major cutbacks. However, given inflation, the allocations in terms of spending power have declined.

In 1976, the 'Indian Health Care Improvement Act' (Public Law 94–437) was passed by the federal government. Documenting the poor health status of the indigenous population, the Act allocated increased budgetary resources to the Indian Health Service. Also, acknowledging the large numbers of indigenous people with unmet health-care needs in urban centres, urban health programmes were authorized.

In 1978, the 'Indian Child Welfare Act' (Public Law 95–561) was passed in response to indigenous people's objections to findings that 25 to 35 per cent of all indigenous children were being raised in a non-indigenous environment. The law specifies that whenever an endangered child who is an enrolled member of an 'Indian tribe' or eligible to become an enrolled member comes before the courts for placement outside the home of the child's biological parents, the child's indigenous government must be notified. Furthermore, efforts must be made to find suitable placement within the child's extended family, or if that is not available within the child's indigenous community. Only when all possibilities of placing the child within an indigenous home have been exhausted can an outside placement be considered.

Also the legislation promotes the concept of helping indigenous communities to develop programmes which would prevent child abuse and neglect and/or help the parents of children at risk to take whatever remedial steps are necessary to provide a more wholesome home environment. There have been many problems in implementing the law, including lack of compliance by some welfare agencies which circumvent the law, as well as lack of resources which would enable indigenous governments to respond more effectively when notified that an indigenous child is at risk (Northwest Indian Child Welfare Institute, 1987).

Also in 1978, the 'Indian Education Act' was passed in an effort to improve the appropriateness and overall quality of formal education for indigenous people by mandating the establishment of local indigenous parents' committees wherever there is a request by ten or more indigenous parents. The law mandates that the parents' committee must be consulted whenever policies affecting indigenous children are under consideration. Their potential authority includes input into the local hiring of teachers and staff as well as budgetary discretion (Bureau of Indian Affairs, 1986). In practice, the degree to which school systems consult with and are responsive to indigenous parents seems to depend upon the assertiveness of the parents, who often must threaten to go to court in order to be heard.

Overall, the effects of self-determination have been very positive for most of those reservations which have contracted to administer their own services.

Cultural heritages

Because of the vast diversity of indigenous cultures as well as the changes which have occurred within cultures as the result of European American influences, the reader is forewarned that every generalization made in this text regarding indigenous cultures needs to be scrutinized critically before assuming its pertinence to any particular group or person.

In fact, the differences between the indigenous cultures have been enormous. For example, using linguistic criteria as a way of measuring common origins, the differences between some of the indigenous language families in North America are as great as between English, Arabic and Russian. Furthermore, within linguistically related populations, there are enormous cultural differences as well, which reflect the needs of migrating branches of people sharing a common language to adapt to diverse environmental conditions. For example, the Kutchin people of Alaska and the Navajo of Arizona both speak Athapaskan dialects, and both are matrilineal in tracing descent. However, over centuries of separation, the Kutchin culture has adapted well as hunters in the frigid tundra above the Arctic circle in Alaska, while the Navajo in Arizona, New Mexico and Utah have adapted to warm desert conditions by becoming pastoral shepherds. In woodland areas surrounding the Great Lakes, Algonquian-speaking peoples, such as the Ojibwe (Chippewa), have lived side by side with Iroquoian-speaking people, such as the Mohawk and Oneidae. The Ojibwe, like the Kutchin, have relied principally upon hunting wild game and gathering of wild foods for survival. Unlike the Kutchin, they are partrilineal rather than matrilineal in their system for tracing descent. Their neighbours, the Mohawk, however, are matrilineal, and while hunting and gathering activities are important, much more emphasis is placed on horticulture. Women are the principal cultivators and the custodians of the land. In this regard, Iroquoian-speaking peoples are similar to many of the Pueblo cultures in the Southwest, such as the Zuni, who are members of the Uto-Aztecan language family (Spencer, 1960).

Although generalizations regarding the indigenous cultures in the United States are inexact, as there are usually notable exceptions for every characterization made, all of the pre-Columbian societies in what is at present the United States relied principally upon foraging (gathering vegetables, hunting wildlife, and/or fishing) or upon simple horticulture (farming with a digging stick or hoe) for their subsistence. Consequently, they do tend to share traits common to foraging as well as simple horticultural societies world-wide (Lenski and Lenski, 1974). Many of these cultural traits survive to this day, with modifications adapted to contemporary living conditions.

One important general characteristic is that there tends to be an absence of inherited differentials in status. Very little in the way of material possessions can be accumulated, and resources which can be acquired, such as horses within the Great Plains societies, are commonly distributed among a wide array of relatives upon the death of the owner. Also, because of the harshness of life in subsistence economies, there are very strong social pressures to share wealth when it is acquired. Among the Ojibwe, for example, much of the mythology instructs the listener about how selfish behaviour ultimately results in the selfish person's coming to a bad end.

To this day, it is considered inappropriate to display ostentatious wealth, and if you have more than your friends and neighbours, you are expected to share what you have. A wide array of cultures have formal 'give-away' ceremonies for redistributing wealth. Unlike European American culture where the individuals honoured are given gifts, indigenous people, such as a bride and groom, present gifts to each other's family members. Status and prestige are acquired as a result of one's achievements and generosity in sharing those achievements rather than from one's family of origin, and political leaders are those who have proved themselves through their accomplishments to be wise and generous. Trusted medical-religious leaders (often referred to as 'medicine people') exhibit these same leadership characteristics in addition to showing evidence of being able to communicate with the spirit world.

All things, animate and inanimate, are believed to have a spirit and an essential place in the balanced order of the universe. Because human beings are dependent upon the natural world for survival, the spirits of all things must be respected, and whenever an animal or plant offers itself to humans to serve as food, clothing, tools and/or shelter, it is important to thank its spirit ritually for being so generous in order that we might live. The principle that 'with all beings and all things we shall be as equals' is embodied in the day-to-day practices of many of the indigenous peoples of the United States. When human affairs go badly, it is commonly believed that the underlying cause is disrespect having been exhibited and/or other imbalances having occurred in the relations of the affected parties with their fellow human beings and/or with the natural environment. Remedies require efforts to restore appropriate balance and mutual respect in relationships.

These beliefs are often mystifying to non-indigenous Americans, who are more inclined to believe in mastery over nature rather than reverence for the natural environment. Consequently, they tend to be unsympathetic when indigenous people refuse to exploit the environment for monetary gain. Also, non-indigenous Americans are inclined to believe that competitive accumulation rather than co-operative sharing is required to survive and 'get ahead' in the modern world.

For indigenous Americans, the principle of mutual respect applies between human beings just as it applies between humans and all other beings within the universe, and mutual respect tends to be the guiding principle in indigenous systems of political governance. No person is considered intrinsically superior to any others, and decision-making tends to be collective. In those communities which are small enough for all adult members to know one another and to consult directly with one another, a simple consensus is sought. In large societies, more complex systems have been developed for selecting spokes-people. As noted earlier, respected leaders emerge because of their accomplishments. Despite stereotypic notions about 'Indian tribes' generated by the popular media in the United States, it is very rare for an indigenous society to rely solely upon a single 'chief'. Instead, councils of respected leaders, particularly elders, are relied upon to make decisions after conferring with one another and with their constituents. Moreover, no leader's power is absolute. Their influence always depends upon their abilities to convince their people of the wisdom of the decisions being made. Decision-making by consensus can be a long and arduous process. Unlike 'majority rule', which oppressively imposes the will of the majority on the minority, every effort is made to forge compromise solutions which respect everyone's interests. Prior to the establishment of reservations, if consensus could not be reached between disagreeing factions, societies could divide and go separate ways under independent leadership. Nowadays, with mobility limited, 'majority rule' is much more common, and conflict between interest groups sometimes festers, rendering some indigenous communities intensely fractionalized.

At the core of the social organization of most indigenous societies are kinship relationships based upon networks. The extended family is far more important in the everyday life of the individual than is usually the case in societies that are urbanized and industrialized. The extended family (which sometimes includes classificatory kin as well as biological kin) forms a mutual support network involving obligations to assist one another by sharing material goods and labour and offering emotional support as needed (RedHorse, 1980). The importance of the extended family is systematically disregarded by the American welfare systems in the United States in that welfare rules, regulations and procedures tend to violate indigenous helping systems. For example, until the 1978 passage of the 'Indian Child Welfare Act', the courts and child welfare agencies chronically displaced indigenous children in alien environments when the most appropriate placement would have been within the extended family (Northwest Indian Child Welfare Institute, 1987).

Demographic profile

A total of 504 indigenous societies are federally recognized by the US government. The 197 'Alaska Native Villages' (which are not strictly speaking 'reservations') are included in this 1986 figure. These 504 societies occupy only about 300 reservations. There is not a one-to-one relationship between reservation and culture. Large cultural groups, such as the Navajo, the Ojibwe and the Sioux (Lakota/Dakota), each occupy multiple reservations, while at the same time a single reservation may be occupied by more than one culture group. Shared usage is due to the federal government's former policies of relocation of indigenous people and consolidation of reservation lands. For example, many Winnebago were relocated from Wisconsin to the Omaha Reservation in eastern Nebraska. Reservations vary in size in the United States from the Navajo Reservation, which is the largest, with nearly 16 million acres of land in three southwestern States, to the smallest, which are less than 100 acres (Bureau of Indian Affairs, 1986). Some have no indigenous people residing in them at all!

The 1990 US Census of Population enumerated 1,959,234 people who identified themselves as 'American Indian, Eskimo or Aleut'. They account for only 0.8 per cent of the total US population. Detailed reports of the 1990 Census for ethnic groups are not yet available. However, findings from the 1980 Census provide relatively reliable indices of current demographic trends. In 1980, only 36.2 per cent of the indigenous population lived inside identified 'American Indian' areas and 'Alaska Native Villages' (including reservations, 24.9 per cent; Historic Areas of Oklahoma, 8.5 per cent; Tribal Trust Lands, 2.2 per cent; and Alaska Native Villages, 0.6 per cent), with 63.8 per cent living outside of 'American Indian' areas. Fully half of all people identifying themselves as 'Indian or Alaska Native' in the 1980 Census resided in metropolitan areas, as compared to three-quarters of the general population. The majority of indigenous people living in metropolitan areas live within the low-income areas of central cities, whereas the majority of all metropolitan residents live in the suburbs (Racial Statistics Branch, 1980).

The location of indigenous urban dwellers in central cities as compared to the suburbs reflects, in part, the fact that indigenous Americans are more likely to be poor than the general population. In the United States, a 'poverty level' income has been defined for the purpose of identifying Americans whose incomes are below the level considered necessary to meet nutritional and other essential needs. In 1980, 28.2 per cent of indigenous Americans lived below the poverty level, compared to 12.5 per cent of the total US population (Indian Health Service, 1991).

The median family income for indigenous Americans was US$13,700, compared to US$19,900 for all Americans (Indian Health Service, 1991). Because indigenous families tend to be larger (4.6 people per family on the average as compared to 3.8 people per family for all Americans), the discrepancies in per capita income are even greater – US$3,600 for indigenous Americans as compared to US$7,300 for all Americans (Indian Health Service, 1991). The percentage of indigenous Americans 16 years and older in the labour force is lower, while unemployment rates are higher – 13.3 per cent as compared to 6.5 per cent (Indian Health Service, 1991). Also, the indigenous population tends to be considerably younger than the

American population as a whole. Given that 32 per cent of the indigenous population was under 15 years of age in 1980 as compared to 23 per cent of the general population (Indian Health Service, 1991), the indigenous wage earner is typically supporting a much larger dependent population.

The relatively young age structure of the indigenous population is attributable to higher birth-rates combined with lower life expectancy. The birth-rate for indigenous Americans was 28.0 per 1,000 population in 1986–88, as compared to 15.7 for all Americans in 1987 (Indian Health Service, 1991).

Life expectancy at birth for indigenous Americans was 71.1 years (67.1 years for males and 75.1 years for females) in 1979–81, as compared to 74.7 years for all Americans (70.7 years for males and 78.1 years for females) (Indian Health Service, 1991). The highest discrepancies between the age-specific death-rates of indigenous Americans and the general population are amongst young people between the ages of 15 and 35 years. The excessively high mortality rates of indigenous people while they are young adults is especially tragic, as it is during these years that people's potential is greatest as providers and parents to young children.

The higher death-rates are indicators that the conditions in which indigenous people live and die tend to be relatively hostile compared to those of other, more affluent Americans. The remainder of this chapter is devoted to looking at the human service needs of indigenous Americans and at the adequacy of the delivery systems in addressing these needs (Indian Health Service, 1991).

CONTEMPORARY HUMAN SERVICE DELIVERY SYSTEMS

Eligibility for services

Not all of the 1,959,234 people in 1990 who identified themselves as being 'American Indian, Eskimo or Aleut' are entitled to receive services through federal programmes for indigenous people. In fact, only 1,102,001 (56 per cent) are considered by the Indian Health Service to be within its 'service population' (Indian Health Service, 1991). The absence of universal entitlement is a serious issue jeopardizing the well-being of many indigenous Americans.

Indigenous people's entitlement to federally funded health and social services is derived principally from early treaties which were negotiated between the indigenous societies and the federal government. There are tremendous political forces in the United States which pressure the federal government systematically to restrict the number of people who have treaty-based rights to services. Policies and practices designed to decrease the numbers of indigenous people having treaty rights have operated at both the societal and the individual levels. Each level is discussed in turn below.

At the societal level, not all indigenous societies negotiated treaties with the federal government and these, consequently, are not eligible for federally funded services. The Lumbee, for example, who number more than 60,000 people and whose homelands are in Robeson County, North Carolina, were already living peaceably with their European American neighbours when the treaty-making era began, and consequently treaties were never negotiated with them. Whereas the living conditions in most indigenous communities are poor, even worse conditions can be observed within many of those indigenous communities which are not entitled to the same services as federally recognized areas – 'Reservations', 'Pueblos', 'Trustlands', 'Tribal Jurisdictions', 'Rancherias' and 'Alaska Native Villages'.

There are also large numbers of individuals whose heritage is from a federally recognized society, who consider themselves 'Indian' and who are discriminated against as 'Indians', but who have become alienated from their communities of origin due to federally initiated restrictions on enrolment (Jaimes, 1988). Historically, the US government imposed a 'one-quarter blood quantum' rule for determining eligibility for 'tribal enrolment'. At that time, enrolment in a federally recognized society was necessary to receive treaty-based services. Subsequent to the 1975 passage of the 'Indian Self-determination Act', many indigenous governments have asserted their rights as sovereign entities to determine their own membership criteria. However, because of the political, economic and social implications of changing their enrolment criteria, many indigenous governments have continued to exercise a 'one-quarter blood quantum' requirement for enrolment. Other restrictive criteria are also sometimes applied. For example, a child whose father is from a matrilineal society and whose mother is from a patrilineal society may not be eligible for enrolment in either.

Present eligibility practices are typically based on cumulative experience and local custom. For example, an indigenous person moving away from his or her community of origin may be welcomed at one health and human services centre for indigenous people but denied services at another. Furthermore, a given individual may be eligible for some services provided at the centre but not for others. The following passage written by the Indian Health Service (IHS) attempts to summarize the plethora of rules, regulations and practices as follows:

> To be eligible for IHS direct services, a person need only be of Indian descent and be regarded as an Indian by the community in which he lives as evidenced by factors in keeping with general BIA [Bureau of Indian Affairs] practices. To be eligible for services not available with IHS's direct care system and which therefore must be purchased through contract care, there are . . . additional requirements.
>
> (Jaimes, 1988, bracketed information added)

Although flexibility has practical advantages, the attendant ambiguities can be a barrier to indigenous people whose eligibility for services is uncertain. It can be particularly uncomfortable for people who do not know their parentage, as when their mother gave birth out of wedlock. The potential embarrassment and stigma of being told that one is not legitimately entitled to services is probably enough to keep many people from asking for help. Furthermore, the granting of services administered by indigenous governments can become political.

Despite the racist nature of 'blood quantum' rules for receiving treaty-based services, Congress has been considering reinstating the requirement that an indigenous person must 'be of one quarter or more Indian or Alaskan Native ancestry', as well as 'be a member, or be eligible for membership in a federally recognized Indian tribe' in order to receive treaty-based services. The immediate effects would be to reduce the service population by 20 per cent (*National Indian Health Board Reporter*, 1986), and the long-term effects could be even more devastating. Given that the United States does not currently offer universal medical care to its citizenry, much of the commentary focuses on the adverse implications for indigenous health care. However, the proposed changes would have similar implications for all human services funded by the federal government in fulfilment of treaty-based obligations.

> The proposed regulation may set in motion a process of ultimate termination, albeit long term and subject to change, of providing organized health care to Indians. If the current demographic trends continue and the regulation is enacted, as time goes on, fewer and fewer Indians will qualify for benefits. Eventually service units

will no longer be justified on the basis of dwindling service populations while an ever-increasing number of Indians will lose their health care benefits. To the Indians, it will represent yet another broken promise.

(Bashshur, 1987)

Restrictions on eligibility for health, educational and human services are a major facet of the very serious identity issues facing indigenous people. The loss of entitlement is not simply a denial of goods and services. For many people, it represents a loss of community and of the types of social support which sustain people emotionally as well as materially during difficult times. In fact, human service practitioners working with indigenous people often attribute the high rates of alcohol and drug abuse, as well as high suicide rates and other indices of despair, to identity problems (Marshall, 1986).

While the sovereign right of indigenous governments to determine membership must be respected, the issue of eligibility for federally funded services could be resolved more humanely by re-defining the service population in the broadest possible terms to include all people of proven indigenous heritage. Many Urban Indian Health Boards as well as reservation-based health and human service centres already serve a wide array of clients from many cultures. Were the federal government to provide sufficient resources, more indigenous centres would have the incentive to open their doors to a wide array of indigenous people needing services. What is often forgotten in these discussions is that many of the people who would prefer to access indigenous human service centres go elsewhere at the same or greater expense to the public coffers. The advantage of permitting such people to access indigenous centres is that the services are tailored to be culturally and socially sensitive to the special needs of indigenous clients. Also, ethnically mixed families can be served as a family unit in a single, co-ordinated setting.

Systemic problems

In addition to eligibility and entitlement issues, endemic problems in the delivery of human services to indigenous people occur because of jurisdictional ambiguities. For example, there tends to be tension in the inter-relationships between indigenously administered human service delivery systems and those provided for the general population. Ideally, there would be co-operation between agencies so as to provide the best possible services to indigenous clients in need.

All too often, however, indigenous individuals seeking human services to which they are entitled are turned away from agencies serving the general public and told to go to the indigenously administered agencies in the area. This commonly occurs, for example, when low-income indigenous people seek medical or dental care, day care, or other costly human services. It also is sometimes experienced by indigenous people requesting police protection. One example of the latter is a county sheriff's refusal to go to a home where there was heavy drinking and domestic strife so as to bring the children into protective custody. His fallacious argument was that doing so would be in violation of the 'Indian Child Welfare Act'.

In addition to real confusion regarding overlapping jurisdiction, some human service providers working within the non-indigenous sector express frustration and resentment about the extra effort that is required to co-operate with indigenous governments. In-service training for non-indigenous human service providers within the public sector has helped somewhat to foster more co-operative relationships.

Not only are there problems in the interface between human service delivery systems in the formal sector, but there are also inherent tensions between formal human service delivery systems and informal helping networks. Indigenous informal helping networks remain extremely important in promoting well-being.

In urban areas where only a portion of one's kinship group may reside, adaptations typically emerge whereby friendship networks are substituted for kin. Many people, when in crisis, depend upon these networks. Formal human service organizations, however, have all too often worked at cross-purposes with these kinship-based indigenous helping systems. For example, until recently, children who were residing with a relative other than a biological parent have often been assumed to be 'neglected' and were vulnerable to court-ordered placement outside the kinship network.

Another example of conflict between systems occurs when indigenous people are penalized by outside agencies for sharing commodity food, housing and welfare benefits with others who are needier than they. One example of such penalization is to ask a single mother on welfare to list the income of all the people within the household where she resides. If she is living with others temporarily until she can afford a house of her own, the fact that their income is counted with hers can lower the amount of benefits to which she would otherwise be entitled. This, in turn, undermines her ability to muster enough resources so as to acquire autonomous housing and live independently.

In general, by usurping functions of indigenous helping systems, modern agencies have undermined these systems' effectiveness in responding to the needs of their members, and unwholesome dependencies upon outside resources have thereby been encouraged. In general, indigenously administered human service agencies tend to be much more sensitive to the importance of working with rather than at cross-purposes against indigenous helping networks.

There are a number of areas where human service agencies organized by European Americans have been in conflict with indigenous cultures. Most fundamental among the points of conflict is that many agencies operate on the implicit assumption that European American culture and forms of social organization are inherently superior to indigenous solutions. Confronted with criticism of their life-ways, indigenous clients tend to become alienated from the agency purporting to address their needs, and patterns of avoidance and/or non-compliance are established.

A corollary source of misunderstanding is that in indigenous societies caregiving relationships between people who are approximately the same age usually entail reciprocity between social equals. It is confusing and alienating, therefore, to be treated in a condescending manner by European American providers. Also, indigenous members of small-scale societies are often ill-equipped to understand and deal effectively with large, impersonal bureaucracies having elaborate divisions of labour. It is frustrating to deal with multiple providers, each of whom specializes in one narrow aspect of the client's problems, who appear to be oblivious of the broader context, and who may appear 'cold' and calculating rather than personable and empathetic.

Also contributing to incompatibilities between external human service agencies and indigenous cultures are misunderstandings generated by differences in the meanings attached to communication efforts (including oral, written and body language), differences in world-view about the causes and treatments of problems (such as discrepant interpretations of dreams and visitations by members of the spirit world), and differences in perceptions of time (including misinterpretation by providers when indigenous clients fail to appear for an appointment 'on time').

The description of human service delivery systems which follows includes services funded and/or offered by the federal government, State governments, reservation governments and indigenous urban organizations. It is of significance to note that eligibility criteria applied by each of these policy-formulating bodies sometimes differ considerably both within and between agencies.

Federal agencies

The two arms of the US government which have primary responsibility for human services to indigenous peoples are the Bureau of Indian Affairs (BIA) and the Indian Health Service (IHS). Each of these will be described briefly in turn, followed by a short overview of other federal agencies offering special services to eligible indigenous people. This is followed with a description of State governments' service delivery systems to indigenous communities.

The Bureau of Indian Affairs (BIA)

The BIA is located within the Department of the Interior and has 'primary responsibility for working with Indian tribal governments and Alaska Native village communities . . . in a government to government relationship' (Bureau of Indian Affairs, 1986). The BIA is hierarchically organized. The central decision-making headquarters are in Washington, DC. The Nation is subdivided into Area Offices serving contiguous States. They, in turn, oversee Agency Offices, which provide direct services to the reservations. Subsequent to the 1975 passage of the 'Indian Self-determination Act', many reservations have contracted directly with the BIA to administer their own services rather than to receive direct services from the Agency Office and its personnel. Wherever contracting has occurred, the number of BIA personnel in the respective Agency Office has been reduced and the moneys funding those positions have been transferred to the indigenously run tribal and/or urban agencies to provide comparable services.

Most of the money received by indigenous governments for human services is appropriated through the BIA; consequently, the BIA has a high degree of discretionary power, which is often resented by indigenous leaders who argue that many of the BIA's funding decisions do not respect indigenous people's priorities and/or are not in indigenous people's best interests.

In real income (adjusted for inflation) the budget of the BIA has dropped considerably. During the first half of the 1980s, the budget remained constant, at approximately US$1 billion per annum with no increments for inflation. In 1986, the appropriation actually dropped by 4.3 per cent to US$964 million so as 'to comply with the requirements of the Gramm-Rudman deficit reduction Act' (Bureau of Indian Affairs, 1986).

Services funded through the BIA are wide-ranging, including economic development, jobs programmes, schools and other educational establishments, housing, natural resource management and conservation services, child welfare services and law enforcement. Some of the human services will be discussed in greater detail in the 'Services Provided' sections below.

The Indian Health Service (IHS)

In 1954, responsibility for health services was transferred from the BIA in the Department of the Interior to the Public Health Service, in what is now the Department of Health and Human Services (Indian Health Service, 1991). This transfer has had positive consequences in that the quality of health services has improved contributing to significantly better morbidity and mortality rates. The services supported through the IHS include primary prevention programmes as well as comprehensive treatment in the areas of alcohol and substance abuse, maternal and child health services, mental health services, injury prevention and treatment, nutritional and dietetic services, dental services, pharmaceutical services, public health nursing services, community health representative and home health aide services, as well as environmental services such as the provision of safe drinking water and sewage facilities. The IHS's appropriation (US$818.2 million in 1986) (Bureau of Indian Affairs, 1986) approaches that of the BIA.

Other federal agencies

From time to time, the US Congress passes legislation charging other arms of the federal government with responsibility for offering services uniquely intended for indigenous people. For example, the Indian Education Office in the Department of Education had a 1986 budget of US$67 million (Bureau of Indian Affairs, 1986).

Also, at times, special agencies are created to address specific problems. An example is the Navajo-Hopi Relocation Commission, whose charge has been to segment the joint use by Navajo and Hopi people of reservation land surrounding Big Mountain in Arizona, which both societies have been occupying. The 1986 budget of US\$22.4 million (Bureau of Indian Affairs, 1986) is intended to relocate families. Often this has been accomplished against the will of those evicted from residences of long standing, and many indigenous leaders, both Hopi and Navajo, protest that the federal government has the ulterior motive of accessing the rich coal deposits under the land surface (KQED Current Affairs Department, 1985).

Other federal agencies, such as the Departments of Agriculture and of Commerce, also oversee funding specifically designated for Indian programmes. For example, the Farmers Home Administration in the Department of Agriculture offers assistance to facilitate industrial, business and community development, and 'The 1986 Housing and Urban Development (HUD) appropriation included a budget authority of approximately US\$372 million for Indian housing' (Bureau of Indian Affairs, 1986).

State programmes

Whether or not a reservation falls under State jurisdiction depends in large part upon whether the indigenous government successfully resisted federal pressures to transfer jurisdiction. In general, indigenous leaders prefer to remain under federal rather than State auspices because the treaties which protect their rights are with the federal government. States are under no obligation to honour these treaties. Given that indigenous people represent only a small minority of the electorate in any given State, their needs are not likely to be considered high among the State's appropriation priorities. In those locations where there is overlapping jurisdiction, there tends to be a plethora of rules and regulations, some of which are contradictory to each other and to indigenous people's needs, and jurisdictional disputes dangerously jeopardize the sovereignty of indigenous governments.

Nevertheless, within those 'open' reservations in which States do have jurisdictional responsibilities, the availability of State resources can provide a significant augmentation to federally supported programmes. In Minnesota, for example, the State subsidizes mental health services within Indian communities, channels some of the housing programme resources for low-income people to the indigenous governments to assure that indigenous people are served, co-operates in the implementation of the 'Indian Child Welfare Act', co-operates in the regulation of hunting and fishing rights, and funds a large, indigenously administered post-secondary scholarship programme. Also, in Minnesota, most but not all the reservations are under State criminal jurisdiction (Ebbott, 1985).

Indigenously administered services

Indigenous governments

Indigenous governments vary in organizational structure. However, most democratically elect representatives as well as a 'chair' or 'chief' to a body commonly referred to as a 'Tribal Council'. This is the policy-making body which is charged with the responsibility of being responsive to its constituents' interests and addressing its constituents' human service needs. In this regard, Tribal Councils also take primary responsibility for regulating their government's relationships with other government agencies, and organizations outside their jurisdiction.

Indigenous governments differ markedly with respect to the services offered under their auspices. The following quotation from an Indian Health Service document is indicative of the proportion of indigenous governments which have opted to take over and administer health services.

> As of October 1, 1990, the Area Offices consisted of 136 basic administrative units called service units. Of the 136 service units, 58 were operated by Tribes. The IHS operated 42 hospitals, 66 health centres, 4 school health centres, and 51 health stations; while Tribes operated 7 hospitals, 39 health centres, 3 school health centres, 64 health stations, and 173 Alaska Village Clinics.
> (Indian Health Service, 1991)

Given that the other human services are often offered in conjunction with health services, these statistics are fairly representative for welfare services as well.

Many indigenous governments have been reluctant to assume responsibility for human services because they fear that 'self-determination' may be a ploy by the federal government to abdicate responsibility for providing treaty-based services. Once indigenous governments have taken over administrative responsibility, they fear that the federal government will cut back on appropriations, thereby depriving the indigenous governments of the needed resources to meet the responsibilities they have taken on. Some other indigenous governments have attempted to contract for services and have failed. That is, due to a variety of mishaps, they went into receivership, and federal agencies had to resume control. In some cases, indigenous governments found that their attempts to offer some unpopular services, such as law enforcement, proved to be political liabilities. Consequently, they returned responsibility to the BIA.

Despite the failures, most of the indigenous governments which have taken the initiative have proved remarkably successful at improving both the quality and quantity of human services offered. The Fond du Lac Reservation in northeastern Minnesota is exemplary. Its service population includes about 3,000 indigenous people who reside on the Reservation, in surrounding rural areas and in the city of Duluth. Its Human Services Division includes multiple components, with many programmes in each component. The following is a partial list of programmes they offer, in addition to medical, dental, public health, nursing and community health representative services (Norgard and Walt, 1991).

Fond du Lac's social service programmes include the following: Family Based Services (offering counselling, assessment, information and referral, transportation, family problem identification and resolution); Child Protection (including child intervention, case management, out-of-home placement supervision and referral services); Families First (short-term crisis intervention); Foster Parent Support (including training sessions and support groups); a Veterans Centre (offering counselling); a Senior Organizer and Advocate (for the elderly); an Indian Women's Advocate (offering support, networking and educational services); a Victim's Advocate (offering a victim's needs assessment, court advocacy, employer information, emergency food information, and other assistance); a Mental Health Programme (offering evaluations and counselling as well as traditional healing techniques upon request); a Mental Health Training Centre where 'second year graduate students from colleges and universities . . . spend three to six months interning with Fond du Lac mental health staff'; Medical Social Services (offering 'assistance in obtaining . . . services offered by other county programmes, help with discharge planning at local hospitals and nursing homes; . . . assistance with social security and disability claims', and help in dealing with major life crises; Vocational Rehabilitation; as well as an Options for Kids and Families programme (in which groups of eight to ten children meet regularly for eight weeks to discuss topics of concern to them). Also there is an Indian Women's Transitional Housing Programme (which helps Indian women and their children achieve self-reliance).

Fond du Lac's Human Services Division also offers the following: Chemical Dependency Programmes: Public Education, Summer Youth Activities, Summer Family Retreats, Outreach, Assessment, In-patient and Out-patient Treatment, Advocacy, Aftercare and Self-help Groups. In addition, the Human Services Division has a Group Home providing 'intensive therapeutic and remedial services over a six to twelve month period of time'.

There are benefits of local control beyond the impressive improvements in quality and quantity of service such as have occurred on the Fond du Lac Reservation with self-determination. For example, professionally educated indigenous people no longer have to leave their community to find suitable employment. Instead, they serve as important role models, giving others the incentive to stay sober and to advance their educations because openings are available doing meaningful and gratifying work in their own community. The overall morale of many indigenous communities is improving. People feel that their government is more responsive to their needs and concerns, and they feel that they have more control over their own destinies. In other words, self-determination at the community level also is translated into more self-determination at the personal level. The dramatic decline in substance abuse which has occurred in many indigenous communities is indicative of an overall social and cultural transformation – a renaissance – facilitated by self-determination legislation, policies and procedures.

The success of indigenously controlled human service delivery systems is attributable to a number of factors. Not only are ethnic barriers removed and trust fostered between providers and their clientele, but also indigenous human service agencies can be remarkably successful at consolidating a wide array of programmes within a single centralized and accessible location. More integrated care is thereby facilitated. Providers are in close communication with one another, and clients are able to receive multiple services at a single, familiar location.

One way that indigenous governments have been able to expand and improve the services they provide is by augmenting existing resources with grants from philanthropic organizations. Indigenous governments, as compared to agents of the federal government, are much more successful in attracting such moneys. This is in part because philanthropic foundations tend to prioritize new and innovative programmes rather than current programmes, and often have policies prohibiting support of federal and State agencies. Also, they are often impressed with an indigenous government's successful 'track record' and demonstrated commitment to improving the life conditions of their service population.

Indigenous urban organizations

Indigenous urban organizations are quasi-governments able to provide many of the services offered by reservation governments as described above. Often they are founded by a grass-roots organization of indigenous urban dwellers who incorporate on a not-for-profit basis. Some are organized to meet a specific need, such as to establish a health centre or an alternative 'survival' school. Others provide a wide array of services, such as food shelves, 'latch key' and day-care programmes, support groups for battered women, and recreational programmes for the elderly.

As compared to Canada, indigenously managed human service organizations are relatively well developed in the United States. This may be one reason why the indigenous mortality rates of urbanized areas in the United States appear considerably better than those in Canada (Kramer, 1991a).

As a result of indigenous people's political and legal challenges to the absence of federally funded services in urban settings, the federal government became sensitized to the need. In 1976, a task force of the American Indian Policy Review Commission recommended the establishment of urban programmes because the needs of urban indigenous people were not being met by existing programmes.

> As Indians, they retain unique rights, based on the federal trust relationship growing from the treaties, that should apply to the individual as well as the tribe. If the tribe is sovereign, then the individuals who make up the tribe are equally sovereign. By providing services based on residency to a part of this group only, the government is in effect coercing people into adopting a particular place to live. Returning to the reservation may be seen as the only way of getting the services to which Indians are entitled but which urban Indians are denied.
>
> It was further argued that federal policies were primary causes of urban migration. If the federal government had fulfilled its trust responsibilities by helping to develop more viable reservation economies, the urban migration would have been unnecessary. The commission also noted that the law authorizing most of the BIA programs, the Snyder Act, directs that programs be provided 'throughout the United States'.
>
> (Ebbott, 1985)

This acknowledgment of the need and obligation was reflected in the passage of the Urban Health Initiative Programme of the 'Community Health Centers Act'. There are currently '34 Urban Projects consisting of 28 health clinics and six facilities providing community services' (Indian Health Service, 1991) funded by the Indian Health Service. Also, the IHS has charged some reservations located adjacent to metropolitan areas to include the city within its service unit. In such cases, the reservation commonly establishes an urban branch to its health and human services delivery system, and all indigenous residents, regardless of whether or not they are enrolled on that particular reservation, are offered services.

The BIA, while offering some services in urban settings, has been relatively resistant to extending its service population, arguing that available resources are already stretched to provide needed services to eligible people living 'on or near' reservations.

SERVICES PROVIDED

The description of services which follows is somewhat arbitrarily subdivided into the following delivery areas: health and medical, economic, housing and education. Each section begins with an assessment of the history and contemporary status of indigenous people with respect to this dimension of well-being. This is followed by a discussion of the strengths and weaknesses of the human service delivery systems in addressing indigenous people's needs. Unless otherwise noted, the people included in these discussions of services are *only* those who are considered members of the service population by the federal government.

Health and medical services

Indigenous life expectancy has been improving in the United States but still lags behind that for all Americans. Looking at discrepancies in mortality by cause, indigenous Americans are at much greater risk than the general American population of death due to such unnatural causes as alcoholism (438 per cent greater), accidents (131 per cent greater), homicide (57 per cent greater) and suicide (27 per cent greater), as well as other 'life-style'-related diseases such as diabetes mellitus (155 per cent greater) (Indian Health Services, 1991). Also, mortality due to tuberculosis is 400 per cent higher, and death due to influenza is 27 per cent greater (Indian Health Services, 1991).

Much of the improvement observed in life expectancy is

attributable to dramatic reductions in infant mortality. It is very interesting to note that the infant mortality rate of indigenous people in the United States has actually dropped below the national rate (see Table 2.1).

In interpreting these data, it is important to note that the infant mortality rates for all ethnic groups in the United States are extraordinarily high for such an affluent nation. In fact, in 1980, male life expectancy in the United States ranked eighteenth in the world (Organization for Economic Co-operation and Development, 1985). This relatively poor performance for the United States can be attributed in part to the low priority given to providing human services for the poor. The fact that indigenous Americans' infant mortality rates have improved so dramatically as compared to those of other racial minorities, especially those of African Americans, is attributable to the treaty relationships that indigenous societies have with the federal government. Indigenous Americans are unique in that their treaty rights entitle them to many health and other social services which are not available to other low-income Americans (Kramer, 1988a).

The dramatic improvements in infant mortality coincide with the administrative take-over of health services by indigenous governments. While continuing to provide medical treatment services, many of these governments have placed new programmatic emphasis upon primary prevention. For example, under self-determination, many reservations have established excellent maternal and child health clinics which include pre-natal care, a well baby clinic, nutritional supplements for pregnant as well as nursing mothers and their infants, and family planning counselling. The programmes are often financed by the federally funded WIC (Women, Infants and Children) programme – which was established to serve low-income people of all ethnicities. Noting that many infant deaths are attributable to accidents, indigenous governments sponsor programmes for loaning infant car-seats to parents of small children. These are but a few examples of new programmes designed to promote health and prevent illness.

Although the improvements in adult mortality rates have not been as dramatic as those for infants, health fairs, sobriety pow-wows, exercise programmes, anti-cigarette smoking campaigns and a wide array of community based self-help support groups appear to be making a positive difference with respect to adolescent and adult health.

The abuse of alcohol and other mind-altering substances is

Table 2.1 Infant mortality per 1,000 live births

Year	American Indians and Alaska Natives	US black	US all ethnicities
1955	62.7	43.1	26.4
1987	9.7	17.9	10.1

Source: Indian Health Service, 1991

considered by many indigenous leaders to be the most serious problem facing their communities. Although the problem remains salient in most indigenous communities, visible improvements have been made in many of those having local self-government. One reason for this is that most people who achieve leadership positions are sober. In the limelight, they become role models for others. In contrast to previous eras, when the human service administrators and providers were outsiders, local members of the community have an incentive to stay sober, as there are responsible jobs available for those who do. Also, in terms of overall morale, indigenous people under self-determination are beginning to have a sense of control over their own destinies. If the indigenous human services system is not meeting their needs, they have a much greater opportunity to complain and to be heard than when the services were administered by a federal bureaucracy. Whereas in the past, the prevailing mood was often of resignation, hopelessness and despair, there is a new air of optimism in indigenous communities. People are developing the collective will to fight alcoholism and other forms of drug abuse, and they are gradually winning the battle. Indices of their success include improvements over the past two decades in death-rates due to accidents, homicide, suicide and cirrhosis, rates which tend to be particularly sensitive to changes in a population's alcohol consumption.

At the same time, the indigenous governments are initiating a wide array of new programmes for helping the victims of alcohol and drug abuse. Residential treatment centres have been established for indigenous clientele on many reservations as well as in urban centres. Group homes and other prevention and treatment services have been developed for youth. Most indigenous governments host Alcoholics Anonymous and Alinon groups.

In indigenous communities, interpersonal violence is almost always alcohol-related. In order to protect women and children from domestic violence, shelters have been established by many indigenous governments. In addition, abused women have organized self-help groups, which are proving to be powerful not only in helping the victims to recover from abusive relationships but in prodding the community to address the problem actively.

One shortcoming of alcohol and drug abuse treatment centres within indigenous communities is that the vast majority of their clientele are men. This is particularly unfortunate, given the risk of foetal alcohol syndrome in the offspring of alcoholic mothers. Where there is an absence of family-based alcohol treatment programmes, single parents must leave their children under the care of others in order to receive residential treatment, and many mothers are afraid of losing their children if they admit they are alcohol-dependent. The establishment of family-based residential treatment centres could enable parents to keep custody of their children, and the family as an interdependent social system could receive appropriate services. Not only would the alcohol-dependent person receive treatment, but other affected members of the family would be empowered with the necessary information to deal constructively with the problem as well.

Another positive development, which is facilitated by local control, is that many of the human services administered by indigenous governments are aided by the counsel and services of indigenous spiritual leaders in the community. Usually these leaders are respected elders. In some communities, traditional religious-medical practitioners ('medicine men and women') are officially attached to the medical clinic, the mental health centre and the alcohol treatment centre, as well as other human service programmes. Although not necessarily utilized by everyone, their services appear to have an empowering influence at both the community and the individual levels.

Economic services

It is important to note that economic well-being is one of the most important factors affecting people's health and well-being in the contemporary United States. Indigenous people are much more likely than the general population to have insufficient resources to attain a physically healthful and emotionally gratifying life-style (see Table 2.2).

Unemployment is high within the indigenous population. In the United States, 13.0 per cent of the indigenous people within the labour market were unemployed in 1980, as compared to 6.5 per cent of the general population (Racial Statistics Branch, 1984).

On reservations, the unemployment rate tends to be even higher. Statistics for 1986 indicate that 29.1 per cent were unemployed. An additional 28.3 per cent of people aged 16 to 65 who are defined as 'able to work' were not in the labour market (Bureau of Indian Affairs, 1989). (Those who would not be considered 'able to work' include students in school, the disabled, people 'who must care for small children', incarcerated individuals and so on.) In other words, less than half the people of employable age are actually receiving wages. With their wages they are not only supporting the young and the aged but over half the adults of employable age as well.

One explanation for these high figures is that indigenous people, like other minorities in the United States, tend to be 'the last hired and the first fired', which causes them to be particularly affected by fluctuations in the economy. A common pattern for indigenous people, especially young adults living on reservations, is to leave their rural homelands to seek employment. If they find none, if the work is seasonal or if they are laid off, they tend to return home until new employment prospects emerge.

Not only is the percentage of indigenous people who are employed lower, but the wages of those who are employed tend to be considerably lower than for other Americans. Amongst those indigenous people living on or near reservations in the United States who are employed, 45 per cent earned less than US$7,000 in 1986 (Bureau of Indian Affairs, 1986).

Despite these discouraging statistics, since self-determination the proportion of indigenous people who are employed has increased as well as the average wages earned. Consequently, the proportion of indigenous people whose incomes are below the poverty line in the United States has been decreasing. Whereas 38.3 per cent of all indigenous people were living below the poverty line in 1970, the proportion was reduced to 28.2 per cent by 1980. By way of contrast, 13.7 per cent of all Americans lived below the poverty line in 1970 and 12.5 per cent in 1980 (Bureau of Indian Affairs, 1986; Racial Statistics Branch, 1984).

Such improvements are probably due to two different dynamics. The statistics may be an artefact of the increase in people identifying themselves as 'Indian, Eskimo or Aleut' in the 1980 as compared to the 1970 Census. However, the improvements are also attributable to the establishment of strict 'Indian preference' hiring practices within federally funded agencies whose principal clientele are indigenous.

Table 2.2 Median family incomes in the United States in 1979 (in US$1,000)

American Indian	13,678
Eskimo	13,829
Aleut	20,313
National (all ethnicities)	19,917

Source: Racial Statistics Branch, 1984

'Under Federal law, a non-Indian cannot be hired for any vacancy if a qualified Indian has applied for the position' (Bureau of Indian Affairs, 1986). At the federal level, 'Almost 80 per cent of the employees of the BIA are Indians' (Bureau of Indian Affairs, 1986). Under self-determination, the percentage of indigenous employees within indigenously administered agencies is often higher. In fact, in many places, a highly significant proportion of the community is employed by the indigenous government.

Another development which has improved the employment prospects of indigenous people under self-determination has been the establishment of new businesses owned and operated by the indigenous governments. These range from operations which extract natural resources off reservation lands, such as oil and timber, to cattle-raising and manufacturing. Also, many indigenous governments currently operate gaming casinos. Given a favourable ruling by the federal judiciary affirming indigenous governments' sovereign rights to operate gambling facilities, indigenous governments have acquired an 'edge' on the market in many localities. Although controversial because of adverse side-effects, such as occurs when indigenous people become compulsive gamblers, gaming operations have provided a windfall of money for many communities, and some of the profits are earmarked for providing human services.

As with other Americans whose family incomes qualify them for public assistance, many low-income indigenous Americans receive Aid for Families with Dependent Children (AFDC), General Assistance (income subsidies), Food Stamps (subsidizing grocery purchases), as well as other means of support. Most indigenously managed human service agencies have social workers to assist people in accessing available services.

Housing services

It should be understood that many indigenous cultures do not put the same premium on having spacious living quarters as do the majority culture. Traditionally, indigenous people have tended to live in conditions which would be considered 'crowded' by contemporary standards. There were a number of reasons for this. A very important one in northern climates is the need to share warmth during the winter months. Another factor, particularly significant among nomadic gathering and hunting peoples, was the need to have dwellings which were mobile and/or easy to erect. There is little hard evidence to support the idea that such physical intimacy in household design is necessarily unhealthy physically or emotionally to the inhabitants.

This has become a serious issue in the implementation of indigenous child welfare policies. In particular, meeting State requirements regarding dwelling size can be an obstacle to the placement of indigenous foster children within their own communities or cultures.

Indigenous people in the United States are also more likely than the general population to live in dwellings which do not have central heating. Central heating is significant, particularly given the high morbidity and mortality rates due to accidents. Many of these are attributable to household fires during the winter months. 'A 1985 inventory of housing on Reservations revealed that 85,843 existing dwellings meet standards and 56,828 are substandard units' (Bureau of Indian Affairs, 1986).

Not only is substandard housing a problem on reservations and in other rural communities, but indigenous people also often live in substandard housing in urban areas. The combination of low income and ethnic/racial discrimination against indigenous people contributes to the difficulties indigenous people have in securing safe housing in urban areas. It is unknown how many indigenous people are among the growing population of homeless in the United States, but most knowledgeable human service providers estimate that the number is disproportionately high.

Most indigenous governments have housing authorities which help their constituents access available resources in order to own or rent housing. Co-operating federal agencies include the Bureau of Indian Affairs (which makes grants to individuals to build or repair homes), the Department of Housing and Urban Development (HUD, a federal agency which has collaborated with indigenous governments to sponsor home ownership and rental programmes for indigenous people on reservations and in urban areas), and the Farmers Home Administration Program (which provides low interest loans to home-builders).

There are a number of difficulties with these programmes. In particular, the bureaucratic 'red tape' required to access these resources poses a barrier, and indigenous people's incomes are often too low to qualify, in any case. Also, because of the poverty of the occupants of low-income housing managed by indigenous governments, they often have extreme difficulty in collecting rental and home-buyer payments. This jeopardizes the indigenous government's credibility with the funding agencies (Ebbott, 1985).

Education services

One must preface any discussion of indigenous education with a reminder of the long history of abusive educational policies of the federal government which caused many indigenous people to distrust school systems. In particular, indigenous children were mandatorily removed from their communities and forced to abandon their cultures in boarding schools operated by the BIA and by missionary organizations. Many public schools continue to this day to be inhospitable to indigenous children. Alienated by a hostile school environment, many drop out as soon as it is feasible to do so. Table 2.3 shows the percentage of the population completing a high school education.

The vast majority (75 per cent) of indigenous schoolchildren in the United States attend public schools. Most of the remaining children attend BIA-supported schools, and only 'a very small number attend private or parochial schools' (Bureau of Indian Affairs, 1986). In 1985–86, the BIA funded 166 elementary and secondary schools, including '56 day schools; 46 on-Reservation boarding schools; seven off-Reservation boarding schools; 57 tribally operated schools'. An additional fifteen dormitories were operated by the BIA for children attending public schools (Bureau of Indian Affairs, 1986).

The 'Johnson–O'Malley Act' was passed in 1934 to help 'meet the special educational needs of eligible Indian students in public schools' (Bureau of Indian Affairs, 1986). The funding is administered by the BIA.

Indigenous culture, language and history have been and continue to be ignored in public schools. Not only do non-indigenous people need to acquire an appreciation of cultural diversity, but indigenous children and adults also have a right to information about their cultural heritage, their history and their treaty rights, as well as about how to deal effectively with social and economic discrimination.

Also, indigenous people have a right to be taught in ways which are epistemologically correct. In general, for example, indigenously controlled schools tend to place a much higher value on good human relations based on reciprocal respect rather than hierarchical or consensual approaches to decision-making, on sharing, and on promoting a family-like feeling of mutual responsibility amongst students, teachers and administrators.

Contrast this with the attitude in most dominant culture public schools, which are clearly hierarchical, where children have fewer rights than adults, and where indigenous children are commonly penalized because they are non-competitive in relation to their peers, sometimes indifferent to their teacher's authority, and different in many other ways. Often, the penalties are subtle, as when a child is simply ignored. At other times, the penalties are blatant, as when a child is chastised and/or assigned to a special class for behaviourally disordered and/or learning-disabled children.

Many indigenous governments and urban organizations sponsor alternative 'survival schools' in an effort to improve the learning environment of indigenous children. A problem faced by these survival schools is that they are often used as a place of 'last resort'. Consequently, as many as 80 to 85 per cent of the students enter the schools with negative attitudes and limited academic skills. Despite the extraordinary challenge, these schools appear to be at least partially successful in their mission.

There is a critical need for more indigenous people to continue beyond secondary school and to enter the professions. Table 2.4 shows the percentage of the population having four or more years of college, and is indicative of the shortage of college-educated indigenous people.

Table 2.3 Percentage of population (aged 25+) with at least a high school education in the United States, 1980

American Indian	56
Eskimo	44
Aleut	39
National (all ethnicities)	66

Source: Racial Statistics Branch, Bureau of Indian Affairs, 1986

In recent years, progress has been made. In 1985, 26,000 indigenous students were enrolled in colleges and universities (Bureau of Indian Affairs, 1986). Of these, 16,000 received BIA scholarships. Also, the IHS offers scholarships for indigenous students pursuing professions in medicine, dentistry, pharmacy, nursing and the allied health professions. These are augmented by other federal and State sources which finance scholarships and other private sources of financing for indigenous post-secondary students.

One of the most promising developments has been the establishment of indigenously operated colleges which are immensely important in reducing the 'bottle-neck' in the educational 'pipeline'. Funded largely through the BIA, there were twenty indigenously controlled colleges in 1986, and the number of students enrolled in these community colleges has burgeoned (Bureau of Indian Affairs, 1986; Kramer, 1991a).

Child welfare services

Somewhat akin to the residential school in terms of the alienation of indigenous children has been the widespread court-ordered displacement of indigenous children into European American custody. Prior to the 1978 passage of the 'Indian Child Welfare Act' in the United States, approximately 25 to 35 per cent of all indigenous children were being raised in non-indigenous settings (O'Brien, 1985). Now control is being returned to indigenous governments, and placement priorities are with extended kin or within another household in the child's indigenous community. These reforms occurred largely because indigenous societies protested against the culturally genocidal nature of child displacement. Also, research on the impact of displacement on indigenous children has documented the negative effects which 'cross-racial' placement has had on the affected children. These children tended to experience severe identity crises

Table 2.4 Percentage of persons (aged 25+) with four or more years of college in the United States, 1980

American Indian	8
Eskimo	5
Aleut	12
National (all ethnicities)	16

Source: Bureau of Indian Affairs, 1986

during adolescence because they were discriminated against as 'Indian' but were culturally 'white'. Knowing little of their rich cultural heritages and not having had opportunities to learn survival skills from a supportive indigenous community, these young people were particularly vulnerable to becoming runaways, attempting suicide, and abusing alcohol and other drugs (Westermeyer, 1979).

Because single-parent families tend to be particularly vulnerable to poverty and related problems, increases in the proportion of indigenous families headed by a single parent are a cause for concern for those single-parent families who are not surrounded by extended family and/or a supportive community. Table 2.5 shows the percentage of families headed by a single female.

It is a common practice in many indigenous communities for children to reside with people other than their parents. There are a number of reasons for this. One is that respect for children and for community means that parents do not 'own' their children, and therefore it is customary to share children whenever the child is happy living with others. Often children will circulate at will amongst a number of loving kin. Another non-traditional reason is that parents seeking employment outside their indigenous rural homelands sometimes feel that their children are better off remaining within their own indigenous cultural milieu rather than having to adjust to an alien environment.

The passage of the 1978 'Indian Child Welfare Act' has been an important step towards improving services to indigenous children and their families. However, there have been multiple problems in the implementation of the Act. Non-indigenous child welfare agencies often disregard the Act, and indigenous governments have insufficient resources to educate adequately and monitor non-indigenous human service agencies. For those agencies which do attempt to comply, there are often an insufficient number of indigenous homes (sometimes because of State licensing constraints) to meet the need for foster care. At the same time, indigenous governments must invest a large amount of scarce resources to employ child welfare workers, find and train foster parents, offer supportive services to families at risk, as well as provide counselling and legal services when abuse and neglect cases come before the courts.

OVERALL ASSESSMENT

This chapter began by summarizing the history of the forces affecting the well-being of indigenous people in the United States. The effects of being conquered, colonized and becoming the hapless victims of political, social and economic forces outside their own control has had dramatic effects on the indigenous people's collective and individual consciousness. A great many indigenous people have been in chronic grief due to the loss of natural resources needed to live with dignity in their homelands, due to the rapid displacement of traditional life-ways, and due to the loss of affirmation acquired from being a valued member of an integrated community. The resulting malaise has exhibited itself in high rates of alcohol and drug abuse and social disorder, including interpersonal neglect and violence, and in high death-rates from unnatural causes, especially accidents, homicide and suicide. Until recently, the human service agencies charged with addressing these negative features of indigenous communities were externally controlled, under funded and of questionable value. That is, despite the good intentions of the personnel, their overall effect was all too often to increase the dependency of indigenous communities on external resources, undermine indigenous helping networks, and generally increase the sense of helplessness and hopelessness of the people these human service agencies were intended to assist.

Despite this pitiful state of affairs, there is another history marked by the extraordinary courage and tenacity of the indigenous people, who have survived despite the negative forces impinging upon their life-ways. Contrary to predictions by authorities at the turn of the twentieth century, who referred to indigenous Americans as a 'disappearing race', the indigenous population is now growing rather than diminishing in numbers. Indigenous governments are regaining lost power and authority, and the overall well-being of indigenous Americans is improving. There is cause for cautious optimism as indigenous people assert increasing control over many of the forces shaping their lives, including the human service delivery systems. In summary, an indigenous renaissance is sweeping the country and transforming lives.

Table 2.5 Percentage of families headed by a single female in the United States, 1980

	1970	*1980*
American Indian	18	23
National (all ethnicities)	11	14

Source: Racial Statistics Branch, Bureau of Indian Affairs, 1986

Many of today's indigenous societies joyfully celebrate at ceremonials their people's tenacity at being able to withstand so many hardships. The celebration of survival is particularly apparent in the sobriety movement sweeping the continent and is explicitly articulated at powwows and other ceremonies. Indigenous cultures have developed strategies enabling them to cope with the changing social environment while keeping many of the strengths of their traditional culture intact. With guidance from the teachings of respected elders, who by definition are survivors, indigenous societies are forging their own solutions to the problems which have plagued them. These often selectively combine elements from both the indigenous as well as the European American culture. Mirroring their societies' adaptations, indigenous individuals are emerging with bicultural identities, but they are not the disintegrated personalities of the past. They are people who have acquired the skills and knowledge to succeed in European American society while at the same time identifying fully with their people.

In the human services sector, this has meant significant transformations in the administration and structure of agencies and the services they provide. The net outcome is a dramatic improvement in the effectiveness of the human service delivery systems and in the overall well-being of the populations they serve. Nevertheless, a host of serious problems remain. Many of the problems stem from inherent tensions between indigenous societies and the federal government. Federal agencies continue to be more responsive to the changing whims of non-indigenous politicians than to the acute human service needs of indigenous people. Consequently, the budgetary allocations for indigenous programmes are chronically inadequate to elevate the standard of living up to the level that middle-class Americans take for granted. Nevertheless, it is remarkable how indigenous governments under self-determination have managed to do so much with so little. The recent progress which has been made in the health, welfare and education of indigenous Americans is a very hopeful sign indeed.

REFERENCES

Bashshur, R., Steeler, W. and Murphy, T. (1987) 'On Changing Indian Eligibility for Health Care', *American Journal of Public Health*, 77.

Berkhoffer, R., Jr (1978) *The White Man's Indian: Images of the American Indian from Columbus to the Present*, New York: Alfred A. Knopf.

Blanchard, E. L. and Barsh R. L. (1980) 'What is Best for Tribal Children?: A Response to Fishler', *Social Work*: 350–7.

Brown, D. (1971) 'Little Crow's War', *Bury My Heart at Wounded Knee: An Indian History of the American West*, New York: Holt, Rinehart & Winston: pp. 37–65.

Bureau of Indian Affairs (1986) *American Indians Today: Answers to Your Questions*, Washington, DC: Department of the Interior.

—— (1989) *Indian Service Population and Labour Force Estimates*, Washington, DC: Department of the Interior.

Champagne, D. (1989) *American Indian Societies: Strategies and Conditions of Political and Cultural Survival*, Cambridge, MA: Cultural Survival, Inc.

Churchill, W. (ed.) (1988) *Critical Issues in Native North America*, Copenhagen, Denmark: International Working Group for Indigenous Affairs, Document No. 62 (Dec./Jan.), pp. 15–36.

Deloria, V., Jr. (ed.) (1985) *American Indian Policy in the Twentieth Century*, Norman, OK: University of Oklahoma Press.

Denevan, W. M. (ed.) (1976) *The Native Population of the Americas in 1492*, Madison, WI: University of Wisconsin Press.

Ebbott, E. (1985) *Indians in Minnesota*, 4th edn, Minneapolis, MN: University of Minnesota Press, pp. 65–74.

Fuson, R. H. (trans.) (1987) *The Log of Christopher Columbus*, Camden, ME: International Marine Publishing Co.

Hertzberg, H. (1971) *The Search for an American Indian Identity*, Syracuse, NY: Syracuse University Press.

'The Honour of All: The People of Alkali Lake' (1986) Williams Lake, BC: The Alkali Lake Indian Band, videotape.

Indian Health Service (1991) *Trends in Indian Health 1991*, Washington, DC: Government Printing Office (300–165/50070).

Jaimes, M. A. (1988) 'Federal Indian Identification Policy: A Usurpation of Indigenous Sovereignty in North America', in W. Churchill, (ed.) *Critical Issues in Native North America*, Copenhagen, Denmark: International Working Group for Indigenous Affairs, Document No. 62.

Johansen, B. E. (1982) *Forgotten Founders: Benjamin Franklin, the Iroquois, and the Rationale for the American Revolution*, Ipswich, MA: Gambit Inc., Publishers.

KQED Current Affairs Department (1985) 'Trouble on Big Mountain', San Francisco, CA: videotaped documentary.

Kramer, J. M. (1988a) 'Infant Mortality Rates and Risk Factors among American Indians Compared to Black and White Rates: Implications for Policy Change', in Winston A. Van Horne and Thomas V. Tonnson (eds) *Ethnicity and Health*, Ethnicity and Public Policy Series, vol. 7, Milwaukee, WI: University of Wisconsin, Institute on Race and Ethnicity, pp, 89–115.

—— (1988b) 'The Policy of American Indian Self-determination and its Relevance to Administrative Justice Issues in Africa', in Peter T. Simbi and Jacob N. Ngwa (eds) *Administrative Justice in Public Services: American and African Perspectives*, Stevens Point, WI: Worzalla Publishing Co.

—— (1991a) 'Advancing Post-Secondary Education in Circumpolar Regions while Respecting Indigenous People's Rights to Self-determination', *Proceedings of the First International Conference on the Role of Circumpolar Universities in Northern Development, Thunder Bay, Ontario, 24–26 Nov., 1989*, Thunder Bay, Ont.: Centre for Northern Studies.

——— (1991b) 'A Comparison of Factors Affecting Native Health in Canada and the United States', *Proceedings of the Eighth International Congress on Circumpolar Health, Whitehorse, Yukon, May 20–25, 1990*, Whitehorse, Yukon: Tundra Publishing Co.

Lenski, G. and Lenski, J. (1974) *Human Societies*, 2nd edn, New York: McGraw-Hill.

Marshall, M. (1986) 'Alcohol Use by North American Indians', *Beliefs, Behaviors, and Alcoholic Beverage: A Cross-Cultural Survey*, Ann Arbor: University of Michigan Press, pp. 109–90.

Meriam, L. (1928) *The Problem of Indian Administration*, Washington, DC: Brookings Institution, Institute for Government Research.

National Indian Health Board (1986) 'HHS Approves Notice on IHS Eligibility Changes', *National Indian Health Board Reporter* vol. 4, 5.

Norgard, P. and Walt, C. (1991) *Human Service Programs of the Fond du Lac Reservation*, Cloquet, MN: Human Services Division of the Fond du Lac Band of the Minnesota Chippewa Tribe.

Northwest Indian Child Welfare Institute (1987) *Cross-Cultural Skills in Indian Child Welfare*, Portland, OR: Parry Center for Children.

O'Brien, S. (1985) 'Federal Indian Policies and the Protection of Human Rights', in Vine Deloria, Jr (ed.) *American Indian Policy in the Twentieth Century*, Norman, OK: University of Oklahoma Press.

Organization for Economic Cooperation and Development (1985) *Measuring Health Care, 1960–83*, Paris, France: OECD, 131.

Racial Statistics Branch (1984) *A Statistical Profile of the American Indian, Eskimo, and Aleut Populations 1980 Census*, Washington, DC: Population Division, Bureau of the Census.

RedHorse, J. G. (1980) 'Family Structure and Value Orientation in American Indians', *Social Casework*, 61(8).

Sanders, D. (1985) *Aboriginal Self-Government in the United States*, Kingston, Ont.: Institute of Intergovernmental Relations.

Spencer, R. F. and Johnson, E. (1960) 'North American Language Families', *Atlas for Anthropology*, Dubuque, IA: William C. Brown Co. Publishers.

Ubelaker, D. (1976) 'The Sources and Methodology for Mooney's Estimates of North American Indian Populations', in William M. Denevan (ed.) *The Native Population of the Americas*, Madison: University of Wisconsin Press, pp. 249–86.

Westermeyer, J. (1977) 'Cross-Racial Foster Home Placement Among Native American Psychiatric Patients', *Journal of the National Medical Association*, 69(4): 231–6.

——— (1979) 'The Apple Syndrome in Minnesota: A Complication of Racial-Ethnic Discontinuity', *American Journal of Psychiatry*, 10(2): 134–40.

3 The Huichol and Yaqui Indians of Mexico

Sandra Luz Navarro Pulgarin

The Indian tribes of Mexico have suffered all types of marginalism since the Spanish era. The Huichol Indians were amongst the few groups which were not greatly influenced by the Spanish Conquest, due to the fact that they fled to the Sierra Madre to live. Today they continue living in the same area, in their same huts, in the same unhealthy environment and they suffer injustices in regard to their civil rights. The Yaqui is a very good example of the Indian who has tried, by means of uprisings and in other ways, to defend Yaqui territory and Indian culture. Huicholes and Yaquis both suffer from marginalization, lack of recognition of their own Indian values and traditional customs, invasion of their territory, and exploitation of their manual labour.

This chapter attempts to highlight the outstanding characteristics of and social benefits enjoyed by the Huicholes and Yaquis and to describe their development programmes, which began only fifty years ago, when the Instituto Nacional Indigenista (INI) was created. This institution aims to implant methods and techniques which permit the development of the Indian community, so as to better the standard of living of all ethnic groups in the country. It is for this reason that INI has acted as an advocate and defender of Indian territory, of bilingual education, of the acknowledgement of Indian rights and of a court where their law cases can be tried, and of other programmes for community expansion.

It has not been easy to accomplish these things. By trial and error in these programmes new ideas have come about, giving better solutions to such problems, so that these ethnic groups can have a higher standard of living.

It is important to point out recent efforts of the INI to include the participation of the Indian community. The INI intends Indians to design and implement programmes according to their needs, with INI assistance.

THE HUICHOLES

Historical antecedents

Some authors claim that the Huicholes are descended from groups of Indians who came from the north and settled in the plains of central Mexico. Others suggest that the ancestors of the Huicholes were Chichimecas, hunters and collectors of Teochichimecas who later adopted the corn cult.

According to Soto Sorio, the Huicholes occupied the greater part of the present territory of the State of Nayarit, but their constant quest for expansion and their necessity to find victims to offer their gods obliged them to live in a constant struggle with their neighbours, especially with the Indians living in the State of Zacatecas (see Map 3.1).

The first encounter the Huicholes had with the Spaniards was in the year 1524, when the conquerors settled near their territory. Nevertheless, it was not until 1531, with Nuño de Guzmán's expedition into the State of Sinaloa, that they were invaded by the

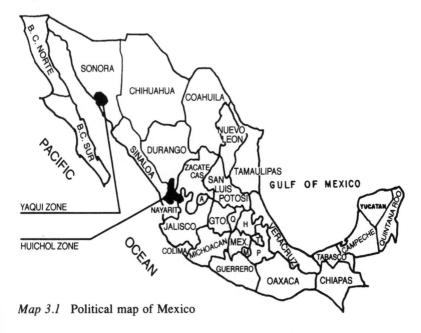

Map 3.1 Political map of Mexico

Spanish army. The Huicholes were obliged to migrate to the north and west of the State of Nayarit, where they found places which were impenetrable, and could not be reached. This geographic isolation allowed them to live independently for nearly two centuries until they were finally subdued in 1722. During this period of independence several Jesuit missions were established. The Huicholes were very disinclined to undertake any social change, and especially to adopt Christianity. In 1767 the Jesuits were expelled because they maltreated the Indians, and in their place Franciscan missions were established. During this period they had very little influence amongst the Indians. This influence was very superficial, even up to the present.

The Huicholes fought against the Laws of Alienation (Desamortización 1856) and for the reclamation of their Indian territories. Later, during the Mexican Revolution (1910–20), groups of Huicholes fought alongside Villista's forces with General Rafael Buelna, in an attempt to obtain their freedom from exploitation and from the mixed-blood Indian invasion.

During the years 1853–54 they started talking about Manuel Lozada, a controversial leader. Some historians consider him a bandit, because he headed an Indian uprising from the district of Tepic, Nayarit, committing several atrocities which made the people of the district panic. However, others consider him to be the opposite: defender of the Indian groups, agrarian leader, and even a hero. Because of their desire to become independent, many groups of Huicholes fought between the years 1860 and 1877 with Lozada's army.

It must be emphasized that the Huicholes have always been energetically opposed to all cultural change. They erect a barrier against everything that is strange to them. There has consequently been very little cultural change, especially in the distant parts of the Sierra Madre Occidental mountains. It is this resistance to change which makes it difficult to establish social programmes and to integrate them into Mexican society and productivity.

In 1895 Lumholtz, an anthropologist, estimated the population to be about 4,500. The census taken in 1930 showed 3,716. A more exact census was the one taken by 'Operation Huicot' (Huichol, Cora, Tepehuano) under the Lerma Plan (PLAT 1970–1877), the main objective of which was to promote the development of the regions near the following rivers: the Lerma, Chapala and Santiago in the States of Jalisco, Nayarit, Durango and Zacatecas. The Huichol population was estimated to be 8,291 (see Table 3.1).

Table 3.1 The Lerma Plan 'Operation Huicot': estimated census

State	Town council	Huicholes
Nayarit	La Yesca	1,447
	El Nayar	2,117
	Ruiz	517
	Rosamorada	100
	Acaponeta	67
Durango	Mezquital	232
Jalisco	Mezquitic	2,711
	Bolaños	1,089
Zacatecas	Valparaiso	11
Total		8,291

Source: Enrique Cárdenas de la Pena, *Sobre las Nubes del Nayar, SCT*, Gobierno del Estado de Nayarit, Mexico, 1988: 74

Table 3.2 Linguistic data

Indian	Population who have spoken the Indian language for 5 or more years	Condition of the Spanish language		
		Spanish language	Do not speak Spanish	Not specified
Huichol	40,777	34,852	5,359	566

Source: *X Censo General de Población y Vivienda*, 1980, Estado de Jalisco, Vol. II, book 14, Mexico, 1984

The Huichol language has its origin in the Yuto-Aztec language. It is closely related to the Nahuatl language. Even though there are some differences in the dialects of various communities, this does not influence speakers'communication with one another (see Table 3.2).

The Huicholes are located in the high ranges of the Sierra Madre Occidental mountains, which has several high peaks that vary between 1,000 and 3,000 metres. The area is located to the north of the State of Jalisco, in the municipalities of Mezquitic and Bolaños, to the east of Nayarit, and to the south of Durango and Zacatecas, where a small number of Huicholes live. The five main communities where the largest Huichol populations live are: Tuxpan de Bolaños, San Sebastián Teponahuaxtlán, Santa Catarina Cuexcomatitlán, San Andres Cohamiata and Guadalupe de Ocotan. These are situated

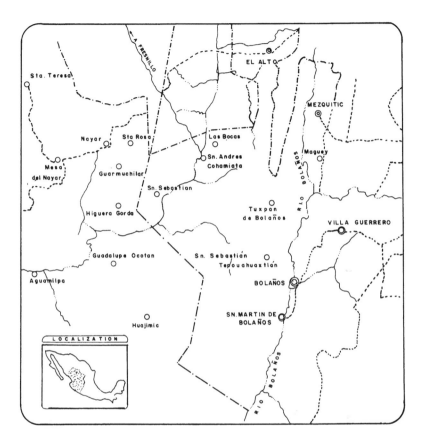

Map 3.2 Location of the Huichol region

within an area of 4,107 square kilometres in which 400 villages are scattered (see Map 3.2).

This region has a marked contrast geographically and its climate is usually cool. Winter is dry in the higher parts and hot in the ravines. The rainy season begins in the middle of June and continues until the middle of October. During this time many villages have no communication with the outside world.

There are great forest areas consisting of pine, oak and cedar, which are susceptible to exploitation. In places like San Andres Cohamiata there are large ranges of areas of pastureland that could be used for grazing cattle, but these natural resources are hard to develop because of poor transportation which consists of walking or by horse between villages. Small planes are used to communicate with outside regions, and there are several airfields, the largest one being in San Andres Cohamiata.

The population

The Huicholes are of medium height – charming, agreeable and very ceremonious. The new generation continues to live in the same places as did their ancestors, conserving their magic world of mysticism and the ceremonies to their ancient gods; deer – peyote – corn. Deer represents food and fertility. They sprinkle the corn seed with the blood of the deer so that the blood will fertilize the seed. It is a sacrifice they offer their gods in order to obtain rain for their crops, good health and long life. Peyote – *Lophophora williamsii Lemaire* – is a small cactus that has hallucinogenic properties, and is used to curb hunger and thirst. It plays an important part in Huichol methods of conserving their art traditions, agriculture and religious beliefs. And as for corn, if they have none, they consider themselves without food even if they have other sources of nutrition.

They have a very extensive mythology, but no supreme god. Their deities are known as 'Grandfathers', 'Father' or 'Mother' and so on. It is very probable that they do not honour all their gods but they do honour the most important, like 'the Grandfathers', 'the Sun God' and the 'God of Fire'. Both of these latter ones seem to be found underground. 'The Aunts' are the four important deities of the rain which are supposed to live in caverns underneath Santa Catarina and the 'Sea God' is represented by serpents. The 'God of Fertility' is considered as a separate entity and its temple is very important.

Indigenous policy

The Huicholes live in scattered villages after their family group tradition, in extreme poverty, without running water, light or other services, in a very unhealthy environment due to their isolated way of life, their lack of integration into Mexican society, the poor community economy and many other factors no less important. From 1576 until the dictatorship of president Porfirio Díaz (1876–1911), the policy towards Indians was one of segregation. This excluded them from the many benefits which the mixed-blood and Creole population enjoyed. Except for the alms they received from religious institutions, they had no other help. After the Mexican Revolution (1910–20), the government tried to help their development. Under this policy we find a few organizations which were started for their protection.

In 1936 a Department for Indian Affairs was created as an institution to co-ordinate programmes that the federal government and the States planned for the indigenous communities as well as to fulfil functions for protection and to obtain benefits for the inhabitants. In 1946 this Department was eliminated, and in its place another Department dependent on the Secretaría de Educación Pública (SEP) was created. This Department was given the title of General Direction for Indigenous Affairs, and in 1948, in answer to the proposals made in the first Inter-American Indigenous Congress, the Instituto Nacional Indigenista (INI) was created in Mexico.

According to President Adolfo Lopez Mateos, the object of this institution was to investigate the problems of the Indians in Mexico, to study and promote the measures considered necessary for the federal executive, to intervene and to function as a consultant for official institutions as well as to work to better the Indian way of life, with the approval of the President (Reed, 1972).

In Mexico there are 56 ethnic groups scattered amongst the different regions. In these groups Co-ordination Centres have been set up by the federal government and the States, with the aim of establishing average social standing, economic and cultural, for the Huicholes. Each Centre works according to the characteristics of the region in which it finds itself. Centres follow the structures and rules imposed by the federal government and develop the following programmes: Health, Education, Forestry, Agriculture, Economics, Social Work, Communication and Transportation. All of these are brought into being by the INI in co-operation with government institutions in the various communities.

The INI founded the Cora-Huichol Co-ordination Centre in 1960, with its base in Tepic, Nayarit. Its principal objective was to satisfy as much as possible the most urgent needs of the ethnic groups. Because of the size of the area and problems in communication, in 1976 the Huichol Co-ordination Centre was established in La Magdalena, Jalisco.

The Cora-Huichol Co-ordination Centre undertakes the investigations concerning the general problems of the region, giving the hierarchy of cause and effect as follows:

Cause and effect
1 Lack of global and integral diagnosis.
   Effect: has as a consequence, a more or less mediocre programme.

2 Little constitutional knowledge of ethnic specifications.
   Effect: An unequal enforcement of justice.
3 Economy of subsistence. Poor agricultural product, extensive cattle-raising regions with small results. Little or no technology in forestry and rich activity in handcraft but poor commercialization.
   Effect:
   3.1 Unemployment.
   3.2 Emigration.
   3.3 Intermediaries.
   3.4 Low income levels.
   3.5 Poor nutritional levels.
4 Lack of respect for its culture, traditions and organizations.
   Effect: The effect can be translated in the communities having no direct participation.
5 Lack of true attention to health.
   Effect: Sickness and death due to poor nutrition, poor living conditions, lack of shoes, clothing and the existence of noxious insects.
6 Education: very low educational level.

Housing

Indian living conditions are extremely miserable. Everyone erects their own homes made of mud, stone or reeds, depending on the region and climate. The roofs are made of thatch. Houses have no windows and only one very low door. Usually the living quarters consist of one room; sometimes two, with a partition to separate kitchen from bedroom. They are round in shape although sometimes they might be square. When there are two or three houses together, they share the same yard. These houses contain no furniture; when the Indians eat, they squat on the ground or sit on logs. Some have small stools made of reeds. They have no tables. They sleep on the floor or on mats. These huts are scattered all over the mountains, some near rivers, others on the sides of slopes. Frequently the Huicholes move from one place to another, and then they construct another hut. They have special ceremonial centres where a few families live. It is here that they gather for their festivals. There is no government programme for housing, only a little help to roof the huts, for which they are given corrugated cardboard.

Education

The educational programmes directed towards the Indian population have developed favourably over the years. The INI and the Dirección General de Educación Indigenista (DGEI) have made the following analysis: in Mexico, after the Conquest, the education imparted to the Indian was controlled by different political currents which were not in the interest of the Indians. These political currents were first, segregation, then incorporation and, finally, integration. With integration has come bilingual and bicultural education, and respect for plural ethnic culture.

In 1911 the Mexican government established rudimentary schools. Its objective was to teach the Indian to learn to read, write and speak in Spanish and to learn basic arithmetic. In 1933 the government founded eleven Indian boarding schools. Its chief purpose was to train the young people in agricultural technology so that they in turn could take their knowledge to the different regions, as necessary. At present there are 32 schools, where youngsters from age 14 to 21 are trained. The objective is to eliminate cultural background and to provide basic education at the elementary school. These boarding schools also train the Indian in different productive skills. Those who attend these schools are interned for the whole scholastic year and can only go home during school vacations. The high cost of maintenance of these schools has made it impossible to expand the programme. There are about 5,300 students attending these schools.

Due to distance, geographical regions like the Cora-Huichol-Tarahumara, where there is a wide dispersion of population, developed an alternative educational system to boarding schools. These are substitute schools called 'shelters'. These schools are situated strategically amongst the widely spread villages. In the beginning they were run by two promoters from the Department of Education, a man, a woman and sometimes a cook. Children remain in these shelters from Monday through Friday and go home for the weekend.

In 1971 five shelters were officially recognized. By the school year 1975–76 they had increased to 629, in which there were 32,500 students. At the time of writing there are 1,250 such schools, with a total of 63,900 Indian children.

Of the 10 million Indians living in Mexico, 3 million are women who are basically in charge of their children's education. The Secretaria de Educación Pública (SEP) and its different departments have elaborated a plan and programme (1988) for educating and training these Indian women. This programme promotes three areas, with the following basic units:

1 *Educational development*: learning their mother tongue, oral Spanish, an intensive course at an elementary school, knowledge of infant care and health care.
2 *Promotion of the family income*: family production, commerce, credits and savings.
3 *Organization of community development*: organizing their community for social benefits and cultural promotion.

These programmes in the Indian communities are co-ordinated by educational promoters, technicians in agriculture and veterinary science, surgeons, doctors and social workers. Each person taking part in these programmes must be highly trained and must be bilingual.

Health

The Huicholes are in a deplorable state of health and are malnourished. The most common illnesses – gastrointestinal and acute respiratory illnesses, skin disease and tuberculosis – are very frequent in these regions.

Health programmes arc carried out by the Instituto Nacional Indigenista (INI), the Secretaria de Salud (SSA) and the Instituto Nacional del Seguro Social-Solidaridad (INSS-Solidaridad). The INI has at its service a doctor and a dentist who serve the Indian villages. The INSS-Solidaridad and the SSA have health clinics; for example, in the surrounding areas of Durango there are twenty medical units and three medical centres. The INI sends its serious cases to the nearest cities. They receive food and shelter from the relatives who accompany them. Although medical fees are very low, some of the patients receive very little benefits from these Institutions. In 1986, at the beginning of the programme called the 'Día Nacional de Vacunación Antipoliomielítica' (National Day of Poliomyelitis Vaccination), in which it was planned to vaccinate all the children of the country in the same day, some villages in the State of Durango and possibly other States had not received a single vaccine or any other medical service during the year.

Traditional Huichol medicine is a practice intimately tied to their way of life and religious beliefs. The Huicholes recognize two types of diseases: foreign or Spanish disease and their native ones. Six diseases are of Spanish origin: measles, whooping cough, smallpox, tuberculosis, the plague and typhoid. The ability of their healers (shamans) to cure these diseases is very limited, so they resort to magic for their prevention. To cure these maladies they resort to ceremonial rituals, medicinal plants and peyote.

Through the training programme for indigenous women, it has been possible to retain many cultural practices and promote actions aimed at maintaining better family health. The programmes are orientated as follows:

1 A re-evaluation of traditional practices in medicine and an ecological equilibrium.
2 A more profitable use of the natural resources found in each region.
3 Better basic hygienic practices.
4 Problems of unwholesome or unhealthy conditions in the communities.

The economy

The fragile economy of the Huicholes rests mostly on their traditional agriculture, based generally on corn, beans and pumpkins. The corn crops are very poor, averaging from 300 to 400 kilogrammes per hectare. Bean crops produce about 150 to 200 kilogrammes per hectare. Another part of their economic activities is cattle-raising. As was mentioned before, they have large ranges of pasture land. Their principal source of family income is from cattle-raising and the selling of cattle to people of mixed blood. Amongst the different groups of Huicholes, they consider themselves either rich or poor according to the amount of cattle owned. The keeping of sheep is basically to produce wool.

Commerce, in the form of marketing, is unknown, but not the buying or selling of cattle or other beasts. In times of drought or in winter, the Indians dedicate their time to the making of beautiful and colourful handcrafted articles. At such times provisions become scarce and whole families have to travel to the coast or to Tepic, Nayarit, to work on tobacco plantations or cut sugar cane. Others find work in their own communities with mixed-blood people or close relatives.

According to the Centro Coordinador de Durango (Co-ordination Centre of Durango), the monthly income per capita is 89,915.00 Mexican pesos (US$31.00), so it is easy to imagine the extreme poverty in which the Huicholes live. It is necessary to mention that the Huicholes are not prone to exhibiting abundance, in either food or clothing. To the Huicholes, a display of wealth is in very poor taste; it is only permitted in their ceremonies.

With the idea of promoting their social and economic development, in 1973 government credit institutions participated in the first economic promotions, such as the fattening of cattle. In 1975 the Banrural Bank intensified this activity in order to help the Plan Huicot, with economic resources from the Crédito Agrícola Bank and the Crédito Ejidal Bank. However, this programme was stopped so as to let each State government take care of the Indian problems in their own district. The government of Zacatecas stopped the programme entirely, as it had no Indian groups in its State. In 1977, Banrural channelled these activities through the Banco del Norte for the Indians in Durango, the Banco del Occidente for the Huicholes of Jalisco, and the Banco del Pacífico Norte for the ethnic groups in Nayarit.

All these activities and work in the mountain regions have taken place in spite of tremendous problems due to poor transportation. In the beginning all food, agricultural seeds, tools, medicines, agricultural machinery, educational equipment, animals (pigs, chickens and so on) were transported by plane. It was not until 1984 that there were roads within the area.

The response of the Huicholes to these programmes has been positive, since it has helped develop their natural resources. At present, the Cora-Huichol Co-ordination Centre of Tepic, Nayarit (INI), has promoted projects for the development of the Indian regions, in co-ordination with the following institutions:

- Secretaría de Comunicaciones y Transportes (SCT)
- Secretaría de Agricultura y Ganaderia (SAG)
- Confederación Nacional de Fruticultura (CONAFRUT)
- Distribuidora Conasupo, SA (DICONSA)
- Secretaría de Recursos Hidráulicos (SARH) and others (see Table 3.3).

Likewise, in Durango and Jalisco they have set up programmes like these, with flexibility to suit the specific region and community.

Political organization and rights

The Huichol Organization has four authorities: governor, judge, captain and deputy marshal. The first two have an assistant, or 'Topil' (police). The captain has as subordinate a sergeant, and the deputy marshal is helped by the Alguareal (police).

Table 3.3 Proposals for projects and general undertakings of the Cora-Huichol Co-ordination Centre, Tepic, Nayarit, 1990

Project title	Executive institution
Rural Roads	SCT
Forest Conservation and Exploitation	INI
Cattle-raising for Meat Unit	INI
Cattle for Double Purpose Unit	SAG
Corn and Bean Planting	INI
Family Orchards	INI
Sheep-raising Unit	INI
Agricultural Unit	INI-SAG
Poultry Unit	INI-SAG
Fodder Crops Unit	DIGER
Land and Water Conservation	SAG
Construction of Water Troughs	SAG
Establishing Orchards	CONAFRUT
Regional Warehouse Construction	DICONSA
Radio-telephone Programme	SCT
Bridge Construction	SCT
Sawmills	SAG
Breeding of Pack Animals Unit	INI
Projects and Surveys	SAG
Commercialization of Agricultural Products	INI
Construction of Irrigation Works	FIRCO
Agricultural Machinery	INI

Source: Cora-Huichol Co-ordination Centre, Tepic, Nayarit, 1990

The governor's decision is final in community matters, and, together with the judge, they preside over cases to be judged. The captain represents the police force and is under the orders of the governor. The deputy marshal is in charge of prisoners. He places all the fines, puts malefactors in gaol and makes the delinquent work on the governor's properties. Every year there is a change of personnel, and this is known as 'cambio de varas' (change of sceptre). With the exception of homicide, the judicial departments are self-governed (quarrels, robberies, offences against parents or authorities, or violation of law and order in the community).

Former governors and the elderly people of the community form a council, and it is they who analyse and decide on matters of importance.

According to lawyer Arturo Alvarez Sanchez from the Tuxpan de Bolaños Co-ordination Centre, the serious infractions against the law in this community are of the following types:

Homicide

The authorities place the culprit in a room where the *cepo* is. This consists of a pole with holes. According to the seriousness of the crime the culprit is tied by a foot or his fingers. After 24 hours he is taken out and hung by both hands so as to publicize his crime. Once he is sentenced by a municipal law he is turned over to higher authorities.

Adultery

The authorities bring in the culprit tied and naked, so he will feel ashamed and will not commit the offence again.

Robbery

He is brought in and, if found guilty, must pay twice the value of what he took.

Witchcraft

The person bewitched, together with the authorities, bring in the witch, who must cure the person he has bewitched. In case he refuses, he is punished in the *cepo* or torture pole.

However, the functions of the traditional authorities have been decreased, in view of the implantation of the national government laws, under which community laws are not recognized, but only the laws regarding citizens. In cases of major crimes, the Indian is judged and sentenced in a language which he does not understand and by laws different from those of his community.

During the Conquest, due to the extreme poverty of the Indians and their ignorance of the law, it was very hard for them to obtain justice unless they could find someone to help them – a lawyer or someone who knew the law and could follow all the steps ordained for the tribunals. Learning of this, in 1541 the Spanish crown ordered someone to be named to protect the Indian before the judges. A few years later a lawyer was named to represent them in all civil or criminal trials. At the end of the century, the monarch tackled the problem, placing lawyers paid by the government at the service of the Indians to help them at the trials. Two lawyers had to be present every day to assist them in civil cases and two lawyers for criminal cases.

The Instituto Nacional Indigenista has established legal departments in which there is always a lawyer available to assist the Indian in all cases of infraction against the law, real or false. Very frequently their violations are due to lack of knowledge of the federal law, ignorance of the language and lack of knowledge of their rights. Within the programme, in defence of the Indian, the INI has helped release 3,224 Indians who have been gaoled (data until 1988).

On 11 November 1989, the director of the programme for the procuration of justice announced that 1,045 Indians had been released and that there were 2,000 additional prisoners. He estimated that the main problem was violations regarding possession of the land, and violation to rights within urban zones. About the latter he stated that, due to the migration from country to city, there were almost 4 million Indians who lived by working as bricklayers, domestic servants or as pedlars without any attention, and very often they suffered violations of their labour rights. Their work is usually underpaid, as their wages are always lower than the established rate. Also, they do not have access to the Instituto Mexicano del Seguro Social, which is the institution that benefits the work force of Mexico in case of illness.

Indian demands can be felt in the Ethnic groups in Mexico. For example, regarding the meeting held in Nayarit the *Mexico Indigenous Review* reports:

In the first days of October they gathered in the common land of the Cora, Tepehuanes, Mexicaneros and Huicholes from Jalisco and Nayarit. Conclusions expressed by the Huichol representative were: respect for their traditions, way of life and customs; and recognition of their cultural form of organization and the need to be recognized constitutionally as Indians with their own characteristics. The meeting approved the initiative to reform Article 40, and a proposal was made for the Indian to be recognized in Mexican society. Also included in such a decree was a proposal for the Indian to participate directly in the political life of the country and in defence of their indigenous interests; to prohibit foreigners from pillaging of their sacred grounds, handcraft and music; to prohibit other religions from weakening their unity and their ancestral beliefs. They also asked for faithful respect of the traditional government structure and for the city council to recognize these governments, a bilingual education that would strengthen the true values and last, prohibition of the settling of mixed-bloods near their ceremonial centre so their

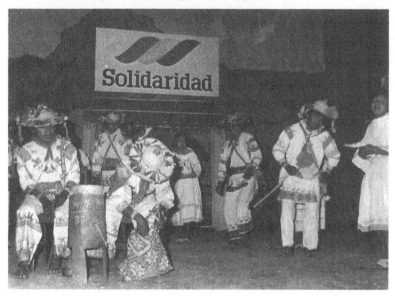

Plate 3.1 'Mitote' Huichol dance
Photo: Victor Madrigal

sacred grounds would not be violated. Also the prohibition of bootlegging of liquor during their festivals. The meeting was closed by Velso Delgado, Governor of Nayarit.

(*El Universal*, 14 October 1988)

Legal status

In Mexico there was no Indian legislation. There was no national law that recognized the existence of ethnic groups in the country. It was not until 7 April 1989 that the National Commission of Justice was established for the Indian communities of Mexico under the Instituto Nacional Indigenista, by the President of Mexico, Carlos Salinas de Gortari, who said:

I take much interest in the proposal of elevating to a constitutional status the acknowledgement of the Indian communities. If any Mexican is entitled to be recognized by the Mexican constitution, it is precisely the Indian.

Since then, the Commission resolved to formulate a proposal where the cultural rights of the Indian communities were recognized constitutionally. The first proposal was made on 8 August 1989. The proposal consists of adding to Article 4 the following measure:

> The Mexican nation has a plural ethnic setting, supported fundamentally by the presence of the Indians of Mexico. The State Constitutions and the Federal Ordinance and laws, both state and city, shall establish a norm wherein it will protect and preserve the development of the language, culture, uses, customs and specific form of social organization of the Indian communities in everything that is not against the present Constitution. This Ordinance shall be of public order and social interest. The law shall establish the proceedings in which the Indian will be assured an effective access to state jurisdiction. In legal trials of federal or local order, in which the Indian is a part, his judicial practices and customs will be taken into consideration during the process and at the time when such cases are resolved.

Agrarian rights

The Indian is organized under a communal regime within a legal status that the Presidency of the Republic has issued, and that has been granted by confirmatory laws of communal possessions. This proves the inalienable right of the Indians to be the legal owners of their territory. It is important to emphasize that the Mexican Agrarian Law does not mention in the Bill anything special about the communal property of Indian groups. It only recognizes Mexican citizens. Article 52 refers to rights to agrarian property which the nucleus of the population acquired and which cannot be mortgaged or exchanged, so that in no case can they be taken away or rented; any act, contract or operation concerning this land is null. The parcel of communal land allocated the Huicholes is approximately 3,000 square metres per adult, which cannot be bought or sold.

In support of these agrarian dispositions the lawyers of the INI very frequently have cases to defend in which they intervene in disputes between mixed-bloods and Indians within their territorial limits. In the case of the Huicholes, even when the Agrarian Reform (1915–35, 1934–40, 1940–58 until the present time) confirmed the communal property to the Indian, the mixed-bloods are always invading their pasture lands and territories, taking advantage of the lack of boundaries between the States of Nayarit and Jalisco. Some inversion projects and plans have been affected because of this problem in Huichol communities.

THE YAQUI

Historical antecedents

The history of the Yaqui tribe is marked by a theme of self-determination and territorial sovereignty which, over the past 400 years, has exposed them to armed struggles against the different political regimes that have been in power in the country. The Yaqui are considered rebels and very resistant ones, which has been confirmed by their long struggles since the sixteenth century until the twentieth century. This tribe is an example of the rejection of external domination.

In 1523, Diego de Guzmán attempted to conquer the Yaquis' territory, and failed. It was not until the beginning of the seventeenth century that Diego Martínez de Hurdaide attempted a second invasion, and he too failed. However, a peace treaty was signed with the Yaqui, which permitted the Jesuit missionaries Andres Perez de Rivas and Tomas Basilio to develop a mission in the area. These missionaries had a strong influence on the group organization, until the Yaqui were dispersed amongst 80 villages. The Yaqui are organized in eight districts along the side of the Yaqui river: Cocorit, Bacum, Torim, Vicam Potam, Rahum, Huiriris and Belem.

There were changes in the means of economic production because of the use of new technology and agricultural machinery. New crops were introduced, especially wheat, and also cattle-raising was started. Because of these changes Yaqui and European elements are mixed together, which changed the old Yaqui culture.

In 1740 the Yaqui rebelled for the first time. The cause of this rebellion is not clear, with some writers claiming that it was because the Jesuits infringed their rights while others believe that the Jesuits failed to cope with their needs as a growing population. This rebellion ended with the execution of the principal Yaqui leaders. From 1741 to 1825 there was peace, and the Yaqui became the dominant group in the northwest of the country.

In 1825, Juan Banderas headed an armed rebellion with the aim of proclaiming the independence of the Confederación India de Sonora (the Indian Confederation of Sonora State), which would bind the Pimas Bajos, Opatas and Mayas. The following year peace was signed. But even with this measure taken, the government initiated a systematic attack against the Yaqui. José María Leyva (Cajeme), a Yaqui leader in 1875, instigated another rebellion with the same goal as before, but he was defeated. This leader again tried to gain independence in 1885, in answer to an ordinance from the federal government to colonize the territory. In 1886, Cajeme was caught and executed by federal troops. Juan Maldonado (Tatabiate), another Yaqui leader, continued the struggle for their land. It was not until 15 May 1897 that a peace agreement was signed with the authorities. However, the oligarchy took possession of a portion of the Yaqui territory, which was broken up into small areas and given away, initiating colonization. For this reason, in 1899 there was a new rebellion, which was immediately stopped by the army.

In 1901, the offensive was again taken by the government of Porfirio Díaz, and many Yaqui were deported to the south of the country (Yucatan, Quintana Roo). Colonization was cleared for foreign owners of large estates, and for nationals.

The Yaqui continued fighting until 1913. Once more, in 1926, President Alvaro Obregón opened 500 square kilometres to colonization, resulting in a rebellion lasting until 1929. Finally, recognition of the Yaqui demand took effect in 1939, when President General Lázaro Cárdenas was in office. Legally, 4,890 square kilometres were authorized as land for the Yaqui tribe. They were also authorized to use 50 per cent of the water from La Angostura dam (now Lázaro Cárdenas Dam) to irrigate their land.

Geographic environment

The Yaqui tribe resides in the southeast of Sonora State in the communities of Guaymas, Bacum, Cajeme and Empalme, in an area of 4,890 square kilometres (see Map 3.3). The climate in the area is semi-desert with very extreme temperatures ranging from 50º Centigrade in summer to 3º in winter. This region has good transportation. The Pacific southern railway runs from west to east and also alongside a part of the highway which runs from Guaymas to Ciudad Obregón. There is a dirt road that crosses the mountains, and there are roads from different communities which connect with the main highway. There are seven bus lines and one truck line, which is the property of a Yaqui company.

Demography and language

After the period of the Yaqui wars, only 4,000 Yaqui were left in the valley. Ortiz's peace helped the Indians to return, and their population increased to 18,000 from 1900 to 1905. But at the start of 1910 the population again decreased because of their deportation to the south

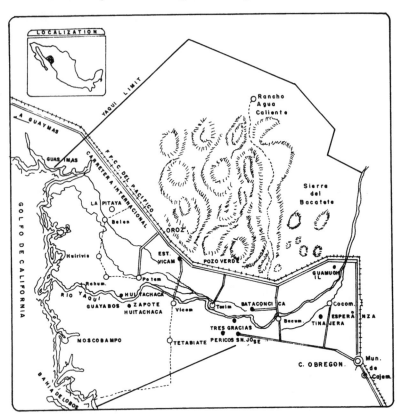

Map 3.3 Location of the Yaqui zone

of the country and movement into the mountain regions, with the result that only 8,500 Yaqui remained in 1930. In 1982 a census was taken in the Yaqui communities by INI and the Dirección Regional de Educación Indígena, which showed a population of 23,444, of which 4,190 were monolingual.

According to Swadesh and Arana, the Yaqui language comes from the Cora-Pima of the Yuto-Nahua group of the Nahaucuitlateco. The Yaqui language is spoken normally within families and between members of the tribe, even in the presence of strangers.

Social and political organization

The basis of Yaqui social organization is the monogamous or patriarchal nuclear family. The chief authority is the father, who is the economic provider, and who also helps in some of the domestic work. He also participates in the informal education of his children, who, from an early age, help in productive labour.

Women take care of the children and the old people, and also help to provide economically, especially in commercial activities. Yaqui women play a very important part in the community, normally intervening in economic, social and political issues.

Yaqui political organization is represented by a civil, military and religious authority. They have a legislative department and a series of norms established for their traditions. Each community authority has a *cobanahua* (governor), a *pueblo yohue* (major town), a captain, a commander, a *Temastimole* (liturgical male teacher), a *Kiyohteryohue* (a liturgical female teacher), and an army, formed by the rest of the community. All of these positions are for life, except that of the governor, who is elected annually, but it is possible for him to be re-elected. They also elect an assistant auxiliary, a general secretary to the governor. The community authorities meet every Sunday in order to review all the judicial cases and also to talk about community problems. If a problem exists in any of the communities, the authorities of the eight communities meet at Potoman.

In the last few years there has been a division amongst the Yaqui groups. On one side you find the *Civilistas* or *Auténticos*, and on the other, the *Governistas*. But even so, if there is a problem from the exterior, they will unite against any aggression.

Housing

The Yaqui house is very simple, generally having a bedroom, a kitchen and a porch. Its structure is very simple. It is made of reed covered by mud, and they plant mesquit on the ground. They have no plumbing at all. The furniture is very poor. Their beds are made of metal or wood, or they sleep on mats covered with cardboard. They have a few chairs, tables and benches and a few cardboard boxes in which to put their clothes. They have little help to improve their living quarters. Only about 50 per cent of the homes have running water or are near a stream or irrigation canal, with the remainder having no running water but occasionally receiving water in tanks. There are no specific programmes for housing.

Education

Educational programmes are similar to Indian educational programmes in the rest of the country. In 1983, of 6,515 Yaqui students in the territory, only 1,408 were taught by Yaqui teachers. According to the Indigenist programme, 5,103 students went to the federal or State schools in the region, but is not known how many of them were Yaqui.

Kindergarten school programmes are run by bilingual members of the tribe. Children from 4 to 6 years attend these schools. The teaching is translated into the Yaqui language.

Teachers are bilingual, but the students do not learn to write, as there is no written form of the language.

Technical Secondary Agricultural Schools were set up by the government in the Yaqui area to help with the urgent needs of the tribe, but very few Indians have profited by this. For example, from 1977 to 1980 only eighteen agricultural technicians and eight livestock technicians graduated. Four boarding schools take care of children from the community who have no means of education, each with 50 students.

Yaqui youths are also awarded scholarships for secondary, preparatory or professional schools. These scholarships are given by the INI in co-ordination with the Dirección de Educación Indígena.

Health

The principal health problem of the Yaqui tribe comes from chronically poor nutrition and a deficient knowledge of personal and community hygiene. The principal causes of sickness are intestinal parasites, malnutrition, and skin and dental diseases. A major health problem is alcoholism amongst the male population, which is strongly tied to their religious culture, because at a very early age the young men take part in festivals. There are three groups of Alcoholics Anonymous, where members of the tribe go for rehabilitation. Drugs and drug dependency are beginning to be problems amongst the young people. There are no existing specific programmes aimed at this problem, only those that exist within the national government.

Medical attention is the responsibility of the social welfare and INI institutions which are in the surrounding area. These institutions have not been able to attack these health problems properly, because of factors such as lack of personnel, and of economic and material aids.

Another way of coping with Yaqui health problems is by their traditional medicine. The Yaqui tribe still retains its magic religious concepts of diseases. They think disease is a disorder in the person,

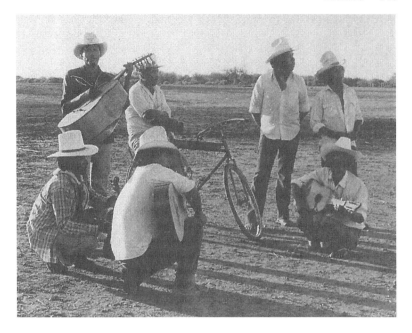

Plate 3.2 Yaqui Indians
Photo: Ana Teresa Lizárraga

provoked by an imbalance in their relationship with their divinity, with the spirits, with nature or with people around them. The first reaction of the sick person and his family is to seek a reconciliation, using rites and natural medicine. There are those who specialize in these traditional practices, for example, people who utilize herbs as medicine or herb doctors, those who set bones, masseurs, and others who use prayers and other cures in general. In Yaqui traditional medicine herbs are widely used; for example, the poplar is used for swollen body parts, while eucalyptus, pomegranate and ashes are employed for respiratory problems. The Yaqui dry and eat a rattlesnake as a cure for many illnesses. There are many other practices that are used in Indian traditional medicine.

The economy

The fundamental activity in the Yaqui economic system is agriculture, in which 95 per cent of the population take part. The products raised in the Valle del Yaqui are soya, cotton, wheat, corn, tomatoes, alfalfa, peas, chilli, fresh vegetables, oranges and lemons. These products are sent to national markets or are used in the community. Of the 4,890 square kilometres of Yaquiland, only 2,000 square kilometres can be irrigated and used for cultivation, while 70 square kilometres have a high concentration of salt, are not level or have no drainage. It is estimated that 400 square kilometres have been invaded by *ejidatarios* (poor farmers) or small landowners. About 2,000 square kilometres can only be used for cultivation of livestock, but the water problem is very severe.

Besides these problems, the Yaqui are confronted with the commercialization of their products and being able to obtain bank credits from agricultural banks. This causes them to rent their land, work for someone else or on their fields. Since 1953, the Yaqui have formed organizations for credit. The groups were formed by ten members, having ten hectares. In 1983 a Comisión de Fomento Agrícola y Ganadera was formed from the Yaqui colony, which was charged with co-ordinating construction for irrigation and provision for running water, and for making agricultural implements available. They were provided with livestock and a transaction for credit operations through the Banco Nacional de Crédito Agrícola, which was established in 1926.

Until 1951 an International Commission was encouraged to aid the development of the Yaqui tribe with all the shares and obligations transferred to the Banco Nacional de Crédito Ejidal, which today is Banco Nacional de Crédito Rural (Banrural). Until 1983 Banrural worked with different groups, integrated by 2,472 members. Each group is represented by a *socio elegado* ('delegate'). In the past three years three shipments of machinery have been financed by this credit bank, but this agricultural improvement failed because of the lack of technology, lack of counsel, vigilance and control, and because of external interests and other factors.

The only forestal activity within the Yaqui tribe is the exploitation of vegetable coal. In 1979 a Union of Coal Products was formed, but it failed because it had no counselship.

The Yaqui livestock activity was fully developed by Jesuit missionaries, and by the time they abandoned the region (1767) the Yaqui had adopted livestock-raising as part of their economy. At present they raise different kinds of cattle, receiving technical counselling from Banrural, SARH and INI.

The Yaqui territory has approximately 60 kilometres of litoral, with great natural resources on its seacoasts. There are two large bays – Lobos and Guasimas – and Los Esteros de la Luna, Palomas, Baira,

Suiti, Camopochi and Algodones. In June 1958 the Sociedad Cooperativa de Comunidades, SCL was founded with 150 members, having an initial capital of 22,500 Mexican pesos. At the beginning of 1972 its name was changed to Sociedad Cooperativa de Producción Pesquera de Rivera Comunidades Yaquis, SCL. Until March 1983 it had on its register 593 active members, and a board of directors was integrated by an administration and vigilant committee and by the necessary commissions. For their activities and functions the Co-operative Society asked for the backing and approval of the authorities of eight communities.

Most of the members of the Co-operative come from the following communities: Oroz, Huitchaca, Potom, Rahum, Huirivis, Belem and Vicam town. They transfer to the fishing camps during the shrimp season, from September to December. Only 20 per cent of these people live permanently there. The Co-operative spends large sums on the construction of temporary houses to accommodate its members during these four months, with the aim of solving this problem. In order to develop and activate fishing, the government instigated a housing project (150 houses). The State government endorses the Co-operative for the fund for popular housing, and the Co-operative made individual contracts with the beneficiaries. According to data for the 1982 season, shrimp production was 129,574,075 kilogrammes, which represents about US$1,304,163.

Indigenist action

The Centro Coordinador Indigenista Yaqui was founded in 1973, and until 1975 it had no systematic programme, but was allowed certain amounts of money for priority or urgent actions. Up until 1982 it kept its organization and its operational programmes were the same as those implemented by the INI in the rest of the country. In 1983, because of a petition by the traditional authority and the INI, a plan called the Plan Integral de Desarrollo Yaqui (Integral Plan of Yaqui Development) was proposed by the tribe, which has seven sectors working. They have developed 59 programmes, which were integrated into 189 projects.

HUICHOLES AND YAQUIS

Both the Huicholes and Yaquis have their own separate cultures, but both have the same high feeling for their ethnic identity and for their religions, which carry over into their activities. In their feasts they make many offerings, and drink, and have music and dancing. Religion is very different between Huicholes and Yaquis. The Yaqui women take a large part in the religious and productive life of the group.

The Huicholes have lived in distant and inaccessible lands for many years, for this reason their development and integration into Mexican society has not been fulfilled. They continue to be proud of their culture, their values and way of life, weaving their typical costumes, and in many instances they prefer that their children have no schooling, because when they acquire a certain amount of education, the children will leave their families and their territory.

The Yaquis today dress in a similar fashion to the Mexican farmer of the north of the country. Their communities have good communications and they have basic services like electricity and running water.

The legislation of the Mexican Republic under the 1917 constitution only recognized the Indian right to the restitution and confirmation of the communal territories. Today, both Huicholes and Yaquis continue to have invasion problems, and also border problems with the surrounding states.

The objective situation in context to the national life is the result of a long historic process, which is expressed in the economic, social and political inequality compared to the different social sectors of Mexico. This inequality can be found in the application of the law, which ignores them, and at other times in a contradiction between legal and institutional practices. The Huicholes and the Yaquis do not have real protection, and in many cases the established guarantees of a positive national right are not applied.

CONCLUSION

The integration of the Huichol and Yaqui tribes, as well as that of the remaining ethnic groups, into national life is not an easy process. The traditional Indian authorities have started a struggle for the acknowledgement and recognition of their values and traditions, within their communities, with the co-operation of the Instituto Nacional Indigenista, which has co-ordinated many programmes of social service for Indian tribes throughout the country.

Mexican government institutions continue to work for a better social welfare system, to improve the quality of life and to defend the rights of these people, who have suffered all types of marginalism during the last four centuries.

REFERENCES AND FURTHER READING

Aguirre Beltran, Gonzalo and Pozas Arciniega, Ricardo (1981) *La Política Indigenista en México, Métodos y Resultados*, vol. II, Colección SEP-INI No. 21, Mexico: Libros de México, SA.

Anguiano, Mariana and Furst, Peter T. (1987) *Colección INI (Investigaciones Sociales No. 3)*, Mexico: Talleres de Colorprint.

Caso, Antonio, et al (1981), *La Política Indigenista en México, Métodos y Resultados*, vol. I, Colección SEP-INI, No. 20, Mexico: Libros de México, SA.

Castro Acedo, Jorge (1990) *Estudio de la Comunidad de Bacum*, Sonora: Servicios Médicos de Sonora.

Centro Coordinador Indigenista del Estado de Durango (1990) *Plan Integral de Desarrollo de la Zona Indígena del Estado de Durango*, Mexico: Centro Coordinador Indigenista del Estado de Durango.

Centro Coordinador Indigenista del Estado de Nayarit (1990) *Formatos sobre el Panorama General de la Región y Formatos sobre la Oropuesta de Proyectos y Acciones Generales*, Mexico: Centro Coordinador Indigenista del Estado de Nayarit.

El Colegio de México (1981a) *Historia General de México*, vol. I, 3rd edn, Mexico: El Colegio de México.

— — (1981b) *Historia General de México*, vol. II, Mexico: El Colegio de México.

Colmenares, Ismael M. et al. (1978) *100 Años de Lucha de Clases en México (1876–1976)*, vol. II, 1st edn, Mexico: Ediciones Quinto Sol, SA.

Departamento de Educación Indígena de Durango (1990) *Programa para la Modernización de la Educación Indígena en el Estado de Durango*, Mexico: Departamento de Educación Indígena de Durango.

Galaviz Tapia Luz, Noemi (1988) *Estudio de los Sectores Tres y Cuatro, de los Servicios Médicos de Sonora*, Mexico: Centro de Salud de Vicam, Sonora.

Gonzalez Martinez, Juan Manuel (1987), *Los Huicholes Ganaderos Prósperos de Jalisco,* Colección INI, Cuadernos de Trabajo No. 8, Mexico: Editorial Libros de México.

Gouy-Gilbert, Cecile (1985) *Una Resistencia India, Los Yaquis*, Colección INI (Serie de Antropológia, No. 71), Mexico: Talleres de Colorprint.

Hernandez, Fortunato (1902), *Las Razas Indígenas de Sonora y la Guerra del Yaqui*, Mexico: Talleres de la Casa Editorial 'J. de Elizalde'.

Inca Rural (1980) *Ley Federal de la Reforma Agraria*, Mexico: Futura, SA.

INI-DGEI-UPV (no date) *Programa de Motivación Autogéstiva para Albergues Escolares*, Mexico: Orígenes y Funciones del Albergue Escolar Indígena.

Instituto Nacional de Estadística (1985) *Geografía e Informatica, Información Estadística del Sector Salud y Seguridad Social, Cuaderno, No. 4*, Mexico: Instituto Nacional de Estadística.

— —(1986) *Geografía e Informatica, Anuario Estadístico de los Estados Unidos Mexicanos*, Mexico: Instituto Nacional de Estadística.

Instituto Nacional Indigenista (1981) *Los Yaquis*, 1st edn, Mexico: Instituto Nacional Indigenista.

— — (1989) *Comisión Nacional de Justícia para los Pueblos indígenas de México*, Mexico: Instituto Nacional Indigenista.

La Barre, Eston (1987) *El Culto del Peyote*, 2nd edn, Mexico: Premia, Editora de Libros, SA.

Lizarraga Silva, Samuel (no date) 'Estudio de Comunidad de Potam, Sonora, Servicios Médicos de Sonora', mimeographed.

Loera Chavez, Margarita (1981) *Economía Campesina Indígena en la Colonia, un Caso en el Valle de Toluca*, Colección del INI, Mexico: Libros de México, SA.

Lumholts, Carl (1986) *El Arte Simbólico y Decorativo de los Huicholes*, Colección INI (Serie de Artes y Tradiciones Populares No. 3), Mexico: Instituto Nacional Indigenista.

McGuire, R. R. (1986) *Politics and Ethnicity on the Río Yaqui: Potam Revisited*, Tucson: University of Arizona Press.

Mexico Indígena (1988) Rev. No. 25, año IV, 2a. epoca, Mexico: Instituto Nacional Indigenista. (Nov.–Dec.).

— — (1989a) Rev. No. 2, Nueva Epoca, Coeditan: Instituto Nacional Indigenista y el Centro de Investigaciones Cultural y Científica, Mexico: Ediciones Arpa (Nov.).

— — (1989b) Rev. No. 3, Nueva Epoca, Coeditan: Instituto Nacional Indigenista y el Centro de Investigaciones Cultural y Científica, Mexico: Ediciones Arpa (Dec.).

— — (1990a), Rev. No. 10, Nueva Epoca, Coeditan: Instituto Nacional Indigenista y el Centro de Investigaciones Cultural y Científica, Mexico: Ediciones Arpa (July).

— — (1990b), Rev. No. 11, Nueva Epoca, Coeditan: Instituto Nacional Indigenista y el Centro de Investigaciones Cultural y Científica, Mexico: Ediciones Arpa (Aug.).

Negrin, J. (1985) *Acercamiento Histórico y Subjético Huichol EDUG*, Mexico: Universidad de Guadalajara.

Plan Integral de Desarrollo de la Tribu Yaqui (1983) Sonora.

Poder Ejecutivo Federal (1989) *Plan Nacional de Desarrollo, 1989–1994*, Colección de la Secretaría de Programación y Presupuesto, 1st edn, Mexico: Talleres Gráficos de la Nación.

Pozas, Ricardo and H. de Pozas, Isabel (1987) *Los Indios en las Clases Sociales de México*, 15th edn, Mexico: Editorial Siglo XXI.

Reed, K. B. (1972) *El INI y los Huicholes*, Colección, SEP-INI, 1st edn, Mexico: Libros de México, SA.

Secretaría de Educación Pública (1988) *Subsecretaría de Educación Elemental, Dirección General de Educación Indígena, Plan y Programa de Educación y Capacitación de la Mujer Indígena*, Mexico: Secretaría de Educación Pública.

Servicios Coordinados de Educación Pública del Estado de Nayarit (1990) *Diagnóstico de Salud de la Jurisdicción Sanitaria de Tepic, Nayarit*, Mexico: Servicios Coordinados de Educación Pública del Estado de Nayarit.

Soto, S. A. (1955) *Los Huicholes*, Rev. Artes de México No. 7, Mexico: (Jan.–Feb.), Cap. No.1.

X Censo General de Población y de Vivienda (1984) 1980, *Estado de*

Jalisco, vol. II, tomo IV, Mexico: X Censo General de Población y de Vivienda.

Zingg, R. M. (1982) *Los Huicholes*, Colección INI, Serie Clásicos de la Antropología No. 12, vols I and II, Mexico: Libros de México, SA.

4 Social welfare of indigenous populations in Brazil[1]

Celso Barroso Leite

ENVIRONMENT

Historical identity of the indigenous population

Discovered in 1500 and settled by the Portuguese, Brazil still has indigenous populations, as happens in virtually all countries of the three parts of the American continent: North, Central and South America.

The author refers to Brazil's 'Indians', a denomination that, applied first to India's inhabitants by the Portuguese navigators of the fifteenth century and then also to those of the territories that, with it, formed the Indias proper – that is, the Oriental lands they explored – was extended later on to the so-called West Indies – that is, the American continent. According to some authors, such greater extension, ultimately improper, resulted from the fact that Columbus and his companions thought, when they arrived in the Americas, that they were arriving in India proper.

Some authors contend that the South and North American Indians, including therefore the Brazilian ones, originated in their own continent; these theories have generally been surpassed by the theory that they descended from Asian, especially Mongolic, populations.

One route most probably followed by their ancestors to this side of the world, in very remote epochs, was the Bering Strait, in the northernmost part of the Americas, from where, in the course of time, the descendants of the earliest migrants slowly came down to the Centre and to the South. We were then in the Glacial Era and, at least during a great part of the year, the frozen waters of the strait formed a natural bridge. Other theories indicate migration from the Polynesian islands, and even from northern Africa and the Mediterranean area.

The present Brazilian indigenous population is very small and its number appears to be decreasing year by year.

We know that, except for the United States, Canada and some small countries which only recently became independent, the rest of the American continent is of Latin and more specifically Iberian origin; more specifically yet, they are of Spanish origin, the only exception being Brazil.

However, it is curious that the indigenous populations of Brazil never reached the level of culture, civilization and development attained before Columbus by the indigenous populations of Spanish America, namely Central America (Mexico and Guatemala), and South America (Peru and Ecuador). Compared with the social organization, economic level, political structure and other aspects of those populations, the Brazilian Indians were in a very rudimentary condition when the Portuguese arrived here.

For some two centuries, the Portuguese were in contact especially with the Indians along the coast, who were not much different from the tribes in the interior. Only later – in fact, after Brazil's independence in 1822, and thus recently in historical terms – the indigenous populations became better known and were found to be distributed in various parts of Brazil and amongst rather different groups.

The differences were not pronounced because in fact all the Brazilian Indians belong to ethnic groups that have a similar origin; but there are sufficient differences from an anthropological perspective to distinguish each group from the others. Nobody knows how many groups existed when Brazil was discovered, but it is estimated that some 150 groups still exist (or 160, or even 200, according to other sources).

The precarious conditions in which Indians live today, beginning with their difficulty in obtaining the necessary means of subsistence, result in each group being composed of a small number of individuals. Although there are some large groups, in several of them the total is only a few dozen persons.

It would then be of little significance to limit discussion to a specific group; therefore the focus here is on the indigenous population as a whole. This overall approach is consistent with the criterion followed by the Brazilian indigenist policy.

Sometimes a special event or situation brings to the foreground a certain group, usually more numerous, or some area inhabited by Indians. In 1988 and 1989, for instance, there was an international movement in connection with questions related to the Amazon

Indians; the media shouted that they were being expelled from their territories by firms and adventurers whose economic expansion would, besides everything else, destroy the Amazon forest, with catastrophic consequences for our entire planet. This wave of ecological paranoia appears to have subsided enough to make it viable to search for a rational and not emotional solution for the crucial problems that really exist in that region.

A group of Indians, the Ianomamis, attracted then, and still attract, special attention. They inhabit an area whose mineral riches lure not only a great number of individual gold diggers but also large firms which built illegal airports there, but these were subsequently destroyed by the government. Coincidentally, these Indians are the object of an interesting study by an American anthropologist (Harris, 1978).

Although there exists today a broad and well-meant indigenist policy, the changes in relation to the past should probably be considered rather formal than real. Brazil has generally dealt with Indians as conquerors; to be dominated, assimilated and suppressed. There have, naturally, been exceptions to this (mainly passing fads and isolated and spurious movements), but the general rule has been, here as in the rest of the world, the oppression by the more powerful of the less powerful. There is in Brazil, as doubtless in any other country with an indigenous population in the sense here utilized, a vast and varied bibliography to this effect. For instance, another American anthropologist writes: 'For those who are familiar with the history of the indigenist policy in other American countries, it is clear that the Brazilian government is trying to institutionalize a type of policy similar to the one practiced in the United States' (Davis, 1978:137).

Brazil also has, as should be expected, and again as in other countries, a voluminous fictional literature in which the Indian is glorified in prose and verse. However, the novels, poems and even a rather famous opera, some of which are really good, naturally do not go beyond the make-believe world where they belong.

Even academic and scientific studies, especially in the areas of anthropology and sociology, often do not have, according to some specialists, the objectivity that should be expected. It is alleged, amongst other things, that some foreign indigenists, sometimes motivated only by the requirements of their university careers, usually write less about the Indians as the human and social realities that they are, than about special aspects of their existence and culture. More explicitly, many works on this complex theme have connotations of an exotic and unique theme that reduce their scientific value.

In any event, there is no doubt that from the beginning the Indians received from the Portuguese, in the colonial period until 1822, the year of Brazil's independence, the usual treatment by the winners towards the losers. More precisely, they were killed, tortured, brought into slavery and exploited.

It is worth noting that such treatment did not differ much from the way the Indians treated other Indians. Even the literature that exalts them sometimes shows that very clearly. Maybe the chief difference is in favour of the Portuguese: contrary to certain tribes, that feasted on the conquered enemies, they were not (and still are not) cannibals.

At least until 1537 it was not known for sure if the Indians were human beings or simply animals. A papal bull of that year decided in their favour – that is, it officially recognized their human condition. However, some dissenting voices were heard.

The condition of being recognized officially as a human being did not free the Indians from slavery, and this only came about almost three centuries later, by means of a law in 1831, when Brazil, already independent, was still a monarchy. All this time the indigenous people were traded, in spite of their fierce resistance, which lowered their value as slave workers.

In this connection it seems proper to note that only after another half century (1888) did freedom reach the African slaves in Brazil and their descendants. The latter also constitute a type of indigenous population in an inferior social and economic condition, although they are not technically considered indigenous regarding social welfare (contrary to what happens in South Africa, where Caucasians and blacks have different social security schemes).

Parallel to this ostensibly negative side, from the arrival of the Portuguese their preoccupation was to assimilate the indigenous populations with whom they came increasingly into contact. Their policy of assimilation, that lasted for centuries, was accomplished by means of catechesis; that is, more precisely, conversion to the Roman Catholic religion. Quite a few authors consider that this criterion for assimilation is improper, but it is also recognized that any alternative would also be precarious.

Some even dispute the validity of the reservations where the missionaries concentrated the catechized Indians or those being catechized. The explicit purpose of the reservations was for their protection and conversion. Quite a few critics of this method contend that it was a disguised form of slavery, since the missionaries, while offering the salvation of the Indians' souls, compelled them to use their bodies in the different chores on the reservation, in at least a disguised form of forced labour.

It appears that the harshness of the Portuguese towards the Indian was such that their treatment impaired the effort to convert the Indians to Catholicism. According to a chronicle of that time, learning from a missionary the delights of heaven for the Christians and the tortures of hell for the heathens, an Indian asked him if the Portuguese went to heaven. In view of the spontaneous affirmative answer, the Indian decided that the conversion did not pay: 'Then I prefer to go to hell.'

Near the end of the Empire, when the Indians had already stopped being slaves, but were, after assimilation, practically qualified only for menial farm work, they suffered the same fate as applied to the other farm workers, the Africans and their descendants. By that time Brazil had begun to replace slave manpower by foreign workers, imported by the government or by private employers with an official subsidy, as a foreign product of interest to the country. This aggravated the social economic situation of both the Indians and the blacks.

With the proclamation of the Republic, in 1889, one year after the liberation of the slaves, Brazil's history entered a new period. However, the important political change again failed to have appreciable repercussions on the treatment of the Indians.

Human beings they already were, since the papal bull of 1537, and in 1831 the Empire had freed them from slavery. But still the Indians did not have the full rights and obligations of citizenship for which they had to wait – and to some extent are still waiting.

Brazil's Civil Code, dating from 1916 and still almost entirely in force, when listing the 'incapable relative to certain acts' included amongst them the Indians, and subjected them to a tutorial regime, to be regulated by special laws and instructions which were to end when they became adapted to the country's civilization. Strictly speaking, such a legal provision does not apply to the assimilated Indians. In practice, however, this new condition is not easy to prove, which sometimes raises problems. The Statute of the Indian (Law 6001, 1973) regulates, among other parts of the indigenist policy, the tutorial regime established by the Civil Code.

Parallel to the social welfare programmes for the Indians and the permanent effort towards their assimilation, which must be slow and progressive, some authors think that the slowness and progressiveness are contrary to the interests and even to the wishes of the Indians.

Statements to this effect are well publicized, and one of the most recent is from the well-known Professor Isaias Raw, of the University of São Paulo, which is the most influential university in the country.

According to Raw, Indian culture must be preserved, but not the Indian. He considers it to be contradictory to treat an Indian with western medicines, but not to bring Indians to the city if they wish to come, and not to give them television sets, because we think this will affect their culture. What we do, then, is to confine the Indians to their reservations, as animals in a zoo, he comments. In his view the attractions of western civilization will lead to the disappearance of the Indians. And he concludes: 'The problem is that we consider it to be proper to preserve underdeveloped people. This is for the Indians a hell of a condemnation' (Raw, 1991).

Ideological and cultural differences

The existence of an overall ideology held by the indigenous populations on whom we are focusing is highly debatable. At most it will be possible, for the purpose of comparison with the population in general, to deal with their customs, life-styles and beliefs – in short, their culture, in the anthropological sense of this term.

Not even there, however, is the comparison easy, because, besides being quite rudimentary, in relative terms, since the early times, the culture of the Brazilian Indians has been greatly influenced by the dominant culture, and vice versa, which makes the borderline between the two quite imprecise.

Obviously, the Indians keep primitive customs distinct from what is usual among the population in general. However, it is also certain that other sections of the population not comprised in the concept of indigenous populations have identical or similar customs.

There have been special cases where the differences were significant. No example would be more expressive here than that of cannibalism, practised by some tribes in the past, but never by any other group of the population. However, the last definite cases of cannibalism occurred centuries ago.

Another example would be that of the tribes that still keep the custom of extending a man's lower lip to unprecedented dimensions, which seems to be a very exclusive peculiarity.

It is well known that indigenous fictional literature contains a great variety and wealth of what at first sight might be interpreted as cultural characteristics. It is also known, on the other hand, that fiction is usually far distant from reality.

In any event, it is extremely difficult to compare the Indians' culture with that of the population in general; and, as pointed out earlier, they may not have a common ideology.

In spite of this conclusion, it should be noted that a great number of suicides has occurred in the same tribe in recent years: 42 in 1989 and 26 in 1990, mostly of young Indians. This tribe lives in a reservation adjacent to a large city. Its 4,000 Indians live there in the most precarious conditions, the foremost being the inevitable and disintegrating contact with the city, which aggravates problems such as alcoholism. According to a Brazilian magazine, the chief cause of these suicides must be the 'cultural massacre' of the Indians, including that by the five religious sects that operate in the region, which are trying to eliminate the remaining vestiges of the tribe's culture by a 'crushing process of catechesis' (*Isto E Senhor*, 1991).

Demography

It is more difficult to present demographic data referring to the Indians than to compare their culture and ideology with those of the rest of the population. That requires, first of all, the definition of an Indian.

The Statute of the Indian mentioned above established the official concept: 'Any individual of pre-Colombian origin who identifies himself or herself and is identified as belonging to an ethnic group whose cultural characteristics distinguish him or her from the national society'. In this connection it should be noted that the point of reference is the discovery of America, not of Brazil.

Under its entry *Indigena* ('Indian'), the Brazilian edition of the well-known French *Larousse Encyclopaedia* indicates a total of 120,000 Indians, subdivided into 140 groups. The encyclopaedia lists, with the respective subdivision, probable population, geographic location and level of assimilation or integration – that is, of their relationship to the population in general. Out of these totals

eleven groups, with 62,000 Indians, live in the Amazon region; 35 groups, with 21,500 Indians, in Central Brazil; ten groups, with 9,500 Indians, in Eastern Brazil; and four groups, with 7,000 Indians, in Southern Brazil.

(*Grande Enciclopedia Delat-Larousse*, 1970)

According to the *Larousse Encyclopaedia* the distribution by level of assimilation is as follows: 34 groups, with 32,400 Indians, remain isolated; 27 groups, with 16,000 Indians, maintain occasional contact with the rest of the population; 44 groups, with 27,600 Indians, can already be considered as assimilated, or accultured (which means that at least in theory they are no longer Indians). This variety of levels of integration, from complete isolation to full assimilation, shows the difficulty in presenting precise demographic data on the Brazilian Indians; and some specialists contend that the Indian seldom reaches the point of full assimilation.

The variety of Indian tribes also occurs in the numerical composition of the groups as mentioned earlier: many have only about 50 individuals, while in the few largest groups this figure rises to about 4,000 to 5,000; and until recently the Ianomamis, mentioned above, numbered over 10,000. It is estimated that only 19 groups have more than 1,000 individuals.

The *Larousse Encyclopaedia*, under the same entry, contains a forecast that many consider gloomy but that for others is promising:

> As a result of the process of gradual extermination of the Indian population since the time of the discovery, a process nowadays fostered by the greater technical might of the pioneer fronts that cross the national territory in all directions, since 1900 some 36 per cent of the groups then known have disappeared. This leads us to believe that, if this rhythm persists, by the year 2000 some 50 of the groups now known will have been extinguished.

However, officials of the area with whom the author has consulted consider the figures of the encyclopaedia quite below the reality. According to officials, an almost equivalent number of Indians have been discovered since, which raises their total to about 230,000, or less than 0.2 per cent of Brazil's total population. They added that any figures referring to Indians are simply estimates, since they have never been precisely counted.

Still in this connection the author must mention that in other sources he also found figures much higher than those cited in the *Larousse Encyclopaedia*: 150,000, 200,000 – and the above-mentioned 230,000. The author also found lower figures: from 70,000 to 100,000, depending in part, as the other figures, on who is considered Indian.

The same problems of documentation of this number of Indians currently applies to the probable number of Indians existing at the time of Brazil's discovery. The *Larousse Encyclopaedia* warns against the obvious difficulty of population estimates, indicating that some historians think the Portuguese discovered about 1 million Indians, but an American anthropologist, Julian Steward, raises this figure to 1.2 million. In other sources, however, the author has found much higher figures: 5 and even 6 million.

SERVICE SYSTEM

During its entire history Brazil does not appear to have succeeded in caring satisfactorily for its Indians. At first it was even doubtful that they were human beings. After their human condition was recognized, they continued to be slaves; that is, little progress was made regarding their social, economic and political status. Freed from slavery, they remained as Indians, which at that time was almost synonymous with the notion of pariah, a near equivalence that, in the view of most specialists, still prevails. This situation implies that it would be more proper to refer to the 'ill-fare' rather than welfare of the Indians.

At least in formal terms the first system of services designated for them was adopted late in the first decade of this century with the creation of the Service for the Protection of the Indians and Location of National Workers (Decree 8072, 1910). This was in fact the crowning effort of a great fighter for the cause of the Indians, Candido Mariano da Silva Rondon, an army engineering officer whom the Congress raised to the position of marshal (basically honorary) in recognition of his remarkable services to Brazil and to humankind.

Rondon's services consisted especially of the construction of telegraph lines and roads, in Mato Grosso, Amazon and in the then territory, now state, of Rondonia, thus designated as a tribute to him. During the many years in which he performed his pioneer tasks in territories densely inhabited by Indians, his natural inclinations and his positivistic ideas about human life led him to become a champion of the necessity of humanitarian and understanding treatment of the Indians, contrary to what was then acceptable as sanctioned behaviour.

It is justifiably customary to include in reference to Rondon the slogan that he obliged his soldiers to observe in their frequent and inevitable clashes with Indians during a great part of his life as a backlands pioneer: 'To die, if necessary; to kill, never'. At least in theory, the same doctrine still underlies Brazil's indigenist policy.

Rondon was the first director of the Service created in 1910, and he tried to introduce into the bureau the ethos, generously summed up in his slogan, with due respect not only for the life but also for the customs, traditions and other cultural aspects of the Indians.

The author again refers to the *Larousse Encyclopaedia*, under the entry *Indigenismo* ('indigenism'). It is said that the objective of this first agency for protection of the Indians in Brazil was to 'solve the serious conflicts between tribes that defended the secular possession of a vast territory and the representatives of the Brazilian society that formed the front line of the interior occupation of the country'. Rondon, who had assumed his new functions without quitting the former ones, was at the head of that front.

The *Larousse Encyclopaedia* comments, in this connection, that the question of the relations with the Indians, thus far characterized by conflicts that often ended with their massacre, had finally reached the national conscience and then 'required measures to save the Indians from extermination and at the same time attend to the need to occupy the national territory'.

In the following year Decree 9214 changed the initial regulations, approved by the decree that had created the Service; and the new text consolidated the guidelines of Brazil's indigenist policy, that had as its highlights – and at least in theory still has – the 'respect to the Indians' self-determination as regards expectations of spontaneous development, based on their own cultural standards', as well as the 'protection of the Indian territories, guaranteed them by means of permanent possession of a collective character'. I continue to quote from the encyclopedia, where it is written, under the same entry, that the pioneering character of the new regulations was later recognized by the International Labour Office. The ILO even recommended its adoption by 'all the countries where it might be necessary to discipline relations resulting from contact with tribal populations'.

Decree 1794, 1939, created, parallel to the Service for the Protection of the Indians, a National Council for Protection of the Indians (NCP). Unfortunately, however, the creation of the NCP did not avoid the fact that both the Service and the Council came to operate far below their important objectives. In fact, the deficiencies of the agencies increased and were aggravated by irregularities of all kinds, which were denounced in a shocking report of a commission of inquiry.

As a result of the reaction to the Commission's report, Law 5371, 1967, authorized the government to unite the Service for Protection of the Indians and the National Council for Protection of the Indians into a new organization called the National Foundation for the Indian, best known by its acronym, Funai. Funai's chief functions are: to establish guidelines for the indigenist policy and see to it that they are applied; to manage the possessions of the Indians; and to promote the provision of medical care to them as well as their basic education, aiming at their progressive integration into the national society. The principles that the indigenist policy must observe include: respect for the Indians and for their tribal institutions and communities; and a guarantee of permanent possession of their territories.

A successor to the agencies it absorbed, Funai has as its chief source of means budgetary (especially federal) allocations. Included today in the Ministry of Justice and with headquarters in Brasilia, Funai is administered by a president and a board of directors.

Funai has regional offices in the areas where Indian groups exist, and it is through them that it performs its functions. These are related to the guarantee of Indian territories, to the medical care of the Indians (some direct services and contracts with other agencies), and to their education (also in Indian languages and in Funai's and other schools, by contract, and scholarships). Funai's regional and peripheral branches comprise six regional offices, 342 Indian posts, 34 Indian homes, 453 wards and 253 schools. At present the total of the Indians attending school is 32,793.

Besides its regular functions, Funai drafted the bill that Congress approved as Law 6001, 1972, the Statute of the Indian, already mentioned. The Statute regulates the legal condition of the Indians as well as of Indian communities, for the purpose of preserving their culture and integrating them gradually and smoothly into the national community. More specifically, the Statute regulates the following matters: obligations of the three levels of government in relation to the Indians; their civil and political rights; the assistance and tutorial regime to which they are entitled; their civil registration; the guarantee of possession of their territories; their inheritance and income; their education, culture and health; their penal accountability and the crimes against them.

This list of the basic legal texts relative to the Indians and therefore regulating the services designated for them must include the federal constitution of 1988. In two long articles it expresses and reinforces what has been said about indigenist policy and protection of the Indians, beginning with the vital questions of 'their social organization, customs, languages, beliefs and traditions' and the guarantee of 'their original rights to the lands they have traditionally occupied', that the government has to demarcate and protect.

Finally, it seems proper to add that the government intends to introduce substantial changes in the indigenist policy, as was officially announced late in 1990. The statement added that one of the changes contemplated relates to the crucial question of the criterion for the demarcation of Indian territories, in view of the frequent conflicts, in this connection, between the Indians and gold diggers, invaders and farmers. Also under consideration is a profound restructuring of Funai. In addition, it is necessary to adapt the Statute of the Indian to the new constitution.

According to recent news releases, there are 544 areas of Indian territories, but only 289 of them are already demarcated, and the area of those not yet demarcated corresponds to more than one half of the total. According to an express constitutional provision, the land demarcation must be completed not later than 4 October 1993.

Assessment

It is well known that in view of the special nature and the inevitable complexity of the social welfare programmes it is extremely difficult to assess their results. The data referring to those included in the programmes, the activities carried out, the expenses involved and so forth provide at best quantitative, statistical notions of what is done and what remains to be done. Even when such data are clear, complete and trustworthy, there remains the other side of the question: its qualitative aspect, which is certainly more important. Nevertheless, it is also known that in Brazil, owing to various factors, for the population in general, including the indigenous populations, these social welfare programmes leave much to be desired.

In the case of indigenous populations the difficulty of assessment is far greater, because the complexity of the services involved is aggravated by the very special characteristics of the populations for which they are designated. In addition to the special characteristics of these populations, there exist other complicating elements, such as their territorial dispersion and the difficult access to most of their major nuclei or groups.

Even before examining the elements of social welfare programmes, one can conclude that the welfare programmes designated for the Brazilian Indians are below the standard of what should be expected; probably much below. And it could hardly be otherwise. The social welfare of the Indians, and in fact everything else that concerns them, depends directly and substantially on the untroubled possession of the lands that belong to them or have been designated to them. This is either explicit or implicit, but always clear, in the constitution, in the Statute of the Indian, in Funai's legislation and in every important document referring to the indigenist policy. The constitution defines as 'lands traditionally occupied by the Indians', that the federal government has to demarcate and protect, 'those indispensable for the preservation of the environmental resources necessary for their well-being'.

Another basic element of the Indians' social welfare policy is their special legal condition that the Statute of the Indian regulates, providing at the same time about civil and political rights. The Statute also regulates the tutorial regime to which they are subject, before such integration is completed – still according to the Statute.

All this forms part of the indigenist policy, that Funai has to draft and, once approved as law, to see that it is applied, observing the principles established by the law that authorized its creation. Besides, Funai is responsible for the medical care for the Indians and for their education, not to mention other services.

The government recognized that the demarcation and protection of the Indians' lands has priority when it announced plans for reformulating the pertinent legislation. But the government initiative, in the search for greater efficacy in relation to the most crucial questions, can certainly be considered as one of the concrete facts of a positive character.

It has been officially stated that Funai's recent co-ordination with the proper agencies of the Ministry of Health is already promoting a real improvement of the health of the Indian populations, or at least of some of them, which is another positive factor. Less precisely, it has also been announced that the government is considering the transfer of Funai's functions in this area to the Ministry of Education. It seems that the extension and depth of the transference have not yet been decided and there is no date set for this transfer of functions.

The reason for the transfer of functions is similar to that of the co-ordination with the Ministry of Health: an effort to extend and improve the Indians' education. To the extent that this purpose is achieved, and the transference is not just a neutral change in the administrative structure of the government, there is a third positive factor.

A fortunate coincidence allows me to make an assessment on the basis of recent comments by the Minister of Justice, currently the highest authority in the government (with the obvious exception of the President of the Republic) in relation to the indigenist policy and therefore to the social welfare of the Indians. A Brazilian representative in an event overseas accused the Brazilian government of genocide against the Indian nations, and the Minister refuted him in a strong newspaper article (Passarinho, 1991). 'It would be to close your eyes to reality', he wrote, 'to assert that the relationship of the Government with the Indian nation is perfect.' And he added: 'Serious and challenging problems exist since Funai's creation, as the Service for Protection of the Indians.' Now comes the passage that supports more directly the author's reservation: 'The very complexity of the anthropological question, in its most universal sense, is in itself a great challenge.' The author also referred to 'elements of disintegration of the Indian culture', amongst which the Minister lists 'the invasion of progress, the expansion of the agricultural frontier, the clash with the conquering Caucasians, the economic interest', all of which since Brazil's discovery, 'with the ensuing conflicts with the pioneers' (that is, the first settlers on Brazilian territory). And the paragraph ends thus: 'The search for riches was a merciless war, lost by the weaker, the unarmed, the Indian.'

It is appropriate to reproduce the entire passage:

> To protect the Indians and their culture is a recent phenomenon in Brazilian sociology, and the results are counted in failures rather than in successes. In fact, Brazilian indigenism, on its present lines, reproduces practices that date from the beginning of this century. In the course of time the programmes lost efficacy and became practically useless. To have a policy with modern concepts, it is necessary to accept this critical vision, that points to anachronism.

According to the Minister, that is what the President of the Republic thought when he 'faced the indigenous question, trying to define its long, painful ways and mapping its solutions'. Trying how?

> First, he identified the Indian question as a question of citizenship by placing it under the Ministry of Justice, where the forum of human rights is located. Thus he broke the backbone of the merely tutorial vision that marks the history of the relations between the whites and the Indians.

These and other facts treated in the article, some of which are already mentioned here, according to the Minister guide 'measures in concrete course that result from the political consciousness of what is necessary, not from pressures' (the author notes: including foreign pressures), 'although their discussion has been opened to the entire community, Indian and non-Indian'.

The polemic tone of the article does not affect its authorized informative contents; and in the author's view the article represents an expressive synthesis of the present Brazilian reality in relation to the question of the Indians, including the measures aimed at their social welfare. The Minister informs us of what is being done and realistically recognizes that, as is well known, there is still a long and difficult way to go. Without promising miracles, the Minister presents a promising prospect.

This assessment does not differ much from the Minister's. If socio-economic conditions in Brazil have not made it possible to provide a satisfactory level of social welfare to the population in general – that is, the non-Indian population – it does not make sense to expect that such a level might have been reached in relation to a sector of the population whose very special conditions enormously aggravate the complexity and the difficulties of social welfare programmes.

Taking the reasoning a little further, it seems safe to conclude that, regarding social welfare, the situation of the Brazilian Indians is very likely as precarious as that of other groups of Brazil's population, which are certainly more numerous and in less favourable conditions regarding social welfare.

NOTE

1. This chapter was written in 1991 and thus may not always contain the most current information.

REFERENCES

Davis, S. H. (1978) *Vitimas do Milagre*, Rio de Janeiro, RJ: Zahar Editores.
Grande Enciclopedia Delta-Larousse (1970) Rio de Janeiro, RJ: Editora Delta.
Harris, M. (1978) *Cows, Pigs, Wars and Witches*, New York: Vintage Books–Random House.
Passarinho, J. (1991) 'Entre a versao e o fato', *Jornal do Brasil*, 13 January.
Raw, I. (1991) 'A elite da cabeca', *Veja*, 23 January (interview).

5 Welfare rules and indigenous rights: the Sami people and the Nordic welfare states

Sven E. Olsson and Dave Lewis

The Nordic countries have aquired an international reputation for their highly developed welfare states, a reputation that has given rise to the notion of a particular Nordic approach to welfare. Indeed the Nordic approach is unique as compared with other advanced capitalist nations in the extent to which social policy has become comprehensive and institutional in effect: the welfare of the individual as the responsibility of the society, and no fixed boundaries between market and state as regards public welfare commitments are recognized (Heckscher, 1984). In fact, the institutional welfare state – in contrast to the residual model – tends to limit and partially to supplant the market as the distributive nexus of welfare. Furthermore, the institutional approach employs the principle of a 'social minimum' whereby all citizens are equally entitled to a decent standard of living, full citizenship rights and equality of status.

The comprehensive nature of Nordic social policy is illustrated by its broad scope of public intervention, a scope defined much more broadly than in most other nations as policy attempts to provide for an extensive range of social needs and to ensure a unified system of social protection. Nordic social policy thus exhibits strong universalistic and solidaristic traits as represented by its intention to integrate and include the entire population rather than to target resources selectively towards particular problem groups. This approach to social policy is seen as an important stabilizing feature of Nordic welfare systems, and also as an illustration that compromise amongst social classes can be achieved and managed to benefit society as a whole (cf. Korpi, 1983; Marklund, 1988).

Nordic social policy has, in short, attempted to maximize citizens' equality of status while attempting to minimize dysfunctional conditions manifest in a capitalist economy, primarily those concerning the distribution of income and wealth. In vesting citizens with the basic right to entitlement, the intention of the institutional welfare state is to effect equitable redistribution throughout society. Hence, the Nordic welfare state should not only be appraised in terms of the elaborate social security and welfare services provided, but also in their capacity to ensure equitable distribution. Yet the occupational orientation and corresponding benefit schemes pose a contradiction to the guiding principle of redistributive equality as such provisions tend to mirror existing distributional inequalities; indeed, a problem that would seem rooted in the theoretical foundation of the institutional welfare state model (Mishra, 1977). And furthermore, for reasons that will become clear in the following sections, a problem that is suspected of particularly placing Sami peoples at a real disadvantage.

The Nordic welfare states of today have each evolved during this century, and by and large since the Second World War, from an old tradition supporting particular cultural values and a more recent tradition of political thought. Elements of the old and new became intertwined with one another to form the societal context within which the welfare state developed and that in which it functions today (Flora, 1986; Graubard, 1986; Therborn, 1986). And although all three Nordic states have developed independently of one another during this century, they have done so in light of a remarkable degree of co-operation between one another; perhaps one of the best indications that they each share largely common cultural and political values.

This values-orientation has not only contributed to the uniqueness of the Nordic approach to social policy, but has also served to temper the welfare relationship that has evolved with respect to the Sami. In essence, this orientation is highlighted by the importance attached to the principles of egalitarianism, local autonomy, individualism, efficiency, the (societal) whole, and social equality (Kuhnle, 1980; Stevens, 1989); principles which, taken together, pose contradictory motives relative to both their intended effect and Sami cultural interests. The promotion of Sami interests in social policy can be said to represent egalitarian principles, yet they are in conflict with and largely diminished by other principles advancing the supremacy of the individual and the societal whole. That is, as the Sami pursue their collective right to local autonomy and social equality they come into conflict with the practical and legal implications of the Nordic welfare states' tendency to extend entitlement solely to the individual. And furthermore, just as the individual is the responsibility of society-as-a-whole, the responsibility of the individual is first and foremost to society-as-a-whole. Nordic governments thus find the Sami's cultural and collective rights orientation very difficult and uncomfortable to accept politically, and hence tend largely to ignore it or make a pretence of accepting it, on the one hand, or, on the other hand, attempt to control it by means of instituting controversial policy measures.

In attempting to examine critically the nature of the welfare relationship which exists between the Sami peoples and all three Nordic welfare states, this chapter focuses upon the origins and impact of government policies relative to the Sami's current state of affairs. Faced from the outset of this task by a void of empirical data with respect to present-day social conditions affecting the Sami, this work is constrained in its capacity critically to appraise policy outcomes on a cross-national, pan-Nordic basis – seemingly not an uncommon problem when attempting cross-national policy analysis from an ethnic relations standpoint (cf. Ginsburg, 1991). With these introductory remarks in mind, we now turn to a description of some of the more salient features which contribute to the Sami's present-day social context.

BACKGROUND

The Sami settlement area

The existing area of Sami settlement, as represented in Map 5.1, is known to the Sami as Samiland or Sápmi. Today, Samiland extends over the entire Fennoscandia Arctic region, encompassing Russia's Kola peninsula and the northern parts of Norway, Sweden and Finland; and stretches southward along both sides of the Klen mountain range dividing Sweden and Norway to the northernmost part of the Swedish province of Dalarna. In the main, Samiland represents the areas north of or intersected by the Arctic Circle and is comprised of the administrative districts of Nordland, Tromsø and Finnmark in Norway, Norrbotten in Sweden and Lappi in Finland; a region of 300,000 square kilometres in area and known more commonly as Nordkalotten or the 'Northern Cape'.

The landscape of Samiland has often been described, both by outsiders and non-Sami residents, as bleak and inhospitable. However, in comparison to other Arctic regions, Samiland has been bestowed with great variety in its natural relief. It varies from a broad, high, barren plateau area straddling the Swedish–Norwegian

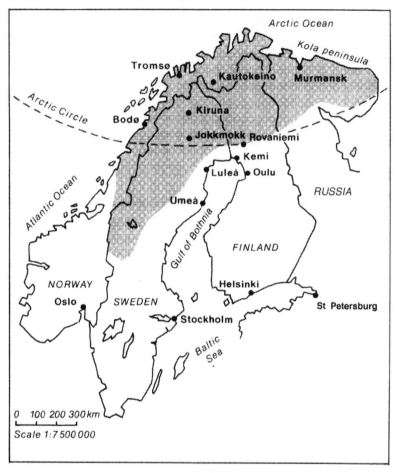

Map 5.1 Sami settlement area
Source: Adapted from Elina Helander (1984) *Om trespråkighet, Umeå*, in
SOU, 1989: 114

border to the glaciated alpine terrain of Sarek (in northernmost
Sweden) and the wide, gently undulating lowlands of Lappi. Much of
Samiland is covered with boreal forest, giving way in the high upland
areas and northern extremities of Finnmark to irregular stands of
birch. Along the north coast and in the uplands above an altitude of
500 metres there is a largely treeless subarctic terrain; on the broad
plateau tundra vegetation predominates, while nestled away in the

deep recesses of its steep slopes are glaciers and snowfields. The main rivers providing southward drainage of the region's landscape are the two Lule rivers, the Mounio, Torne, Ounas and Kemi; all converging upon the head of the Gulf of Bothnia. The largest rivers draining northward to the Arctic coast are the Tana and Alta, both emptying into the sea amidst the fjords and peninsulas of Finnmark.

Population

Nordkalotten represents 31 per cent of the total area of Norway, Sweden and Finland, although its 1988 population of 930,000 people represents only 5 per cent of the total tri-national population for the same year (Nordic Council of Ministers, 1990). Hence, Nordkalotten is quite a sparsely populated region with a population density of 3.1 persons per square kilometre. The largest population centres in the region are Tromsø and Bodø (Norway), Kiruna and Luleå (Sweden), and Kemi and Rovaniemi (Finland); accounting for approximately one-third of Nordkalotten's population. Overall, approximately two-thirds of the region's population is of an urban character, and one-third rural.

Nordkalotten has experienced declining natural increases in its population since 1960 when it recorded a natural increase of 1.3 per cent; by 1970 natural increase had dropped to 0.8 per cent, in 1980 to 0.4 per cent, and in 1988 to 0.35 per cent (as compared to a natural increase of 0.5 per cent overall for Finland, Norway and Sweden). Compounding this negative trend has been a similar but more recent trend of population loss to the region; that is, since 1980 Nordkalotten's population has declined by some 10,000 people (in sharp contrast to the period 1971–80 during which time the region's population increased by almost 25,000 people).

The most often cited estimate of the present Sami population is that of 60,000 people, of whom approximately 35,000 reside in Norway, 17,000 in Sweden, 5,000 in Finland, and 2,000 in the Soviet Union (Nordic Sami Institute, 1990). Those Sami people residing in the Nordic countries represent approximately 5 per cent of the total population in the main part of their settlement area (that is, the Nordkalotten region).

The greatest concentration of Sami people occurs in Norway's northernmost county of Finnmark, where approximately 20,000 Sami live, half of whom are concentrated in four main settlement areas; those being Kautokeino, Karasjok, Tana and Nesseby. These centres are known as Sami communities, communities in which Sami people represent the majority of the population. Sami people also form the majority of the population in Utsjoki, Finland, and represent a significant proportion of the populations of Jokkmokk and Karesuando in Sweden, and Inari in Finland (Swedish-Sami National Federation, 1987). It has been estimated by the national Sami organizations of Norway and Sweden that as many as 5,000 Sami people have emigrated from Samiland since 1960, 80 per cent of whom have migrated either to Oslo or Stockholm in roughly equal proportions (thereby placing both capital cities in a direct challenge with Kautokeino for the title of largest Sami community). However, most of this out-migration has been balanced by a relatively high and stable natural increase of the Sami population (as compared to the declining natural increase of the region's Scandinavian population) during this period.

Industry, natural resources and the regional economy

Samiland contains a vast wealth of natural resources in the form of minerals, timber, reindeer, fish and hydro power. Iron-ore extraction is the predominant feature of the regional mining industry; while of secondary importance is the mining of copper, lead and zinc. In 1987 there was a total of 36 active mining and quarrying operations scattered in small pockets throughout Nordkalotten from the Kiruna-Malmberget district of central Nordkalotten (in Sweden) to the northerly and northernmost reaches of both Finland and Norway. As an example of the region's tremendous mineral wealth and output, Sweden ranked as the world's sixth largest exporter of iron ore in 1988, iron ore accounting for a full 1 per cent of its income earnings from exports; and 90 per cent of Swedish iron-ore exports originated from mines in the Kiruna-Malmberget district. In 1987, mining and quarrying activities in Nordkalotten supported a workforce of 6,650 strong.

Agriculture, forestry and fishing resources are also of significant importance to the Nordkalotten economy. Taken as a whole, these sectors supported more than 45,000 persons in 1980, or approximately 10 per cent of the region's total workforce. Reindeer husbandry is the most significant agriculture-related activity in the region, as farming is of local rather than national importance. It is almost exclusively a Sami enterprise and as such continues to hold a dominant position in Sami society, supporting as many as 6,000 Sami people and hundreds of others in related services and enterprises throughout Samiland at large. At present the reindeer industry comprises approximately 750,000 stock, ranging over vast tracts of northern territory (Nordic Sami Institute, 1990). In Sweden, for instance, reindeer breeding areas currently utilize approximately 35 per cent of the country's total territory.

Fisheries are important, especially to the small coastal communities of north Norway. During the early 1980s, there was a workforce of approximately 10,000 persons engaged in the fishing industry, while thousands of others were employed in related fish-processing plants and ship-repair services (John, 1984). Most of Samiland's landscape is covered by boreal forest, thus representing another valuable natural resource for the regional economy. The forests provide feedstock for the manufacture of paper and other wood products; manufacturing industries which together accounted for more than 12,000 jobs in Nordkalotten in 1987.

Hydroelectric power represents another of Nordkalotten's great natural resources, the full potential of which at present remains unrealized. Indeed, it is the hydropower of Samiland's fast-flowing rivers upon which Norway, Sweden and Finland each depend to supply their significant demand for electricity. In Norway, for instance, as much as 25 per cent of its total energy supply in 1988 was derived from hydroelectric power, while, in the same year, hydroelectricity provided about 15 per cent of Sweden's total energy needs, and roughly half that amount for Finland (Nordic Council of Ministers, 1990).

Nordkalotten is indeed a storehouse of natural resources, but it lacks a balanced economy, for it is first and foremost a region of export, particularly with regard to iron ore and hydroelectricity. Employment has declined throughout the region since 1960 resulting in unemployment rates of at least twice that of the national averages. Nordic governments have, over the past 30 years, unitedly attempted to counteract both the export bias and declining employment by encouraging the development of a strong regional manufacturing sector. Such efforts have, to an extent, been successful, as partly indicated by the region's relatively large manufacturing sector workforce which accounted for almost 50,000 jobs and represented about 12 per cent of the total regional workforce in 1987 (Nordic Council of Ministers, 1990). Yet there remains an overemphasis on the extraction, refining and export of primary goods and raw materials; in part an indication of the physical constraints that limit and restrict more effective regional development policy, most notably Nordkalotten's geographic isolation and harsh climatic conditions. Hence, industry continues to perceive the region's main economic function and utility as that of a storehouse of natural resources which, in turn, has resulted in the occurrence of much conflict between the Sami and Nordic governments over questions of ownership, utilization and management of the region's finite resources (cf. Paine, 1984).

SAMI CULTURE: AN OVERVIEW

History

The Sami peoples are thought to have originated from what is now the northeastern region of Russia, yet their precise origins and routes of earliest migration remain points of contention amongst scholars (Nesheim, 1977). However, archaeological discoveries along Norway's northern Arctic Ocean coastline indicate that the Sami, or their direct descendants, have occupied the present-day area of settlement for at least 10,000 years. Two thousand years ago the Sami inhabited a vast territory which included all of present-day Finland, coastal areas around the Gulf of Bothnia, and the coastline along both the Atlantic and Arctic Oceans from what is now central Norway northward to the White Sea in Russia.

The Sami were, from the beginning, a seasonally nomadic people; their livelihood based upon hunting, fishing and gathering. At the time of initial (or early) contact with Scandinavians immediately prior to the Viking Age (in the eighth and ninth centuries), Sami society was flourishing. Seasonal migrations occurred along specific coastal or inland water routes, between more or less permanent settlements and in small family units of three to five members. As contact was made with Scandinavians to the south and Russians and various other cultures to the east, trade developed simultaneously. The coastal Sami traded the oils and skins of marine mammals, eider down and furs; while the inland Sami traded mainly in large quantities of furs. The Sami area of occupation was very sparsely populated and may have supported only a few thousand people. Hence, as contact intensified with Scandinavians, the Sami were unable to hold what had once been their traditional occupancy areas, and were forced northwards and away from the more temperate and productive coastal areas along the Atlantic and around the Gulf of Bothnia (Nesheim, 1977).

By the late fifteenth and early sixteenth centuries Scandinavian colonization of the north was fully under way. There was a concerted effort on the part of Denmark (then ruling Norway) and Sweden (then ruling Finland) to convert the Sami to Christianity. Sami spiritual leaders (known as *noaiddit*), were widely persecuted, for it was they who held together their communities under the onslaught of missionaries. They were compelled to renounce their old religion and to surrender their sacred drums to the missionaries who converted them. The Sami were also obligated to pay tribute, first to powerful landholders and then to the crowns of Denmark and Sweden; and were faced with the further loss of lands as wave after wave of Scandinavian pioneers were lured north by the states' promises of exemption from taxes and military service.

The obligation of tribute with which the Sami were forced to comply was at the outset satisfied by the Sami's payment of furs in exchange for substitute foodstuffs. By the beginning of the seventeenth century, however, the rules of tribute had changed and the Sami were then required to make payment in the form of dried fish and tame male reindeer; a direct state intervention in the Sami's indigenous food sector. This had dire consequences for the Sami whose population had, in the hundred years since supplementary foodstuffs were introduced by the state, increased in excess of what could be supported within the traditional hunting and gathering system. The larger Sami population resulted in the overexploitation of the indigenous food supply (particularly wild reindeer, moose and other wildlife stocks), which, when coupled with the subsequent royal prerogative of exacting tribute from this same overexploited food source, led to the decay of traditional Sami livelihood. Indeed, it has been argued that the disintegration of the Sami hunting and gathering society occurred at this particular point in history (that is, early in the seventeenth century), and that it was caused by state intervention in the Sami's social mode of production, obviating the need to develop new social relationships based on new modes of production (Lundmark, 1982).

The Sami's response to these changing conditions was not a uniform one; rather, it is possible to identify at least three main responses to these changing conditions (Aarseth and Björklund, 1987). One such response was the emergence of a coast-Sami culture based mainly on off-shore fishing and supplemented by agriculture; a second response was the emergence of an inland-Sami culture in which agriculture was supplemented by hunting, fishing and some reindeer herding; while a third response saw the emergence of a nomadic Sami culture drawn originally from both the coastal and inland groups, and mainly occupied with taming, tending and herding reindeer. The transformation of the coast and inland-Sami variants from hunters and gatherers to farmers and fishermen led to the replacement of earlier seasonal migrations to a life-style based on permanent settlement. With the advent of reindeer nomadism, the communal relationships once characteristic of traditional Sami society became an adapted feature of reindeer nomadism, as small groups of families (known as the Siida) came to tend and follow a particular, permanent reindeer herd, migrating with it between the various seasonal pastures.

Although these cultural transformations were responses to intensified contact and conflict with the Scandinavian cultures (and serve as vivid indications of Sami society's remarkable resilience), they did little to curtail the impact of increasingly dominant and disruptive forces on Sami culture in the seventeenth and eighteenth centuries (cf. Dahlström, 1967, 1970, 1974a and 1974b). Indeed, the missionary-led crusade to Christianize the Sami and the Sami's obligation to pay tribute to the colonizing nation-states continued unabated. Moreover, the obligation of tribute became a tactic used by the nation-states to justify and promote their territorial demands amongst one another, particularly in areas of the far north. Thus Sami people in the far north were obligated to pay tribute to three different nation-states at the same time – an inequity which existed for almost a hundred years (Nesheim, 1977). It was not until 1751 and 1826 that border demarcations were settled, first between Denmark–Norway and Sweden–Finland, and then between Norway and Russia.

The convention of 1751 establishing the boundary between Norway and Sweden–Finland was of particular importance to the Sami. In addition to finally rationalizing the obligation of tribute, the convention also included an accord which recognized the presence of the Sami and their right to use and occupy lands in the north regardless of national boundaries. Known as the Lapp Codicil and often referred to by the Sami as the Sami Magna Carta, the accord was developed as an instrument of international law governing matters of citizenship, title to land and water, neutrality in war, and internal administration and justice (Swedish Sami Rights Commission, 1986). Of particular importance to the Sami was the demarcation of a Sami occupancy and utilization zone, north of a prescribed boundary, within which the Sami were granted exclusive rights to hunting, fishing and reindeer herding.

In 1809, less than 60 years after the enactment of the Lapp Codicil, Sweden lost possession of Finland to Russia, which led to adverse consequences for the Finnish-Sami. In the wake of Russia's rule over Finland, the once exclusive rights of the Sami to hunting, fishing and reindeer herding were extended to all Finnish citizens – Sami and non-Sami alike (Siuruainen and Aikio, 1977). During the latter half of the nineteenth century, Norway and Sweden implemented a number of measures to strengthen the reindeer-Sami's utilization and occupancy rights. These new measures went further than those already included in the accord of 1751 by establishing a cultivation limit for the purpose of reserving territory to the north and west of the limit exclusively for the Sami (Nordic Sami Institute, 1990). Following the introduction of these strengthened measures, Norway and Sweden drew a formal distinction between reindeer-herding and non-reindeer-herding Sami; a distinction which conveyed to reindeer-Sami exclusive utilization and occupancy rights to grazing lands, hunting and fishing. This distinction, and the corresponding vesture of rights only to reindeer-Sami, remains valid today. In contrast, the reindeer-Sami in Finland have never benefited from such occupational safeguards (Aikio, P., 1987).

Today, the cultivation limit remains in effect only in Sweden and, as such, the Swedish reindeer-Sami peoples are acknowledged to have the strongest rights above this limit; that is, the strongest land rights amongst all reindeer-Sami peoples (Swedish Sami Rights Commission, 1986; Aikio, P., 1987). However, such a limit had little, if any, practical effect against the accelerated Scandinavian colonization of Samiland during the period 1880 to 1920 (cf. Lapping, 1986). Sparked by renewed Nordic government inducements of free land and exemption from taxation and military service, Scandinavian settlement expanded throughout Samiland during this period. In Finland, for example, settlement was aided by the state's expropriation of all lands outside village boundaries in Sami-occupied territories, and the subsequent conditions set out for both agricultural and non-agricultural land use (Siuruainen and Aikio, 1977). A series of Reindeer Grazing Acts were adopted in Norway and Sweden during this period to regulate land use and to manage conflicts between reindeer husbandry and other land-use activities related to settlement. Hence, the centuries-old pattern of expansionary settlement repeated itself once again; encroachment followed by conflict leading to the expulsion and northward migration of the Sami.

Around the turn of this century, Nordic states employed new tactics to fracture Sami society further and to assimilate the Sami culturally; tactics that, over time, have proved most effective, especially in the case of the near-total assimilation of the coast-Sami in Norway (cf. Paine, 1957, 1965; Eidheim, 1977; Björklund, 1982). The Norwegian Parliament enacted a new law in 1902 which decreed that only those who could read and write Norwegian, and who could use Norwegian on a daily basis, were entitled to become landowners in northern Norway (Enoksen, 1982). The Sami were expected to adopt a Norwegian family name as a precondition for landownership. The reindeer-Sami in Sweden were effectively denied the right to vote in municipal and national elections unless it could be demonstrated that they were tax payers; and Sami peoples throughout Samiland were generally under-represented in local government and alienated from the political process. Furthermore, the reindeer-Sami in Norway and Sweden were effectively segregated from both the non-reindeer-Sami peoples and the Scandinavian majority by the Lapp Administration. This agency not only administered and enforced the Reindeer Grazing Act, but was also responsible for providing education and various welfare services to the reindeer-Sami peoples (Sjölin, 1982). Along with the Lapp Administration, school and church became powerful instruments of assimilation as Nordic languages became the official languages of both instruction and worship; and the declared aim of both institutions was culturally to transform the Sami into proper Norwegians, Swedes or Finns (cf. Kaddik, 1989; Otnes, 1970; Küng, 1970).

Language and communications

Samisk is the language of the Sami people, and belongs to the Finno-Ugrian family of languages which consists of, amongst others, the Baltic Fennic languages. Samisk has three main dialects comprised of as many as nine subdialects (Keskitalo, 1981; Aikio, M., 1987). The three main dialects are East, Central and South Samisk; each generally referring to that area of Samiland where it is spoken (see Map 5.2). The borders differentiating the three main dialects correspond to Sami settlement patterns over the centuries and occur completely independent of Nordic nation-state boundaries. The differences among them are significant enough that they can be referred to as three different languages. Sixty to seventy per cent of all Sami people speak Samisk and, of the three main dialects, Central Samisk is the most widely spoken and is dominated by the North Samisk subdialect. The North Samisk dialect is spoken by about 80 per cent of all Samisk-speakers (Keskitalo, 1981). East Samisk and South Samisk are spoken in areas where Sami people often represent a minority of the population and thus both have declined in usage during this century. The minority Sami populations in these eastern and southern areas have generally switched to speaking the language

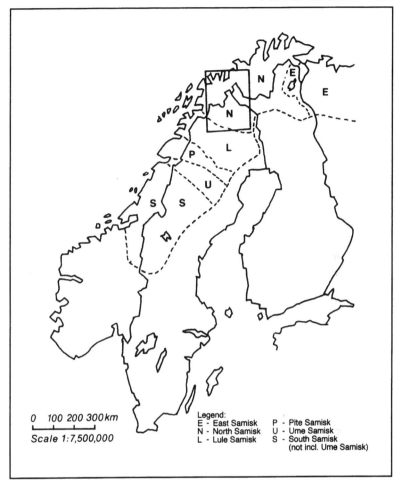

Map 5.2 Samisk language and dialects
Source: Adapted from Elina Helander (1984) *Om trespråkighet, Umeå*, in SOU, 1989: 114

of the majority (that is, Finnish in the east, and Swedish or Norwegian in the south).

All Samisk dialects contain a rich vocabulary in which to describe and relate natural features of their immediate environment. Each dialect possesses many very precise words to describe land, water and snow. There is also a rich and varied vocabulary associated with seen the rapid and steady encroachment of modern loan-words from the various Nordic majority languages, thus threatening the integrity of the Samisk languages and making their intra-Nordic use that much more difficult (Aarseth and Björklund, 1987). The integrity of the North Samisk subdialect has been greatly strengthened since 1980, when Finland agreed to join with Sweden and Norway to institute a common North Samisk orthography. This was an important development as it facilitates a higher degree of Nordic co-operation in fields of literature and communication and provides the majority of Samisk-speakers with a uniform written language. It also represents a catalyst for more recent Sami demands to have Samisk recognized as an official language within their area of settlement, and particularly with regard to the provision of education and other public services.

Communications serve as a medium for the expression of Samisk among the Sami by way of various print and broadcast media. In Norway, three Sami newspapers are published; one on a weekly basis, another twice weekly and the third on a monthly basis. Sweden and Finland each have one monthly newspaper. All five Sami newspapers receive public financial support and also rely to a lesser extent on subscription and advertising revenues. Sami radio and television programmes occur regularly on public broadcast networks in all three Nordic states, primarily within the Nordkalotten region. Each country supports special publicly funded Sami production units which create regularly featured Sami programmes, and which actively collaborate with one another. In the late 1970s and at various times since then, there have been discussions amongst the three Nordic states regarding the establishment of a pan-Nordic Sami broadcast production centre, but such an initiative has yet to be realized.

Cultural expression

Print and broadcast communications represent only one instrument of the Sami's cultural expression in this modern era, for the Sami have a wide repertoire of traditional forms of expression which pre-date the advent of print and broadcast communication media. Perhaps the most popular of these traditional media is that of yoiking, a distinctive form of narrative singing which embodies the Sami's rich oral story-telling tradition. The oral story-telling tradition has always played a central role in Sami culture, and Sami music (particularly yoiking) is a part of this tradition. Yoiking is a way of telling stories, recalling events and people, or describing nature; and it is a tradition that continues today after enduring a long history of suppression and near-extinction at the hands of Scandinavian missionaries, state churches and education authorities. Even today in Kautokeino, Sami children are forbidden to yoik during school hours. Moreover, in addition to its long-held traditional significance, the custom of yoiking today symbolizes to the Sami the renaissance of Sami cultural values which began in earnest during the 1960s and continues today. The yoik has become a source of inspiration for modern Sami folk-songs and other forms of music.

The Sami cultural renaissance has also witnessed the birth of a vibrant Sami literary society. Several modern-day Sami authors have left their mark of late, perhaps most notably among them Nils-Aslak Valkeapää, who became the first Sami to be awarded the Nordic Council's prestigious literary prize, in 1991. Most of the original works of Sami authors have been in Samisk, and much of it was then translated into Swedish, Norwegian and Finnish. Modern Sami literature has renewed the old tradition of story-telling while also providing a treasury of both modern and traditional Sami folklore. Other examples of modern-day adaptations of the Sami's story-telling tradition are those of Sami theatre, now flourishing in all three Nordic countries, and of Sami cinematography, which first achieved popularity in 1987, with the production of a feature-length film entitled *The Pathfinder*, based on old Sami legends and nominated for an Oscar award as Best Foreign Film.

To the Sami, handicraft and art embody cultural expressions which are largely one and the same. Everyday items, many of them still in use today, not only had a practical function but were also designed to be aesthetically pleasing. The drum of the *noadi*, for instance, was not only a musical instrument but also an artist's image of the worlds of men and gods. The traditional outer garment of the Sami (known as the *kolt*) is not only functional and warm, but is also a beautiful example of textile art with distinctive embroidery work and bright, patterned colours. Handicraft and art continue to be seen by the Sami as important elements of cultural expression, as indicated in part by the present-day existence of arts and crafts training centres in both Kautokeino and Jokkmokk, Sweden. Sami leaders also see the production of Sami arts and crafts as a significant component of the expanding tourist trade and, as such, an important contribution to Sami economic development.

Present-day livelihood

Today, typical Sami primary enterprises based on reindeer husbandry, agriculture and fishing provide only a limited and declining number of people with a means of living. What was once a vital and self-sufficient livelihood is now a livelihood dependent upon capital accumulation, wages from paid employment, and income from social security and other government sources. This in large part is due to the modernization of typical Sami livelihoods through a process of capitalization, concentration of ownership and increased mechanization. For the Sami, modernization has resulted in the emergence of a relatively large surplus workforce (Aarseth and Björklund, 1987), the dimensions of which cannot be defined at present due to methods of data collection and reporting employed by the Nordic states. Much of this surplus workforce has been absorbed by wage employment within either the primary Sami enterprise sector or other labour-market occupations.

Although employment is declining in the primary Sami enterprises, such occupations still represent a significant base of employment for pan-Sami society. As noted above, reindeer husbandry directly supports as many as 6,000 Sami people and hundreds of others during the autumn and winter seasons. However, a family must possess at least 300 reindeer to provide a basic level of income which would not necessitate supplementation (Ornstedt, 1991; Aarseth and Björklund, 1987). Hence, many reindeer-herding families throughout Samiland are in the position of having to secure supplementary incomes by way of herding for others, fishing, logging, berry-picking, direct sale of handicrafts, or from paid work in the fishing industry and slaughter-houses. Fishing is still an important occupation in districts inhabited by the coast-Sami people and is often combined with meat and dairy farming and other forms of supplementary income through wage employment. Coast-Sami farmers are among the principal suppliers of milk to the dairy industry in Finnmark, and there is also a relatively strong inland-Sami farming community in the Utsjoki district of northwestern Finland.

Income from wage employment in non-Sami economic sectors represents the overall dominant source of incomes for Sami people. Indeed, it has been estimated that 90 per cent of the Sami labour force is engaged in the dominant, non-Sami economy (Burger, 1987). Although the type of employment available varies considerably from one area to another, jobs in forestry and mining are fairly common and represent modest sources of employment income for the Sami throughout Samiland. Jobs in the manufacturing and service sectors have attracted Sami workers to the region's main population centres. The service sector plays a particularly important role in providing employment to Sami workers in fields of construction, road maintenance, health care, education and social services, and tourism. Sami people are also entering the professional sector of the labour market in increasing numbers as health professionals, teachers, engineers, lawyers and administrators.

Income obtained from wage employment also varies considerably. Those earning the highest incomes are, of course, the skilled and professional workers often employed in public service or manufacturing. Reindeer herders, forest and mining workers also earn large average incomes, but their employment is usually seasonal. The lower-paid groups include farmers, fishermen and some of the reindeer herders.

Income levels aside, however, Sami workers are faced with limited employment opportunities due to the rather one-sided and under-developed economic conditions prevalent in most Sami districts (Aarseth and Björklund, 1987). Those employment opportunities which do exist are usually of a temporary or semi-skilled nature. Furthermore, it has been noted that Sami workers are simply more likely to be unemployed than non-Sami Scandinavians (Burger, 1987). In parts of Sami-occupied northern Finland, for instance, unemployment rates are usually 33 per cent during the long winter season (Siuruainen and Aikio, 1977). Hence, although Nordkalotten is the Nordic region most prone to unemployment, it is the predominant Sami districts within Nordkalotten that face the highest unemployment rates. Those Sami and non-Sami workers affected by unemployment must then rely upon a range of universal social security benefits, outlined below, to support their livelihood.

Social and political organization

The Sami today are one people living in four nations, and hence are subject to the laws and institutions of the particular country in which they reside. Traditionally, Sami society was organized into self-sufficient, co-operative units known as the Siida. The Siida system was governed by an assembly (known as the Norraz) composed of one person from each member family, and its primary function was to regulate and appropriate hunting and fishing rights amongst its members. The Norraz also exercised judicial authority in matters of social deviance and performed a distributive function in allocating the Siida's surplus, ensuring primarily that its poor and sick were secure. Today, however, the Siida system of social organization is of relevance only to the mountain or reindeer-Sami peoples living in Finnmark and throughout northern Sweden; and exists only in a culturally modified form, its traditional lines of authority usurped by the dominant legal and administrative systems of the Nordic states.

Moreover, history indicates that the Nordic states have utilized their national legal and political institutions to assimilate the Sami forcibly (Dahlström, 1974a and b; Eidheim, 1985). Of particular significance in this regard is the policy of Norway and Sweden of dividing Sami peoples into two main occupational groupings according to their association or non-association with reindeer. Those classified as reindeer peoples are vested with certain inalienable legal rights to land, fishing and hunting; and those considered as non-reindeer peoples are treated as ordinary Swedes and Norwegians. Furthermore, status as reindeer peoples is reserved for those individuals whose nuclear family has been engaged in herding and, in the case of Sweden, for those who belong to one of 43 specially designated Sami settlements. Hence, reindeer-Sami peoples represent a very small and tightly controlled minority within pan-Sami society, and number about 2,500 people in each of Norway and Sweden, and perhaps another 1,000 in Finland (Nordic Sami Institute, 1990).

In short, the principal effect of the Nordic states' concerted attempts to assimilate the Sami has been to create subcultural cleavages along occupational lines within pan-Sami society. For the vast majority of the Sami population this has meant being denied the basic right to enjoy, develop and disseminate its own culture and language. The Sami people have been relegated to a minority status in which Samishness has become synonomous with reindeer herding while other forms of cultural expression have been repressed or simply not tolerated. This minority status has given rise over the past 40 years to a Samish Movement, the primary goal of which has been to achieve Sami cultural autonomy within Nordic society (Eidheim, 1977; Ingold, 1976).

As shown in Figure 5.1, the Samish Movement is comprised of a number of Sami interest organizations each promoting the social, cultural and economic interests of Sami populations in all three Nordic countries, and it has been augmented recently by the formation of a Sami organization in Russia. The Movement's overall guiding principle is that of pan-Sami society being a cultural, linguistic, economic and political unit which transcends the boundaries of four nation-states (Baer, 1982).

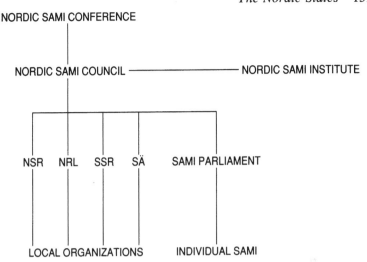

NSR = National Association of Norwegian Sami
NRL = Sami Reindeer Herders' Association of Norway
SÄ = Same-Ätnam (Swedish Sami League or Alliance)
SSR = National Association of Swedish Sami
The Sami Parliament = elected body for Finnish Sami

Figure 5.1 The Samish Movement

'The Sami, one people' is the motto of the Nordic Sami Council, an umbrella organization established in 1956 by national Sami organizations from all three Nordic countries to foster co-operation and unity among the Sami peoples. The aim of the Council is to promote the economic, social and cultural interests of the Sami in a manner compatible with the wishes and constraints of the Sami minority in each country. The Council meets at least once per year and is composed of twelve members. Representation on the Council is evenly divided along lines of national affiliation, and is expected to represent the pluralistic nature of the pan-Sami society from an economic and cultural standpoint. Members are appointed to the Council for terms of three years by delegates to the Nordic Sami Conference, a proceeding held every three years and attended by 60 delegates representing national Sami organizations from Norway and Sweden, and the Sami Assembly in Finland (see Figure 5.1). Like representation on the Council, representation at the Conference is evenly divided along lines of national affiliation with attention given to subcultural (that is, occupational) considerations.

The Council has instituted a comprehensive, 50-point political action programme designed to unify its various constituent member organizations in their struggle for Sami cultural autonomy. This programme, adopted by the Nordic Sami Conference in 1986, sets out numerous demands (directed at each welfare state) for the recognition and realization of the Sami's collective rights. In essence, this campaign for collective rights is highlighted by its aim to secure (on behalf of pan-Sami society): the right of self-determination; rights to land and natural resources; social and cultural preservation; community economic development and safeguards to protect typical Sami livelihood activities; formal involvement representation at the Nordic Council; and the Nordic states' acceptance of international standards for the treatment of indigenous peoples. Although the Nordic states have generally been at odds with the Council's campaign for collective rights, they have at least recognized it as the legitimate representative of the Sami peoples, and provide direct financial support through the Nordic Council of Ministers. The council is also a founding and active member of the World Conference of Indigenous Peoples (WCIP) established in 1975.

The mission and mandates of the two national organizations in each of Norway and Sweden reflect the plurality of pan-Sami society from both a cultural and economic perspective and, as such, they generally perform complementary tasks to each other. Thus, relations between national organizations in each country are marked by a high degree of co-operation and consensus building. At the risk of presenting an over-simplified picture of Sami national political organization, the particular needs and interests of the reindeer-Sami in Norway and Sweden are represented by the National Federation of Norwegian-Sami Reindeer Breeders (NRL) and the Swedish-Sami National Federation (SSR), organizations which have both been in operation for over 40 years (cf. Svensson, 1976). The broader social and cultural interests of Sami society in each nation are represented by the Norwegian Sami National Federation (NSR) and in Sweden by Sami-Atnam.

The Sami Assembly in Finland was established in 1975 in response to an earlier government commission report which received the general support of Finnish Samis, and which sought to overcome the social and political fragmentation that had previously characterized the organization of Finnish Sami society. The assembly serves as a (non-constitutional) representative body composed of twenty members, directly elected to three-year terms by a registered Sami electorate, organized into a small number of constituencies that correspond to areas of Sami occupancy. Although the assembly lacks constitutional powers and serves only as an advisory body to central government, it has unified the plural elements of Finnish Sami society and thus helped to strengthen Sami influence in the decision-making process. Furthermore, it has increasingly assumed the role of service-provider formerly performed by government agencies and, as such, is seen by some members of Finnish Sami society as being an important first step towards Samish cultural autonomy. However, such a viewpoint is indeed a controversial one, as many Sami see the Assembly in its existing form as little more than window-dressing on the part of Finnish government authorities; that is, to mask their alleged intentions of undermining basic Sami rights and further exploiting Sami lands and resources (Aikio, P., 1987).

In 1989, a second Sami Assembly was established in Norway. The Norwegian Assembly has been vested with limited decision-making powers pursuant to the Sami Act (1987) to safeguard and develop the Norwegian Sami's language, culture and livelihood. However, the limits imposed upon the Assembly's decision-making powers have, from the outset, generated considerable controversy as in the case of the Finnish example (cf. Smith, 1987; Stordahl, 1987). Perhaps as a result of this ensuing controversy, and other Sami concerns as regards the Assembly's electoral procedures and composition, the Assembly has yet to be formally recognized or accepted by the pan-Sami peoples as a constituent body of the Nordic Sami Council.

The Nordic Sami Institute has been described as a modern attempt to create a cultural Sami institution outside of the central administrative organs of the state. Its enabling philosophy is that of aiding pan-Sami society in effectively adapting to change; that is, from the starting point of extending and incorporating a Sami world view through which Sami values and knowledge form the core. Founded jointly by the Nordic Sami Council and the Nordic Council of Ministers in 1974, the Institute is a semi-autonomous institution involved in areas of education, research and cultural development on behalf of the Sami peoples. Based in Kautokeino, the Institute is directed by a ten-member board of whom seven are appointed by the Nordic Sami Conference and three by the Nordic Council of Ministers. Administratively, the Institute is organized in three sections: (1) languages and culture; (2) livelihood, environment and rights; and (3) education and information. It is financed by the five nations belonging to the Nordic Council of Ministers.

ORGANIZATION OF NORDIC SOCIAL WELFARE SERVICES RELATIVE TO THE SAMI

Administration and financing

In general, the administration and financing of services relative to the Sami is organized hierarchically from one level of government to another; that is, local (municipal and county), central and pan-Nordic. Services as regards the Sami can be further classified into two categories: the institutional (that is, social security and welfare services); and the non-institutional, or special, services.

Local government services

Today, welfare services are by and large extended to Sami individuals in the same way as they are to the majority population in each of the Nordic states. Most services are provided to individual Sami persons through the auspices of municipal or county-level government. These include a wide variety of health and other personal social services, social assistance, education and occupational training, and housing (Olsson, 1990). The Sami are not entitled to any extraordinary benefits or exemptions as regards the administration of local welfare services, for they must satisfy the rules of entitlement in the same way as members of the majority population. Furthermore, the administration of local services as regards the Sami remains the sole responsibility of local government authorities and not the Sami themselves.

Services provided to Sami individuals by local and county governments are financed through local taxation, grants from central government and direct charges for services (Gustafsson, 1988). Local income and property tax is paid by all persons (Sami and non-Sami alike) to the municipality in which they are registered residents. Local taxation is levied on a flat-rate basis, the rate fixed by each municipal/ county council. Rates vary considerably from community to community according to population size and extent of public service infrastructure. In Sweden, local income tax covered (on average) about 41 per cent of municipal and 62 per cent of county council expenditure in 1985.

Grants from central government are intended to provide municipalities and county councils with general financial support, to encourage the expansion and maintenance of special local government services, and to equalize differences in the costs entailed in providing local government services. This last point is of particular importance to the Sami as the purpose of tax equalization policy is to enable each municipality and county council to maintain a standard level of local government services, regardless of their tax revenue base. In Sweden (and probably Norway and Finland also), the largest tax equalization grants are paid to northern municipalities and county councils where Sami people reside. Once again in the case of Sweden, grants from central government in 1985 accounted on average for about 26 per cent of municipal revenue and 18 per cent of county council revenue. Charges for 'hard' services such as electricity, heating, water and sewerage are intended to cover the actual costs of providing them; while charges for 'soft' services such as day care, health and other personal social services, and housing, cover only a portion of actual costs. Charges for services (and other items of revenue) accounted in 1985 for approximately 30 per cent of municipal revenue and about 21 per cent of county council revenue in Sweden (Gustafsson, 1988).

Central government services

Other services from which Sami benefit are those administered by central government authorities. Central government services (relative to the Sami) fall into two main categories: those being institutional services (that is, social security) for individuals, and special (non-institutional) services to protect and enhance Sami society in each of the Nordic states. The former category applies to all Nordic citizens and residents (that is, Sami and non-Sami alike), and includes such institutional measures as unemployment security, health and occupational injury insurance, parents' and children's allowances, and pensions (Olsson, 1990). As with the administration of local government services, individual Sami persons must satisfy the rules of entitlement for social security benefits in the same way as others.

It is with regard to the organization of central government special services that the Sami are able to exert a limited yet expanding influence over the kinds of goods and services, and level of provision, that have come to be accepted as constituting elements of their collective right to cultural autonomy. In Norway and Finland, Sami special services are co-ordinated by a Secretariat for Sami Affairs responsible in Norway to the Ministry of Local Government and to the Ministry of the Interior in Finland (Nordic Sami Institute, 1990; Aikio, P., 1987); and both secretariats have the responsibility of overseeing the activities of the Sami Assembly in each of their nations. The Sami Assembly was established in Norway and Finland to improve the representation of Sami needs and concerns to central government authorities; and to provide Sami society in both nations with an enhanced but limited measure of autonomy in the conduct of its cultural affairs.

In the case of the Norwegian Sami, for instance, the Sami Assembly have limited decision-making powers pursuant to Norway's Sami Act 1987; its decision-making authority limited mainly to the allocation of funds for Sami cultural activities and organizations. The Sami Act 1987 would also seem to promote – in a limited manner – the Sami people's collective interests in relation to conflicting or competing interests of dominant Norwegian society. For instance, the Act requires that other public bodies should consult the Sami Parliament prior to making decisions that come within its scope, and the Act also provides for the option of the Sami Parliament to appeal directly to the appropriate public authority if its interests are being threatened. In contrast, the Sami Parliament in Finland functions strictly in a limited advisory capacity, having no decision-making authority (Aikio P., 1987). However, both the Norwegian and Finnish Sami Parliaments perform a key function of appointing Sami representatives to a variety of government councils and committees active in various social, cultural and economic aspects of Sami affairs.

In Sweden, Sami special services are organized vertically from government department to department, as there is no single government agency concerned with the comprehensive provision of such services (Swedish Sami Rights Commission, 1989); that is, no single agency that cuts horizontally across the numerous vertical lines of service administration. Hence, in the case of the Swedish Sami, there exist two avenues to influence the organization of central government services relative to their own needs. The first approach, similar to that of the Norwegian and Finnish Sami, entails the appointment of Sami representatives to a variety of government councils and committees active in various aspects of Sami affairs. The second approach is unique amongst the pan-Sami and involves the utilization of an officially constituted Ombudsman against Ethnic Discrimination. The Ombudsman is positioned at arm's length from central government to ensure that Sami interests and the interests of visible minorities as may or may not be reflected in policy of the day are upheld, and to arbitrate policy-related conflicts as they arise (cf. Office of the Ombudsman, 1990). Moreover, Sweden may soon follow Norway's lead in amending its constitution to include a clause recognizing the Sami's right to exist, enacting a Sami Act, and establishing a Sami Assembly and vesting it with limited decision-making authority (Swedish Sami Rights Commission, 1989).

Services provided by central government are financed by general state revenue raised through value-added tax on most goods and services, special levies on certain goods and services, state tax on personal incomes, payroll charges to employers and self-employed, and state property tax. State revenue relative to Sami special services is primarily directed toward supporting Sami education, cultural development and reindeer husbandry.

The promotion of Sami education services in Norway and Sweden is organized by Sami Education Councils and funded directly by the Ministry of Education in each state. The Norwegian-Sami Education Council is wholly composed of Sami representatives appointed by the Sami Assembly, and serves in an advisory role to the Ministry of Education. The nine-member Swedish-Sami Education Council is comprised of a majority of Sami representatives appointed by central government on the advice of the two national Sami organizations; and has the responsibility of managing and overseeing the administration of six separate (compulsory-level) Sami schools offering a distinctly Sami cultural education in complement to the regular public-school curricula. In contrast, the Norwegian-Sami Education Council is largely concerned with developing and integrating Sami educational resources mainly for the use of Sami children in Norwegian public schools (Nordic Sami Institute, 1990). Sami cultural development in Sweden is financed by an annual state grant and funds from the Sami Fund. The Sami Fund also provides grants in support of reindeer husbandry and Sami organizations. The Fund is governed by an executive committee composed of six members, three of whom are Sami representatives nominated by the national Sami organizations (Swedish Sami Rights Commission, 1989). The executive committee advises central government of the amount required for distribution from the Sami Fund; and its administrative arm, the Cultural Delegation (composed of three members of whom two are Sami representatives), decides how grants from the Fund for Sami culture and Sami organizations are to be allocated. The Cultural Delegation also distributes the state grant for Sami culture from the Ministry of Education and Cultural Affairs.

The financing of Sami cultural development in Norway is mainly the responsibility of the Norwegian Cultural Council through its administration of the Norwegian Cultural Fund (Nordic Sami Institute, 1990). The Council's involvement in preserving and promoting Sami culture has been facilitated through the establishment of a joint expert committee for Sami culture. The joint committee is comprised of a number of specialized subcommittees each having limited authority to administer funds to foster a wide variety of cultural activity in literature, oral traditions, folk music, cultural conservation and so on. Sami cultural development in Norway is also financed by other central government agencies, including the Ministry of Local Government, the Ministry of Church and Cultural Affairs, the Development Fund for Reindeer Herding, the Ministry of the Environment, and the Ministry of Children and Family Affairs; and by those northern counties and municipalities having a significant Sami population.

The administration of reindeer herding in Sweden, Norway and Finland falls under the mandate of each nation's Ministry of Agriculture; and the principal legislation regulating the conduct of reindeer herding varies in effect from nation to nation. In Sweden, the Reindeer Herding Act 1971 extends the right to engage in reindeer herding exclusively to the Sami; and only to those Sami who are members of one of the 43 distinct reindeer-Sami villages designated as herding districts under the Act. This Act also regulates the nature and scope of reindeer-Sami rights to land and water; rights which were further clarified and strengthened by the landmark judgement of the Swedish Supreme Court in the Skattefjäll dispute (between reindeer-Sami and the central state) in 1981 (Swedish Sami Rights Commission, 1989).

The Norwegian Reindeer Herding Act 1978 takes a somewhat different approach from that of the relevant Swedish Act in stipulating that within the designated Sami reindeer territory, the right to engage in reindeer herding applies only to those Sami whose parents or grandparents have been herders (Nordic Sami Institute, 1990). Hence, in this regard, Norwegian legislation differs from that of the Swedish in two important respects: first, the Norwegian Sami's reindeer herding rights are tied only to family lineage (and not to village membership as in Sweden), and second, Norwegian legislation permits a limited non-Sami involvement in reindeer herding outside the designated Sami reindeer territory. As in Norway, reindeer-herding legislation in Finland applies to a designated territory within which reindeer herding is granted particular rights to land and water, and protection (or compensation) from competing land uses. However, unlike the relevant Swedish and Norwegian legislation, the Finnish legislation neither entitles the Sami to exclusive herding rights nor to any form of special legal status in relation to Finland's non-Sami reindeer-herding majority.

The formal organization of reindeer management in all three Nordic countries is arranged in hierarchical order from national to regional (namely, county) to district level; the two upper levels fulfil key advisory and regulatory functions, while the district level represents the legal and administrative interests of local reindeer herders. The district level in each nation is composed of numerous boards (in the case of Sweden and Norway) or voluntary associations (in the case of Finland) elected annually by the reindeer herders themselves. There are 86 district boards in Norway, 43 in Sweden, and 12 associations with a majority of Sami members in Finland.

In Norway and Sweden, the operation of district boards is financed through agreement between the state and the respective national reindeer organizations, which, in turn, distribute funds to each of the district boards. Furthermore, both Norway and Sweden have established formal instruments by which to compensate Sami districts financially on an annual basis for the loss of grazing areas due to encroachment of competing land uses. These compensation funds (known in Norway as the Sami Development Fund and in Sweden as the Sami Fund) are directed towards the development of reindeer husbandry, Sami culture and Sami organizations; and are administered in Norway by the Sami Assembly, and in Sweden by a committee of government-appointed Sami representatives. In Finland, the operation of voluntary district associations is principally financed by fees from compulsory membership levied per head of reindeer, and income from the auction of unidentifiable (that is, as regards ownership) reindeer found at separations (Ingold, 1976).

Furthermore, both Norway and Sweden provide direct production subsidies to individual reindeer herders (Ornstedt, 1991). The Swedish and Norwegian governments have also provided direct financial compensation to individual reindeer herders for losses of stock and grazing lands due to radioactive fall-out of the Chernobyl nuclear accident of April 1986, and for costs that herders continue to incur as they adjust to the long-term consequences of Chernobyl.

Pan-Nordic co-operation services

The organization of services relative to the Sami's individual and collective interests is also evident at the Pan-Nordic level. Such services are developed and financed through the Nordic Council (composed of the five Nordic states and led by a Council of

Ministers), and generally take the form of multi-lateral agreements and special initiatives resulting from the high level of inter-governmental co-operation fostered through the Council of Ministers. As individuals, Sami persons benefit from a number of Nordic Council co-operation agreements, including those relating to a common Nordic labour market and co-operation on social security and health care.

The aim of Nordic co-operation as regards the Sami's collective interests is to preserve and promote the culture and livelihood of pan-Sami society. This aim is principally pursued through the mandates of various Nordic Council agencies and through the activities of the semi-autonomous Nordic Sami Institute (for research) and the autonomous Nordic Sami Council. Both of the latter organizations are financed by the Nordic Council but are accountable to pan-Sami society for their activities.

Welfare services in profile

Regional development and labour market programmes

Regional economic development policy in Norway, Sweden and Finland is mainly intended as an instrument to reduce unemployment levels in those regions experiencing various degrees of economic hardship due to structural changes and other problems. Economic development in the Nordkalotten region is facilitated by each of the three nations taking initiatives independent of the others, and through active pan-Nordic development co-operation. National initiatives principally occur in concert with the commonly shared goal of full employment and associated active labour-market policy. These initiatives include programmes intended to increase employment by encouraging the start-up of new industries or the expansion of existing operations, and programmes intended to maintain existing employment levels through wage subsidies, aid to occupational training and skills upgrading, and labour-force mobility assistance. National initiatives in support of Nordkalotten's development also entail improvements to regional infrastructure; that is, transportation and communications networks, and public services as regards health care, education and housing.

At the pan-Nordic level, active development co-operation plays an important role in supporting the economic development needs of the Nordkalotten region as a whole, and the distinct needs of pan-Sami society in particular. The former is mainly facilitated through the auspices of the Nordkalotten Committee and involves practical initiatives to improve the region's comparative advantage in sectors considered of key importance to the region's development prospects; those being education, research and design; manufacturing; and tourism (Nordic Council of Ministers, 1990). The particular development needs of pan-Sami society are addressed by the Nordic Sami Institute, the Nordic Cultural Fund, the Nordic Co-operation Agency for Sami Culture and Reindeer Husbandry, and the Nordic Agency for Reindeer Research. In general, these agencies are involved in applied research and project development activities, the outcome of which is expected to address practical concerns and particular obstacles to the effective development and improvement of the Sami people's livelihood (cf. Nordic Sami Institute, 1990).

Social security

Social security in Norway, Sweden and Finland consists of social insurance, social assistance, and Nordic conventions on a common labour market and social security. Social insurance schemes can be arranged in four categories: unemployment security; health, sickness and occupational injury insurance; pensions; and parents' and children's allowances. Social insurance is, by and large, both compulsory and universal in effect with the notable exception of unemployment insurance schemes in Finland and Sweden, which are voluntary and administered by trade-union-affiliated insurance societies. Furthermore, social insurance generally provides for high income replacement levels (in the order of 60 to 100 per cent) and other generous cash benefits. It is financed to a greater or lesser extent by a combination of general tax revenues from central governments and employer-mandated contributions. Welfare expenditures are financed in this way to spread the financial responsibility in a solidaristic manner across society rather than to tie benefits to individual contributions.

In addition to a basic pension and subsidized housing through income-tested rent allowances, most of the retired receive an earnings-related superannuation pension. For those gainfully employed, maternity benefits correspond to income replacement levels for sickness, while entitlement periods vary from 20 weeks in Norway to one year in Sweden. Fathers of new-born infants in Sweden are also entitled to claim the maternity benefit in place of mothers. Universal child allowances exist for children under age 16 and are replaced by school allowances for all students up to age 19.

Eligibility for benefits under all income replacement schemes is contingent upon employment. For those not receiving a regular income, an inferior scheme based on a daily flat-rate allowance is provided. The extensive nature of all the Nordic welfare states' social insurance systems has meant that relatively few people need to seek social assistance. As part of the municipally operated social assistance programme in each of the Nordic states, housing allowances are provided for those in need. In Sweden, a specially designated central government transfer was allotted to those municipalities having a sizeable Sami population in support of local social assistance programmes. The state discontinued this policy in the mid-1970s, however, under significant pressure from national Sami political organizations which found the practice culturally and socially stigmatizing.

Intertwining the social security nets of all three Nordic countries are a number of Nordic Council co-operation programmes which serve to enhance labour-market opportunities and social security provisions for citizens of one Nordic country living and working in another Nordic country. Chief among these various pan-Nordic co-operation programmes is the Nordic Convention on a common labour market, consisting of a series of agreements instituting a common labour market for professional and technical occupations. An important supplement to the common labour market is that of the Nordic Convention on Social Security established in 1982. The key aim of the social security convention is to provide those Nordic citizens living or working in another Nordic country with social security on equivalent terms to that which citizens of the host country are entitled. Furthermore, the social security convention extends special medical assistance to citizens of one Nordic country during the course of a temporary stay in another Nordic country.

Public services

Social security in Norway, Sweden and Finland is augmented by a broad range of welfare services. Of particular relevance to the Sami's welfare is that of the universal and comprehensive provision of education, health care and housing services.

Education

All parents in each of the Nordic countries are obligated to enrol their children in nine years of compulsory and comprehensive education (beginning at age 6 or 7), following which young people themselves can choose to continue their education for up to three years (in upper secondary school) and then proceed to some kind of further or higher education. Prior to children reaching compulsory school age, all parents are entitled to enrol their children (beginning at the age of 6 months) in municipally operated pre-school education programmes. Such programmes mainly consist of day nurseries charged with the dual responsibility of children's day care and cognitive development; and special attention is given to the provision of language training for children beginning at age 4 (Stenholm, 1984). For the Sami in all three Nordic countries, the matter of language training has meant a concerted campaign to establish Samisk-language nursery-school programmes in several municipalities where there is a sufficient Sami population base to support them. Sami nursery-school programmes are currently operating in as many as eight Norwegian municipalities with financial aid from central government (Nordic Sami Institute, 1990); while in each of Sweden and Finland perhaps only half this number of municipalities support such programmes.

Samisk-language programming at the pre-school level in Finland has been aided by an amendment to the Kindergarten Act 1982, granting Sami parents the right to have their children (at age 6) provided with a kindergarten education in Samisk (Nordic Sami Institute, 1990). Furthermore, in Sweden, Sami parents need only make a straightforward request of the appropriate pre-school administrator, and their children will receive Samisk-language tutoring for at least two hours per week by a Samisk speaker paid by the municipality. (This language service is also available on demand at the compulsory and upper secondary school levels, and forms part of Sweden's national education policy directed at recent immigrants and adopted in the early 1970s.)

At the compulsory school level, Sami parents in both Norway and Sweden have the option of enrolling their children in either a regular public school or one of the small number of specially designated Sami schools in each country. Upon completion of compulsory school, Sami students in northern Sweden and Finland may attend special Sami residential schools located in both Jokkmokk, Sweden, and Inari, Finland; or alternatively, enrol in a regular gymnasium (that is, upper-secondary) school. The residential school in Jokkmokk, for example, offers four accredited lines of study in Sami handicrafts, reindeer management, environmental science, and general studies (with a focus on one of computer science environmental science or Samisk language). Upon completion of compulsory school in Norway, the Sami students of Finnmark have the option of attending either a regular gymnasium in Karasjok which specializes in the teaching of Samisk language, or a vocational school in Kautokeino specializing in reindeer herding, construction and mechanics.

Higher education in the Nordic countries is also organized on a comprehensive basis, and, like health care, the organization of higher education services in the Nordkalotten region is largely integrated with that of each country's national system. For instance, there is a national university situated either within or in rather close proximity to each of the northern regions which comprise Nordkalotten; that is, the University of Tromsø (Norway), and the universities of Umeå (Sweden) and Oulu (Finland). Each of these universities offer multi-disciplinary programmes in Sami studies in addition to a broad range of course offerings in the natural and social sciences, humanities, business and education. Furthermore, each of these northern universities support full medical schools complete with teaching hospitals. In addition to university institutions there are a number of university colleges and vocational training facilities throughout Nordkalotten. Of particular utility to the Sami in this regard are the specialized Sami teacher-training programmes in Kautokeino and Bodø (Norway), Luleå (Sweden) and Rovaniemi (Finland), and the National College of Reindeer Herding also located in Kautokeino. In recent years there has been a marked improvement in further training opportunities in Sami arts and crafts as reflected, in part, by the availability of such programmes at Alta College (Norway), the Nordic Sami Institute in Kautokeino and the Sami residential school in Jokkmokk (Nordic Sami Institute, 1990).

All education services in the three Nordic countries are free of charge to citizens and permanent residents. For the most part, education expenditures are financed through central government general tax revenues, and to a lesser extent by the municipalities and counties through local taxation. Sami compulsory schools in Sweden are financed solely by the state through the auspices of the Sami Education Council. Education expenditure in all three countries has increased considerably in recent decades and, during the 1980s, represented either the second or third largest social welfare programme expenditure in each country (Olsson, 1990; Kuhnle, 1986; Alestalo and Uusitalo, 1986). Furthermore, it is the central governments that establish national education policy which local education councils and municipal authorities are required to follow, including that concerning prescribed curricula guidelines. Higher education services are fully administered and financed by the central governments.

Health care

In all three Nordic countries central government is responsible for ensuring the adequacy of universal health-care services. The provision of most medical services, however, is the responsibility of local government; particularly as regards hospital care, long-term institutional care for the elderly and invalid, psychiatric care and community public-health services. County councils provide health and dental services to all residents within their boundaries, and services are generally free of charge although Swedish health services have a small user fee in force. The largest share of health-service costs are financed through local taxation.

Today, life expectancy at birth in the Nordic countries is amongst the highest in the world, while the infant mortality rate ranks amongst the world's lowest (Duffy, 1989). Such indicators represent but two of numerous other favourable health outcomes common to health status in the Nordic countries, and are attributable in part both to the high standards of living – amongst the highest in the world – and the manner in which health-care services are organized. As regards the organization of health-care services relative to the Sami, the three countries have each followed the practice of largely integrating their northern health-care delivery systems with that of the respective national system. An example of this integration with respect to the northern regions of each of the three Nordic countries was the establishment of medical schools complete with teaching hospitals. Furthermore, the high level of northern service integration with that of the Nordic states' national health-care systems stands in marked contrast to that of other nations with indigenous populations (for example, Canada and the United States), which have established separate health-care delivery systems for their indigenous peoples (cf. Weller, 1989). The integration of services for the whole northern population in each of the three Nordic countries reduces the tendency of service overlap and other administrative problems.

Housing

Central government has, since the Second World War, controlled housing finance in all three Nordic countries, and has thus been able actively to influence the pricing and distribution of the housing stock, thereby minimizing the role of the private market. Moreover, Nordic housing policy is directed at housing production both with respect to types of construction and, above all, maximizing volume. However, while Norway sought to ensure distributive equity between various owners and renters through a combination of rent allowances and guaranteed low-interest public loans, Swedish and Finnish housing policy has favoured private home-ownership through generous tax deductions; the effect of which has been that Norway has developed the most equitable housing policy with respect to distribution.

Housing policy in the three Nordic countries has also been directed towards the benefit of the Sami. During the 1960s and 1970s, considerable effort was made to increase the volume of permanent housing and thereby to alleviate what had been a problem of overcrowding among some Sami households (Aarseth and Björklund, 1987; Ruong, 1967). Immediately following the Second World War, the Finnish government faced up to the major task of resettling and providing adequate housing to several hundred Skolt Sami who migrated to Finland's northern Lake Inari region from the Kola peninsula which Finland was compelled to cede to the Soviet Union at the close of the war. However, unlike the housing conditions faced by other Sami peoples in the Nordic countries, the Skolt Sami have experienced problems of overcrowding and housing of an inferior construction quality (Ingold, 1976). The Skolt Sami are not alone in their experience of overcrowding, because overcrowding due to housing shortages in Finland is estimated to be almost four times greater than that of the average of the other Nordic countries (Esping-Andersen and Korpi, 1987).

Public support of housing supply and distribution in all three Nordic countries is organized and administered by central government, and is financed through general taxation and other means, including tax credits and tax deductions. Municipalities are principally involved in the administration and distribution of rental allowances to residents on fixed or low incomes, and must adhere to eligibility guidelines set by central government. Municipalities are also involved in the supply side of the housing market through their general land use planning mandate.

Adequacy of Nordic welfare-state development relative to the Sami

All three Nordic countries have developed during this century into nations amongst those enjoying the world's highest standard of living. In the process, they have become highly developed institutional welfare states, particularly with respect to the development of social programmes, universal coverage and income security. Poverty in the absolute sense has been erased through economic growth and welfare-state initiatives in relation to regional development and full employment.

Nordic welfare-state development has, however, been dogged by the question of adequacy in light of the advent of fundamental welfare reforms during the post-Second World War period. In general terms, this question concerns both the level and equitable distribution of benefits, and, as regards the Sami in particular, it concerns the realization of pan-Sami society's collective right to cultural autonomy and the kinds of goods and services that constitute elements of this collective right.

Adequacy of social security

With respect to the adequacy of social security, income maintenance in all three Nordic countries is generally of a compulsory nature and based on the twin principles of insurance against income loss and benefits in accordance to earned income. Furthermore, social security has been augmented by extensive public commitments to a wide range of welfare services in fields of education, health care, housing and other sectors. Unfortunately, it is only possible to advance some general remarks as to the adequacy of social security in relation to the Sami's social welfare needs. First, the system of income maintenance in all three Nordic countries is commonly marked by exceptionally liberal conditions of eligibility, universality of coverage in the main, and a method of financing based, by and large, on public and employer-mandated contributions intended to uphold principles of redistribution and social solidarity. In addition, the marginal significance of means-tested social assistance (relative to the importance of other income maintenance schemes) is indicative of both the systems' comprehensiveness and the extent to which citizenship rights have been institutionalized as regards income maintenance benefits (Olsson, 1990).

Second, although earnings-related income security schemes in all three Nordic countries are often lauded for their relatively high benefit levels and universality of coverage (cf. Palme, 1990), they also pose a contradiction to the guiding principle of redistributive equality, as benefits tend to reflect and enshrine existing distributional inequalities. And although distributional inequalities have been addressed to a greater or lesser extent within the income-replacement schemes through the application of an array of income-tested supplementary benefits intended to improve the financial security of low-income groups, the adequacy of such provisions (undermined by the effects of changing public-welfare commitments and reforms to tax policy) remains open to question. Indeed, criticism of the Nordic welfare states' income security system has focused, on the one hand, upon its distributional inequalities, and, on the other, upon conditions of increasing poverty and a tendency towards polarization among societal groups; that is, between those who have, and those who do not have sufficient economic means and who must endure increasing economic hardship (Marklund, 1988).

Numerous qualitative assessments indicate that, in light of the Sami's limited employment prospects and the underdeveloped nature of Sami-district economies, the Sami peoples are one such group afflicted both by distributional inequalities and increasing poverty (Aarseth and Björklund, 1987; Burger, 1987; Beach and Nobel, 1981; Siuruainen and Aikio, 1977; Ingold, 1976). These conditions, when combined with Sami out-migration and the centralization of services in a small number of main centres in the north, represent a serious threat to the well-being of pan-Sami society. Unfortunately, it is difficult to comment further on the nature of social conditions affecting pan-Sami society, and the adequacy of welfare in responding to such conditions, due to lack of empirical data presently available as governments simply do not collect it; not least perhaps because public authorities in the Nordic countries find the ethnic nature of such data politically uncomfortable to manage.

Third, it has been argued that social inequality in Nordic society has not only an ethnic dimension to it, but also a spatial or regional dimension particularly with respect to the north (Weller, 1989; John, 1984; Kuhnle, 1980). These regional disparities are borne out, in part, by such social indicators as unemployment rates in the north of at least twice (and in some instances four times) that of the corresponding national rates, and northern mortality rates generally being the highest in each of the three Nordic countries. Moreover, the capacity of local government to address these and other social inequalities is rather limited due to the inadequate redistribution of national economic resources. Although public policy in each of the three Nordic countries ensures that all municipalities receive equal per capita financial allocations, it fails to achieve equality or equivalency in the provision of health and social services among municipalities because needs and resources are different in different parts of each country. Thus is the case particularly with respect to the northern regions.

In addition, there is the everyday likelihood not only that different municipalities have different needs, but also that those needs might be appraised and addressed differently in different communities. And while this particular dilemma may be interpreted as yet another inadequacy of public policy, it more precisely stems from the Nordic nations' long ideological tradition (as discussed above) of stressing the fundamental importance of local autonomy. Hence, it is not so much an inadequacy of welfare-state policy as it is a case of two competing ideological forces (namely, social equality versus local autonomy) rivalling each other for supremacy. At some point in time, when socially unacceptable levels of inequality prevail among various communities, the virtue of local autonomy is likely to give way to the acceptance of the need for central government intervention to assist in correcting social inequalities (Kuhnle, 1980); as would appear to be the case with respect to the provision of Sami housing and educational services.

Adequacy as regards Sami cultural autonomy

The adequacy of Nordic welfare-state development relative to the realization of the Sami's collective right to cultural autonomy is noticeably deficient. Each of the three welfare states have generally paralleled one another in their development having evolved from a largely common, and typically Scandinavian ideology. In addition to the longstanding tradition of local autonomy, this ideology has been framed upon the twin tenets of egalitarianism and social equality on the one hand, and that of individualism and a profound orientation towards the whole, on the other. These competing influences have represented fundamental obstacles to the development of Sami cultural autonomy, for they have each contributed to the limited perspective of Sami minority rights held by non-Sami, Scandinavian policy-makers and society at large. Of particular effect in this regard has been the dual Scandinavian expression of individualism and societal wholeness, leaving little space for the Sami to express or develop their own collective cultural interests. In essence, the Nordic welfare states have provided social security to Sami individuals with the intent of ensuring them a parallel standard of living to that of the Scandinavian majority while, simultaneously, tending to diminish both the importance and realization of the Sami's collective rights to protect their culture (Nobel, 1991; Beach and Nobel, 1990; Smith, 1987; Beach and Nobel, 1981).

The Nordic welfare states' limited perspective of Sami minority rights is further constrained, particularly with respect to the popular view in Swedish and Norwegian societies, by the notion that Samishness is synonymous with reindeer herding. This view dates back to the mid-nineteenth century and was instrumental in bringing about both the monopolization of reindeer herding by the nomadic segment of pan-Sami society, and the perpetuation of the majority's view of Samishness through its codification in law and public policy. The institutionalization of this stereotyped view of Samishness has created deep cleavages within pan-Sami society, leading to extensive intra-cultural conflict along both occupational and subcultural lines. Moreover, this stereotyped view has contributed to profound inter-cultural conflict as the Samish Movement campaigns simultaneously to advance the rights of the Sami not only as individuals but, more importantly, to further their collective rights as both reindeer pastoralists and a people (Nobel, 1991; Lasko, 1987).

With the advent of Sami Assembly in both Finland and Norway, however, there would appear to have been some recognition on the part of the respective states of the Sami's collective right to self-government. The issue now for the Finnish and Norwegian Sami appears to be that of the extent to which their self-governing powers are truly authoritative, and to what extent the institution of the Sami Assembly will permit them to exercise control over their own social, cultural and economic affairs. As for the case of Sweden, it has become clear that the present system for administering Sami affairs is grossly inadequate. The Office of the Ombudsman for Ethnic Discrimination is understaffed, under-resourced and thus unable to effectively fulfil its dual role as the custodian of Sami and immigrant legal interests (Nobel, 1991). Furthermore, the Swedish Sami Rights Commission submitted its comprehensive report on Sami rights and self-government to central government in 1989, calling for the implementation of a semi-autonomous Sami Assembly and a number of other legislative reforms, including the adoption of both a Sami Act and, more importantly, a constitutional amendment recognizing the Sami's collective existence within Swedish society. However, these and other recommendations have yet to be endorsed by the government; a state of affairs causing much alarm and frustration amongst Swedish Sami political leaders (Åhrén, 1991; Nordling, 1991).

SUMMARY AND CONCLUSION

This chapter has attempted to introduce readers to the rather complex social relationship that exists between the Sami peoples and the Nordic welfare states. Moreover, it has attempted to highlight a number of salient contradictions between the provision of welfare within the framework of the citizenship rights perspective, and that of welfare intended as a means to support the minority rights of an indigenous people. Key to readers' understanding of this contradictory relationship is a basic appreciation of the Nordic welfare states' ideological underpinnings as presented in contrast to both the historical and cultural basis upon which the Sami's drive for cultural autonomy is built. All three Nordic countries were shown to have evolved into highly advanced welfare states, and as having fashioned an approach to welfare unique to all advanced capitalist countries in the extent to which it has become both comprehensive and institutional in effect.

Yet with respect to welfare intended as a means to support the cultural interests of an indigenous people, the experience of all three Nordic welfare states was shown to have been just the opposite. Indeed, the general approach of the welfare state has been to promote the Sami's rights as individuals by simply upholding their existing occupational and welfare rights, thereby seeking to preserve Sami intra- and inter-cultural *status quo* relations. In contrast, the Sami of course are determined to secure their collective and cultural rights, and see the welfare-state approach to policy-making as rooted in the colonial past. In short, it represents the institutionalization of their subordinate status in Nordic society; an ethnic-based form of social control equating to institutional racism. Hence, as the chapter has attempted to show, the Sami as individuals might have benefited materially from this welfare relationship, but there should be no doubting that its principal by-product has been that of dividing and stripping the Sami peoples of their cultural identity.

By way of concluding, it would be appropriate to consider some of the future implications of this welfare relationship to the Samish Movement's goal of cultural autonomy. Indeed, of the three Nordic welfare states, only Norway has recognized the Sami's right to exist as a distinct minority population. Norway amended its constitution in 1988 to include special mention of the Sami, recognizing the need to preserve and develop their language, culture and way of life (Nordic Sami Institute, 1990). However, although the amendment defines an administrative role for the Sami through the enactment of the Sami

Act 1987, it fails to codify the Sami's collective and cultural rights in the process.

Norway would appear to be taking other steps to strengthen the Sami's position in Norwegian society through its recent adoption of Samisk language legislation intended to put Samisk on an equal footing with Norwegian (that is, mainly within a specifically defined administrative district), and its recent signing and formal commitment to the International Labour Organization's Indigenous and Tribal Peoples Convention 1989 concerning international standards for the treatment of indigenous peoples. And while Finland appears poised and about ready to follow Norway's lead with respect to constitutional recognition, language rights and acceptance of international standards (Finland, 1991), Sweden appears to be lagging behind on all counts and has officially declined to commit itself to the ILO convention (Sweden, 1991). Furthermore, while Norway and Finland have taken concrete action to streamline the administration of Sami affairs, Sweden's policy-making process continues to be bogged down by the sum of inaction and occasional piecemeal initiatives that regularly feature objectives conflicting against one another (Nobel, 1991). Hence, in light of these recent policy developments, it seems that Sweden – once the unequivocal standard-setter of Sami affairs – has become the proverbial spoilsport of an otherwise progressive trend towards the realization of Sami cultural autonomy amongst the Nordic states. Indeed, this assessment has been advanced by Sami leaders of late (*Dagens Nyheter*, 1991).

The evolvement of progressive Sami policy represents only one side of the Sami's quest for self-determination, albeit a very critical one. On the other side there is the matter of Sami intra-cultural relations. In this regard, the key to the long-term interests and success of the Samish Movement in its campaign for cultural autonomy is its capacity to organize and enhance Samish cultural identity such that all Sami peoples can embrace it. This will necessarily involve the effective promotion of a range of cultural emblems in addition to that of reindeer husbandry which, to many of the Sami, represents the cultural and economic lifeline of pan-Sami society. There are many other Sami, however, who tend not to attach as much importance to reindeer pastoralism as a cultural symbol, and who view the reindeer itself as being a more prominent emblem of Samish culture than that of reindeer pastoralism. Yet the prominence of reindeer husbandry interests within the Samish Movement sometimes tends to preclude its fullest consideration of other social, cultural and educational concerns. This has led some within the Movement to call for the separation of reindeer husbandry issues from that of Samish cultural concerns in general.

A final consideration with respect to the future of the Sami–Nordic welfare-state relationship is that of the nature of popular public opinion; after all, public opinion is likely to play an important role in signifying changes in the current state of affairs of Nordic social policy relative to the Sami. With this in mind, the Samish Movement has always committed itself to maintaining an active public profile. However, in the absence of a major social, political or environmental issue to galvanize public opinion, the Sami's relatively small, dispersed and mainly northern population base poses a significant dilemma to maintaining a high public profile on a continual basis. Issues of importance to the Sami are rarely featured in the Nordic nations' southern-concentrated media, and the Sami generally perceive Scandinavia's southern-concentrated population to be largely ignorant of or, at best, indifferent towards Sami cultural interests.

Hence, the outcome of a randomly conducted survey of nearly 1,000 Swedes, initiated by the Nordic Sami Council in 1990, came as a pleasant surprise to Sami leaders. The result of this survey indicates that there is strong public support, particularly among southerners, for the advancement of Sami cultural and collective interests, and that there appears to be much less opposition towards the realization of Sami rights among northern Swedes than Sami leaders had previously suspected (*Dagens Nyheter*, 6 October 1990). These survey results, although representing a favourable appraisal of the Sami's position with respect to Swedish public opinion, raise many unanswered questions. Chief among them is whether or not such findings could be replicated in Norway and Finland, and, moreover, whether the Sami can translate their apparent public support into effective gains in the political and policy-making arena.

ENDNOTE

Parts of this chapter grew out of observations and interviews conducted by Dave Lewis in various locations throughout northern Scandinavia in 1983–84, and most recently, in 1991 as part of his ongoing research at the International Graduate School, Stockholm University, Sweden. The authors wish to thank the Letterstedf Foundation, which provided a grant for this research.

REFERENCES

Aarseth, B. and Björklund, I. (1987) *The Sami People*, Tromsø: Tromsø Museum/University of Tromsø.

Åhrén, I. (1991) Chairperson, Swedish Sami National Federation, Personal communication, Stockholm.

Aikio, M. (1987) 'The Finnish perspective: Language and Ethnicity', in A. Pletsch, (ed.) *Ethnicity in Canada: International Examples and Perspectives*, Marburg/Lahn.

Aikio, P. (1987) 'Experiences Drawn from the Finnish Sami Parliament', in *Self Determination and Indigenous Peoples*, Copenhagen: International Work Group for Indigenous Affairs (IWGIA), Document No. 58.

Alestalo, M. and Uusitalo, H. (1986) 'Finland', in P. Flora, (ed.) *Growth to Limits: The Western European Welfare States since World War II*, vol. 1, Berlin and New York: Aldine de Gruyter.

Anderson, B. (1983) *Imagined Communities*, London: Verso.

Aubert, W. (1970) 'En nationell eller social minoritet', in A. Küng (ed.) *Samemakt! Valfard till dods eller kulturellt folkmord?* Stockholm: Raben & Sjogren.

Baer, L. A. (1982) 'The Sami – An Indigenous People in Their Own Land', in B. Jahreskog (ed.), *The Sami National Minority in Sweden*, Stockholm: For the Legal Rights Foundation by Almqvist & Wiksell International.

Beach, H. and Nobel, P. (1981) *Reindeer Herd Management in Transition*, Uppsala Studies in Cultural Anthropology, Stockholm: Almqvist & Wiksell International.

—— (1990) 'Sverige behover en ny samepolitik', *Nordens Tidning*, no. 2: 6–9.

Björklund, I. (1982) 'What About the Coastal Samis?' in B. Wahl, (ed.) *The Sami People and Human Rights*, Oslo: Charta 79.

Brox, O. (1966) *Hva skjer i Nord-Norge. En studie i norsk utkantpolitikk*, Oslo: Pax.

Burger, J. (1987) *Report from the Frontier*, London: Zed Books.

Dagens Nyheter (1990) Samerna har starkt stod', 6 October, A-8.

—— (1991) 'Samepolitiken kritiseras hart', 13 June, A-19.

Dahlström, E. (1967) 'Samerna i det svenska samhallet', *Sociologisk Forskning* 4.

—— (1970) 'Samerna och den svenska kolonialismen', in A. Küng (ed.) *Samemakt! Valfard till dods eller kulturellt folkmord?* Stockholm: Raben & Sjogren.

—— (1974a) 'The Lappish Minority in Sweden', *International Journal of Sociology* (fall/winter, 1973–74): 110–46.

—— (1974b) 'Den samiska minoriteten i Sverige', in L. Svonni, L. (ed.) *Samerna – ett folk i fyra lander*, Stockholm: Prisma, pp. 102–40.

Duffy, D. (1989) 'The effects of Sweden's corporatist structure on health policy and outcomes', *Scandinavian Studies*, 61 (2–3): 128–45.

Eidheim, H. (1977) *Aspects of the Lappish Minority Situation*, Oslo: Universitetsforlaget.

—— (1985) 'Indigenous Peoples and the State', in F. Brøsted *et al.* (eds) *Native Power*, Oslo: Universitetsforlaget.

Enoksen, R. (1982) 'Dividing up Samiland', in *The Sami People and Human*

Rights, in B. Wahl, (ed.) *The Sami People and Human Rights*, Oslo: Charta 79, pp. 12–16.

Esping-Andersen, G. and Korpi, W. (1987) 'From Poor Relief to Institutional Welfare States: The Development of Scandinavian Social Policy', in R. Erikson, *et al.* (eds) *The Scandinavian Model: Welfare States and Welfare Research*, London: M. E. Sharpe.

Finland Ministry of Justice (1991) *Draft Universal Declaration on the Rights of the Indigenous Peoples*, Helsinki: Ministry of Justice.

Flora, P. (ed.) (1986) *Growth to Limits: The Western European Welfare States since World War II*, vol. 1, Berlin and New York: Aldine de Gruyter.

Ginsburg, N. (1991) 'The Wonderful World(s) of Welfare Capitalism', *Critical Social Policy*, 11 (1).

Graubard, S. (ed.) (1986) *Norden – the Passion for Equality*, Oslo: Norwegian University Press.

Gustafsson, A. (1988) *Local Government in Sweden*, Stockholm: The Swedish Institute.

Heckscher, G. (1984) *The Welfare State and Beyond: Success and Problems in Scandinavia*, Minneapolis: University of Minnesota Press.

Idevuoma, P. (1970) 'Om statens formynderi over samerna', in A. Küng (ed.) *Samemakt! Valfard till dods eller kulturellt folkmord?* Stockholm: Raben & Sjogren.

Ingold, T. (1976) *The Skolt Lapps Today*, Cambridge: Cambridge University Press.

John, B. (1984) *Scandinavia: A New Geography*, London: Longman.

Kaddik, A. (1989) *Samediakonen berattar*, Umeå: Svenska Missionssallskapet Kyrkan och Samerna.

Kangas, O. and Palme, J. (1989) *Public and Private Pensions: The Scandinavian Countries in a Comparative Perspective*, Stockholm: Swedish Institute for Social Research, Occasional Papers, No. 3.

Keskitalo, A. I. (1981) 'The Sami People in Finland, Norway and Sweden', in A. Pietila, A. (ed.) *Education of the Samis in Finland*, Helsinki: Finnish National Board of General Education.

Korpi, W. (1983) *The Democratic Class Struggle*, London: Routledge & Kegan Paul.

Kuhnle, S. (1980) 'National Equality and Local Decision Making: Values in Conflict in the Development of the Norwegian Welfare State', *Acta Sociologica*, 23 (2–3): 97–111.

——— (1986) 'Norway', in P. Flora, (ed.), *Growth to Limits: The Western European Welfare States since World War II*, vol. 1, Berlin and New York: Aldine de Gruyter, pp. 117–96.

Küng, A. (ed.) (1970) *Samemakt! Valfard till dods eller kulturellt folkmord?* Stockholm: Raben & Sjogren.

Lapping, M. B. (1986) 'Between Swede and Saami: The Reindeer Herd Rationalization Law', *Scandinavian-Canadian Studies*, 2: 129–35.

Lasko, L. N. (1987) 'The Importance of Indigenous Influence on the System of Decision-Making in the Nation-State', in *Self Determination and Indigenous Peoples*, Copenhagen: International Work Group for Indigenous Affairs (IWGIA), Document No. 58, pp. 73–84.

Lundmark, L. (1982) *Uppbord, utarmning*, Lund: Utveckling, Arkiv.

184   Social Welfare with Indigenous Peoples

Marklund, S. (1988) *Paradise Lost? The Nordic Welfare States and the Recession 1975–1985*, Lund: Arkiv.

Ministry of Finance (1991) *The Swedish Budget*, Stockholm: Ministry of Finance.

Mishra, R. (1977) *Society and Social Policy*, London: Macmillan.

Nesheim, A. (1977) *Introducing the Lapps*, Oslo: Tanum-Norli/Norsk Folkemueseum.

Nobel, P. (1991) *Ombudsman, Office of the Ombudsman against Ethnic Discrimination*, Stockholm: Personal communication (March).

Nordic Council of Ministers (1988) *Cooperation Program for the Health and Social Affairs Sector*, Copenhagen: Nordic Council of Ministers.

—— (1990) *Yearbook of Nordic Statistics 1989/90*, Copenhagen: Nordic Council of Ministers.

Nordic Sami Council (1986) *The Sami Political Program*, adopted by the 13th Nordic Sami Conference, Finland: Utsjoki.

Nordic Sami Institute (1990) *The Sami People*, Norway: Kautokeino.

Nordling, S. (1991) Chairperson, Sami-Atnam, Stockholm: Personal communication.

Office of the Ombudsman against Ethnic Discrimination (1990) *De fyra forsta aren – en redovisning* (cf. Samefragan), Stockholm: Office of the Ombudsman against Ethnic Discrimination.

Olsson, S. (1986) 'Sweden', in P. Flora (ed.), *Growth to Limits: The Western European Welfare States since World War II*, vol. 1, Berlin and New York: Aldine de Gruyter, pp. 1–116.

—— (1989) 'Sweden', in J. Dixon and R. Scheurell (eds) *Social Welfare in Developed Market Countries*, London and New York: Routledge.

—— (1990) *Social Policy and Welfare State in Sweden*, Lund: Arkiv.

Ornstedt, B. (1991) Administrator, Ministry of Agriculture (Reindeer Affairs), Stockholm: Personal communication (March).

Otnes, P. (1970) *Den samiske nasjon*, Oslo: Pax.

Paine, R. (1957) *Coast Lapp Society I*, Oslo: Universitetsforlaget.

—— (1965) *Coast Lapp Society II: A Study of Economic Development and Social Values*, Oslo: Universitetsforlaget.

—— (1984) *Dam a River. Dam a People? Sami Livelihood and the Alta/Kautokeino Hydroelectric Project and the Norwegian Parliament*, Copenhagen: International Work Group for Indigenous Affairs (IWGIA), Document No. 45.

Palme, F. (1990) *Pension Rights in Welfare Capitalism*, Stockholm: Swedish Institute for Social Research (14), Akademitryck.

Ruong, I. (1967) *The Lapps in Sweden*, Stockholm: The Swedish Institute.

Siuruainen, E. and Aikio, P. (1977) *The Lapps in Finland*, Helsinki: Society for the Promotion of Lapp Culture, No. 39.

Sjölin, R. (1982) 'The Sami in Swedish Politics', in B. Jahreskog (ed.) *The Sami National Minority in Sweden*, Stockholm: For the Legal Rights Foundation by Almqvist & Wiksell International, pp. 77–88.

Smith, C. (1987) *The Sami Rights Committee: an Exposition*, in P. Aikio, 'Experiences Drawn from the Finnish Sami Parliament' in *Self Determination and Indigenous Peoples*, Copenhagen: International Work Group for Indigenous Affairs (IWGIA), Document No. 58, pp. 15–55.

Stenholm, B. (1984) *The Swedish School System*, Stockholm: The Swedish Institute.

Stevens, R. (1989) 'Cultural Values and Norwegian Health Services: Dominant Themes and Recurring Dilemmas', in *Scandinavian Studies*, 61 (2–3): 199–212.

Stordahl, V. (1987) 'Sameting and Sami Committees: A Useful Political and Administrative Solution for the Sami in Norway?' in *Self Determination and Indigenous Peoples*, Copenhagen: International Work Group for Indigenous Affairs (IWGIA), Document No. 58, pp. 57–70.

Svensson, T. G. (1976) *Ethnicity and Mobility in Sami Politics*, Stockholm: Deptartment of Social Anthropology, Stockholm University.

Svonni, L. (ed.) (1974) *Samerna – ett folk i fyra lander*, Stockholm: Prisma.

Sweden, Department of Labour (1991) *Skrivelse om ILO's konvention om ursprungsfolk och stamfolk i sjalvstandiga lander*, Stockholm: Department of Labour.

Swedish-Sami National Federation (1987), *Samer*, SSR, Umeå: Swedish-Sami National Federation.

Swedish Sami Rights Commission (1986) *Samernas folkrättsliga stallning*, SOU 1986: 36, Stockholm: Ministry of Justice, Allmänna Förlaget.

—— (1989) *Samerätt och Sameting*, SOU 1989: 4, Stockholm: Ministry of Justice, Allmänaa Förlaget.

—— (1990) *Samerätt och Samiskt språk*, SOU 1990: 91, Stockholm: Ministry of Justice, Allmänna Förlaget.

Therborn, G. (1986) 'The Working Class and the Welfare State', in P. Kettunen (ed.) *Det nordiska i den nordiska arbetarrorelsen*, Helsinki: Finnish Society for Labour History.

Weller, G. (1989) 'Health Care in the Northern Hinterlands: Canada, Scandinavia and the United States', *Scandinavian Studies*, 61 (2–3): 213–30.

6 The Gypsies and the social services in Spain

Carmen Carriga

The Gypsies as a population group have been poorly studied and little is known about them in depth. This general disregard contrasts with the extreme and rebuking nature with which people talk about them and the use of stereotypes which are widely employed. The 'Gadjes' (a Gypsy expression to describe the persons not belonging to their ethnic group) have a conditioned image of the Gypsies, based upon topics which demonstrate a great lack of knowledge of Gypsy culture. The same phenomenon can be observed amongst the Gypsies respecting the Gadjes. The prejudices are reciprocal, as we shall see.

This lack of knowledge is evident when one considers the lack of historical written sources about the Gypsies' background, which otherwise might have given us some knowledge of their life, as it was led and interpreted by them. The oral traditions of the Gypsies, on the other hand, do not add to this lack of knowledge. The Gypsy culture, as with many other popular ways of life within the Gadje world, has never been a 'learned' culture.

The paradox is presented when, having lived and shared their lives for many years, one realizes that little is known about them as a whole and that you may only know the particular community with whom you have lived. It is very difficult to generalize, due to the diversity of the existing Gypsy groups.

A history and description of the culture of the Gypsies is presented from the information and analysis which is thought to be most relevant and which might allow us to know life inside the Gypsy community a little better, without extrapolations conditioned by ethnocentrism and from an understandable and respectful attitude towards the multi-cultural forms that characterize our society. I make extensive use of the ethnographic work of Teresa San Roman.

I present afterwards Spanish laws regarding social services and also the way in which they treat the subject of the ethnic minorities, and especially the Gypsy minority are described. An evaluation is made of some of the procedures and their adequacy that characterize the social intervention programmes which are being implemented in Spain with reference to the Gypsies.

THE HISTORY AND CULTURE OF THE GYPSIES

Spanish Gypsies are different from those in many other countries, and there are very few myths about their origins. In other countries, like France and England, there are many legends describing the origin of the Gypsies, explaining in one way or another how they fled from their lost land and the ways in which they started to disperse throughout the world. In general, they located their point of departure in Egypt (a name which does not refer to the country by the Nile, but to 'Gypte', a Gypsy neighbourhood in Modon, Peloponnese), but this depends on their knowledge and the Gypsy group they belong to. In other stories, one may hear about their coming from Hungary and India.

The most common hypothesis, shared by the majority of contemporary authorities, is that which is related to their linguistic origin. Their language, Romany or Romano, has been the base from which to start the search of their remote past. Their language is Neoaric, of the sort which is found in the northeast of India. From linguistic evidence, it is supposed that they left that country around AD 1000. They followed two routes, one, through Central Europe, and the other through Western Europe, after having passed through North Africa.

In Spain, after crossing the Pyrenees, they appeared at the beginning of the fifteenth century, and were mentioned in several documents, which indicate their penetration in small groups, captained by 'dukes' or 'lords'.

The history of the Gypsies in Spain can be divided into three periods. The first period is the fifteenth century, and covers their entry into Spain. Their arrival was well prepared, and they often brought letters of introduction from European royalty and the ecclesiastical hierarchy with them, who presented them as Christian pilgrims, penitents on their way to Santiago de Compostela. Claiming their privileges as pilgrims, they obtained favours which facilitated their entrance to and settlement in Spain.

The second period, called the 'persecution period', starts at the beginning of the sixteenth century and lasts up to the 1780s. Having abused their privileges and refused to adopt a sedentary life, this period is characterized by abundant documented legislation, the purpose of which was either to integrate the Gypsies into the common life of the country, or to ensure their complete disappearance. This dilemma is mentioned in the first Pragmatic Law of Medina del Campo signed by the Catholic Monarchs in 1499.

The third period extends from the end of the eighteenth century (the Pragmatic Law of Charles III, in 1783) until the present day. Specific legislation regarding Gypsies disappears after they obtained the same obligations and rights as other Spaniards. Their massive sedentarization started, which has been accelerating in pace since the beginning of the twentieth century. The period, however, is characterized by the discrepancy between the recognition of the Gypsy as a Spanish citizen under the law and the prejudice which, in fact, continues to operate. The reality of today does not meet the objectives of the official statement of the Pragmatic Law of Charles III in 1783, namely that Gadjes can drop their prejudices against the Gypsies, and the Gypsies can abandon theirs against the Gadjes. These are prejudices that, in general, remain amongst the authorities themselves, on whom a fundamental part of the process of acceptance of the Gypsies on terms of equality to other Spaniards depends.

We do not have statistical information which can reliably tell us of the number and distribution of Gypsies – neither in the world, nor in Europe, nor in Spain. Gypsies around the world, who appear in the bibliography about this subject, number about 1 to 9 million persons, and those of Spain about 200,000 to 400,000. It is worth mentioning that the census of this population has not been well conducted. It has only been carried out arbitrarily, or only in small communities. The task is no doubt one of extreme difficulty, if we bear in mind that Gypsies are very unstable in relation with their place of residence, and that individuals may conceal their Gypsy origins, in order to avoid problems.

The classification of the Gypsies into different types has been accomplished based upon a linguistic perspective. There are many authors who have dedicated their work to this subject. However, for the present purpose we shall classify the Gypsies by their own criteria. In Spain, there are fundamentally two types of Gypsies, each clearly differentiated: the Hungarian Gypsy, being the minority; and Gitanos. In this chapter we shall focus on the latter. (In fact 'Gitano' is the Spanish word for 'Gypsy', and only Gypsies themselves internally distinguish between the two types.)

The Gypsies are subdivided into Betics, Castilians, Catalans,

Basques, Extremadurans and Portuguese. Although these names may refer to the place of origin of the different groups, their distribution does not exactly correspond with the geographical area indicated by them. Both types, Hungarians and Gypsies, have very marked differences in culture and while the Hungarians speak Romano, the Gypsies use a nearly disappeared dialect, Calo.

Calo is maintained in a very imperfect way, not only respecting its morphology or syntax, but also when relating to the conservation of the vocabulary. It is almost only used in situations where the Gypsy wants the Gadje to be ignorant about what is being said. Apart from the very limited vocabulary which is usually employed, they use the language of the country or area in which they live as the common vehicle of communication amongst themselves. However, the Hungarians, or at least some of them, basically speak Romano, using the language of the country or region where they stay only as a means to communicate with the Gadjes.

Between the Gypsies and Gadjes there is mutual suspicion. No doubt this feeling is ambivalent, and while Gadjes despise Gypsies, at the same time they fear them, think that they are ignorant, and consider them to be able to cheat them if they want to. The Gypsy, on the other hand, admires certain qualities of the Gadje, such as how to speak, write and read well and being able to live in certain peace, as well as for their potential to gain fortune and power. But the Gadje is despised in moral matters, such as not wishing to have any children, being selfish with their family, sending their children to a boarding school and their old people to a home for the elderly, and so forth, and essentially for being less clever than the Gypsies, who are able to cheat them. Both stereotypes are very rigid and it is difficult for each group to rid themselves of the stereotypes 'imposed' by others.

Gypsies of the different types, such as those of the great Hungarian groups and the Gypsies themselves, recognize that they are different. Sometimes members of a given type consider that those from the other group are not Gypsies at all, while on other occasions they state that the other type are 'the true Gypsies'. On the other hand, certain differences between Catalan or Castilian Gypsies, and so on, result in some of these subtypes only having relations within themselves (Castilian and Extremadurans, Catalan and Betic). These differences indicate that some of these subtypes are incompatible and in this case very often a total ostracism of the other group takes place, or even denial that the others are Gypsies at all. In addition, class differences permeate the different levels, nearly as much as the differences between the types of Gypsies.

Kinship groups form a great part of the organization patterns for the social structure of these Gypsies. Individual relationships are marked by the relationships between the family groups.

The Gypsies are firmly organized in patrilineal groups over four or five generations. These lineages as corporate units are totally independent from one another. Several lineages might have a positive relationship, due to neighbourhood or marriage relationships. The lineages might also break off social relationships and become enemies even in subsequent generations.

Family lineages are dispersed, and the localized lineage sector in a certain geographical area is the basic unit for co-operation, while the total lineage gathers to defend themselves, celebrate weddings or the birth of a new member or the death of another. Usually they stay dispersed in extended families. In such a group the Gypsy finds his home, his everyday relationship, his help and daily co-operation, although a Gypsy might belong to a specific lineage, that of his mother, for defence, protection and co-operation.

Gypsies marry young. Though the wishes of the young person are taken into consideration, the parents are responsible for seeking a mate for their child. For this reason, the capacity of a man to earn a living for his family is appreciated, also his capacity to defend the family and it is regarded as important that he is not a habitual consumer of alcohol or drugs and is not a gambler. In a woman, what counts most is that she is a virgin until marriage, her fidelity to her husband, her ability to take care of children, her ability to look after the family on her own when necessary and her tidiness and efficiency in housework. Gypsy marriage is monogamous. Intralineal endogamy is often practised, as well as endogamy with the association of two or three lineages.

The marriage is regarded as unique, with only one ritual, which deals with the woman's virginity and its delivery from her family to her husband's family. However, there are other forms of marriage which, though not officially recognized, are generally consented to as second marriages due to widowhood, divorce or desertion by the husband.

Gypsies have their own traditional rules regarding law and morality. The law of the Gadjes is something Gypsies grudgingly accept, but only sometimes share. The most serious offences for the Gypsies are theft, fraud or swindling another Gypsy, passing information to Gadjes, abandonment of the family, insulting the dead and sexual abuse.

The exercise of authority among Gypsies is a function which comes from experience as well as knowledge. Thus, authority is usually upheld by older men, who individually receive the title of *tio* ('uncle'), when he is about 40 years old. The older man who is sane and has the needed physical strength is the one who is obeyed. The Gypsies clearly distinguish between respect and authority: the oldest man is respected, even if he does not belong to the same family, but only if he does is it possible for him to give orders and see them fulfilled. However, there are other forms of acquiring power such as health, support from the Gadjes, the numeric force of the lineage to which one belongs and the prestige earned resulting from personal behaviour.

Family matters are solved within one's lineage, according to their old people. The problems which might arise between two lineages are solved in three ways: first, peacefully, amongst the elders of the two lineages; second, by force, especially if it is a blood offence or one against the dead; third, through judges, who are old, respected men who know the Gypsy law, and who are often supported by a strong lineage, without any interest in any of the groups involved and accepted by both parties to act in the matter. The judgment is discharged according to the rules stipulated by Gypsy law, and these are traditional, never written. As a consequence, only in certain matters is there individual responsibility. On the contrary, the offence committed by a person is nearly always the responsibility of the family. The punishment does not fall upon one individual, but on his lineage. The individual juridical personality is very poor, and this limits his or her capacity to make an individual decision.

It is important to keep in mind that Gypsy law is frequently based on a principle of objective, not subjective, guilt; that is, the offence is sanctioned, not the intention. The main punishments are physical aggression, ostracism and expulsion from the territory.

Finally, it is important to mention that the dead play an extraordinarily important part in Gypsy life. Gypsies maintain with the dead the same relationship that they had when they were alive, and the dead are able to punish the serious offences of their descendants and dependants whom they might have punished in life. Therefore, some offences have supernatural punishments, such as illness, visions and possession.

One should remember that in great part we have presented cultural patterns to which individual behaviour has not always adapted. There are patterns to which behaviours correspond more or less suitably. Social change is breaking many of these models, but some new ones are emerging, valid for new situations. In other cases only emptiness is left, the loss of identity, which made a young Gypsy exclaim:

We are in a mess, all is changing and we do not write down a single word . . . – you know – everything is only said in words. We only know our traditions because our father was told by his father and so he told us. . . . It is difficult to repeat always the same things in the same way . . . nowadays it is very difficult to know what is a true Gypsy.

At present, in Spain the sedentarization of the Gypsy population is nearly complete. Its mobility, though, is still in general higher than that of the rest of the population. The existence of important Gypsy nuclei in several parts of the state is known. However, we have to face the problem of a deep ignorance related to the most elementary topics. We do not know their number, their location in rural and urban areas, general demographic aspects related to this population, conditions under which they live, their degree of acculturation and marginalization, or their level of use of and access to the general welfare services which are at the disposal of the whole population.

Beginning in the eighteenth century, the great majority of the Gypsy population settled progressively in towns until a massive sedentarization was produced in the surroundings of the industrial cities at the beginning of the twentieth century. This process came to an end almost at the conclusion of the Spanish Civil War. From then, a process of gradual disappearance of the traditional wandering Gypsy work has taken place: cattle raising, the distribution of manufactured objects in remote rural areas; and the sale of iron, copper, brass and basket handicrafts. These activities declined until their almost total extinction, with the industrialization of the countryside, better communications and commercial expansion. The Gypsies (as many other non-Gypsies) live in the larger cities, where they set up marginal activities for the economic and labour system of the society in which they live: scrap dealing, itinerant sales, and the selling and buying of used objects, and so on. The growth of the cities propels them towards the suburbs, away from the centre of the city. During the 1960s, the consequences of economic growth finally reached (relatively) the Gypsy population, who started to work on many tasks considered formerly to belong to the Gadje. They started to enter the labour system and initiated an unusual movement towards acculturation and social integration. Many have learned to write and read, to send their children to schools and to install water and electricity in their huts. They demand pavements, they visit the doctor, they list themselves in the Civil Register and above all, they start a strong and steady fight to obtain housing at the same time as they regulate their juridical situation.

This tendency is frustrated by the impact of the economic crisis and consequent unemployment, so that there exist now, and will exist henceforth social expectations and needs which now are much more difficult to attain. This is the critical point at which Spain and the Gypsies now find themselves. Spain has reached a point where a change is needed in order to incorporate the rising expectations and needs of the Gypsies, or the situation might deteriorate if the necessary institutional supports are not found in a quick and intelligent way, in the short as well as the long term. In fact, at the present time we find greatly deteriorated situations amongst some Gypsy groups. Unfortunately, a considerable number of them are affected by delinquency, prostitution and drugs. New contradictory phenomena are emerging in traditional Gypsy culture. For some people, these are the only ways out from their restricted situations.

INTRODUCTION TO SOCIAL SERVICE LAWS AND THEIR TREATMENT OF THE GYPSY MINORITY

With the promulgation of the Spanish constitution in 1978, a lengthy stage of political dictatorship ended. From a centralized and uniform state, the constitution configured a state with social and democratic rights, which recognized Spain as a nation amongst nations and guaranteed 'the right to the autonomy of the nationalities and regions' which integrate 'the indissoluble unity of the Spanish Nation' (Article 2).

In this way, with the restoration of parliamentary democracy, the historic nationalities and the regions became 'autonomic communities', having access to different forms and degrees of self-government or administrative decentralization. Seventeen autonomous communities exist in Spain at the moment, with different degrees in the exercise of the transferred laws by the central government, in order to fulfil the respective Statutes of Autonomy. This explains why in Spain there exist sixteen different laws regarding the social services (one autonomous community has not yet promulgated any law on this subject, at the time of writing), that attend the situations and characteristics of each community and regulate the supplies and services that the different public entities designate to specific public sectors. The variety of considerations in these sixteen laws is determined by the ambiguousness of the constitutional text when trying to determine precisely what is meant by 'Social Services' and how these should be structured. In this way the constitutional text is minimalist and allows the legislative organs of each autonomous community a wide margin of initiative and creativity. As supposed, in spite of the existing differences, the main guidelines throughout are quite similar. In fact, the Law 7/1985 of 2 April regulated the 'Basis for the Local Regime' and in its Article 18, legislated the competence of the local councils respecting Social Services. In 1987, a plan for 'Public Administration's Basic Help by Social Services' was passed, as a result of the agreement reached between the autonomous communities and the central administration and as an expression of the coherence of the different laws within the Social Services.

In Spain the Social Services are understood, and specified in some of its laws, as the sort of help designated to the realization of genuine and effective equality amongst the citizens and groups inside the society and their participation in the community. In the Spanish state, a public system has been instituted in the Social Services, directed towards guaranteeing access of all citizens to the help which contributes to the achievement of a better quality of life and social welfare.

The Social Services, thus, are the expression of a conception of Social policy understood as:

> the use of means that the public sector extracts from the private sector, in order to produce a series of goods and services of a collective utility, which would not be produced in the same range, nor distributed in a proper social way, if its supply were regulated by the mechanisms of the market.
>
> (Generalitat de Catalunya, 1984)

The Social Services are ruled by a series of general and specific principles, including:

- equality,
- solidarity,
- liberty,
- universality,
- responsibility of public power,
- normalization of services,
- globalization/personalization,
- participation,
- decentralization.

The naming and order of appearance of such principles varies, depending on each law. As a whole, the general order is reflected in those already mentioned.

According to the political majority power in the respective Parliaments of the autonomous communities, the introduction of these principles as the recognition and promotion of the social initiative can be observed (private initiative without any aim of profit). But sometimes the political majorities of the Parliaments consider private initiatives just as instruments, which it becomes necessary to co-ordinate firmly.

The ethnic minorities are looked upon as part of the Spanish Laws for Social Services and are considered as targeted sectors of performance for the public power. All the laws mention the principle of universality of the social resources and exclude any discrimination. Some laws specify that they will promote the social integration of ethnic minorities, conserving their values and specific ways of life, while others anticipate the creation of specialized Social Services for ethnic minorities, so that their specific problems can be dealt with, always taking into account their own identity. Others treat Gypsies specifically at different levels. We will look more closely at these.

The Andalusian Law 2/1988 of 4 April, regarding Social Services, Chapter III, 'Specialized Social Services', Article 11.5, mentions the Gypsy community as a sector which needs specific help and contemplates this as an ethnic minority 'with the goal of promoting performances that in a real and effective way may generate their social equality with regard to the rest of the Andalusian citizens, paying special attention to it, given the numeric and cultural importance of the Gypsy community'.

Before this, there already existed in this autonomous community an 'Office of Studies and Applications for the Gypsy Community', created on 7 October, 1985 by order of the Social welfare and Work Department (now the Health and Social Services Department). In this disposition the 'secular marginalization in which the Gypsy people find themselves, as well as their great number in Andalusia' was confirmed. By the same Order the government of Andalusia concluded 'the firm compromise to use all possible means, in order to achieve the removal of all obstacles which generate the present situation and to attain the life conditions for the Gypsy people equal to the rest of the Andalusian citizens, respecting and promoting their own cultural background'. Amongst others, this office was assigned to consult and assess, promotional grouping functions and to follow up the 'general and specific programmes directed towards the Gypsy community'.

The Community of Extremadura promulgated the Law of Social Services 5/1987, of 23 April. Article 14.1, concerning 'Specialized Social Service for Ethnic Minorities', states that:

giving all the citizens the same rights, having in mind historical and cultural differences, will be especially relevant to the Gypsy community and any other minority resident in Extremadura. The objective is to reach social equality, having in mind the right to receive education; to promote the consciousness amongst the minorities of the task which they can perform towards their own welfare and directed to lessen the differences amongst life resources compared with the rest of the population, as well as trying to eliminate discrimination in the working sector due to racial reasons.

The region of Murcia, through the Law of Social Service 8/1985, of 9 December, section VIII of the 'Social Service for Ethnic Minorities', Articles 47 to 50, directs specific attention 'to the Gypsy community and other ethnic minorities', with the objective of generating 'a real and effective equality' amongst the citizens and with the purpose of eliminating 'institutional or social discrimination' and favouring 'the integration of the Gypsy community and that of other ethnic minorities, recovering, respecting and spreading their cultural values'.

The Generalitat of Valencia, in the Law of Social Service 5/1989, of 6 July, established for that community under Title II, Article 4, 'preferent intervention' of 'the ethnic minorities', considering that they are 'lacking groups of citizens, who require a specific attention so that their access to the normalized system of the services is obtained'.

The Gypsies are not specifically mentioned in this law, but in 1985 by a Decree of the Department of Work and Social Welfare 913/1985, of 4 February, the 'Commission for the Study, Development and Promotion of the Gypsy People' was created. This Commission was to 'co-ordinate all the actions of the Generalitat for the total incorporation of the Gypsy people into the society, recognizing the historical debt that the majority society has to the Gypsies, recognized as a people, even by the United Nations'. This Decree actualized another one from 20 February, 1979, under which the 'Service for the Defence and Development of the Gypsy People' was created. Finally, through a new Decree (49/1988, 12 April), the Decree of 1985 was annulled, and a new 'Commission for the Study, Development and Promotion of the Gypsy People' was created. During this new stage, the commission was assigned the functions of protection and warrant of the jural status of the Gypsies, levelling it to the same position of that of the rest of the subjects inside the jural order, the defence of their labour interests, the promotion of activities for the conservation and development of the Gypsy cultural inheritance, the study of the equality of their situation, including adequate housing, the promotion of a health policy (a special Hygiene Plan was created) and the promotion of Gypsy institutions.

As may have become obvious, the legal situation within the Spanish state is very varied. There are laws that are intended to avoid any type of marginalization. It is implicitly set out by the law that any discrimination should be avoided; and that for this purpose nothing would be more effective than the establishment of the full standardization of the Social Services within the law itself, not the creation of special services for any marginal group or for the ethnic minorities of the population. Attention to these elements of the population within the Social Services, apart from those established for the rest of the population, would in itself be discriminatory. Some specific resources could be made available to Social Centres for the benefit of the whole population, especially directed to needed collectives, and for this purpose specific procedures are sometimes programmed, but it would not be suitable to create special Social Services. We believe that some of the present laws in Spain are adequate in this respect.

On the other hand, some authorities contemplate a special situation for the Social Services respecting the Gypsies, given their numerical and cultural importance within, for example, Andalusia, and others have changed their goals, converting a 'Service of Defence and Development of the Gypsy People' into a 'Commission for the Study, Development and Promotion of the Gypsy People' (for instance, in the Community of Valencia). Merely to specify these different situations may give an idea of one of the most controversial subjects there are to be found in Spain.

AN APPROACH TO SOCIAL INTERVENTION PROGRAMMES

As mentioned above, in the section on the history of the Gypsies, there no longer exist specific laws directed against them in Spain. However, and in spite of the recognition that the Gypsies are equivalent to any other legally recognized persons, situations of inequality have continued to exist up to the present between Gadjes and Gypsies, as total equality before law has not yet been granted. Gypsies are especially vulnerable, taking into account the absence of social acceptance of their labour and their lack of permanent residences.

This observation is even more justified when the laws of the Social Services are accurately analysed. Only if we take a closer look at the treatment which the Gypsies receive by means of the laws that affect them specifically, may we learn that the present situation still partly continues to be the same as in former years. This we may observe in some legal texts, including expressions such as: 'promote procedures which might generate in a real and effective way, their social equality respecting the rest of the citizens', 'considering the equality of rights, within the respect for differences, due to historical and cultural reasons' and 'the elimination of institutional or social discriminations'. Such phrases (present even in legal texts) reveal situations of real inequality in which Gypsies in Spain still find themselves, in spite of all the laws which have been passed and work which has been done. The shortcomings in such plans become obvious: they have not focused on the fundamental variables upon which the suitable formulation of the problem and its possible solutions depend.

For a better understanding of the work performed in Spain with the Gypsies, it is necessary to go back to the times previous to the present democratic regime. From 1960 up to the present, both private and public institutions and individuals with their own initiatives have been concerned with Gypsy affairs, in locations which are basically urban and located in the slums and peripheral areas of the city.

In spite of some remarkable efforts at co-ordination (especially those carried out by organizations belonging to the Catholic Church), these interventions can be said to have been disconnected and have led only to despair. Some efforts were made to set up such initiatives on a better constructed, more rational basis, but they did not receive enough support, above all in the public sector, and especially when trying to solve such problems on a large scale.

The most systematic task was carried out by the Catholic Church during those years, by means of two organizations: the Office for Nomads (the Gypsy Office), and Caritas, both at a national and at a diocesan level. The task of the Church, though started as a charity, crystallized in some places into more comprehensive, long-term programmes, such as the establishment of labour co-operatives or support for the development of housing, with the intention of promoting community development – these were professional and not simply charitable. Many professional organizations, still at work, were initially formed in developing such programmes. However, from the end of the 1960s and perhaps because of the failure of its objectives – being simultaneously religious and social (those plans for the 'Promotion of the Gypsy People', as they were then called) – the Church withdrew from this area of service, decreasing its efforts and presence considerably.

At this same period, other private organizations and persons made great voluntary efforts, and played important roles, but these also declined. Some of the persons who realized these tasks are at present civil servants, and the administration has also adopted many of the programmes of the Catholic Church and private bodies, then in existence.

From the latter part of the 1970s many small associations formed by Gypsies appeared, as a direct or indirect consequence of the above activities. They fought for the incorporation of their people into society, with the same rights as the rest of the citizens, but also with the right to remain Gypsies.

Some local councils also produced procedures and concrete programmes which had their origins either in others carried out by private bodies, or in the problems of city life, such as begging or rehousing of slum dwellers, now made possible by urban growth or the remodelling of urban areas.

This whole epoch ended up in a situation in which the different public and private developing programmes, to a greater or lesser degree, depended on the financial support of the administration's collaboration of budgets, but in general without any co-ordination between them, with disorganization and the frequent abandonment of these programmes.

At present, as it has been seen, the situation is different. The administration legally assumes public responsibility for the bettering of the life conditions and welfare of all the citizens, especially those who are less fortunate. Amongst the latter, without doubt, are the majority of the Gypsies.

At the present time several programmes of social intervention are being carried out by several administrations with the Gypsy people, but groups and voluntary persons and private bodies remain present, and these benefit themselves to some extent from official financial support. During the last two years I have had a direct relationship with eight of these programmes. Most of them are part of the Integrated Action Plans. They are organized by several responsible administrations (autonomous governments and local councils), corresponding to different departments (Social Services themselves, Education, Health, Urbanism, Employment, and so on).

It is impossible to make an accurate analysis of these programmes in this chapter. One cannot fail to notice the obstacles one may find when trying to generalize about the Spanish situation in this matter.

The programs are often wrongly placed due to lack of information and, therefore, of the reality to which they apply, and also due to hidden objectives of the promoters of the plans, linking them to different goals (elections, political factors, social coexistence conflicts, administrative pressures and land speculations). Sometimes the contrary happens: a well-placed programme, inspired towards serious work, only turns out to be so in appearance, because it has nothing to do with what is actually being done. These programmes may be thought of as being presented in order to obtain a good image, and may lead to misunderstanding by those who are unaware of what is being done and rely on what is being said and written. Nevertheless, we find that many of the professionals and volunteers, who actually work or collaborate in the different programmes, are professional persons and perform their actual task well, irrespective of the planning. In general, we could say that we have an impression of the administration as being more interested in 'getting rid of' the problems than in trying to solve them. Fortunately, there are always exceptions.

A good deal of lack of co-ordination exists, both in the programmed procedure between the different administrations of the same area, and between the different departments of the same administration. Not many weeks ago, an autonomous administration published in the local press a misinterpreted and damaging information about a Programme of Integrated Actions, which was performed by the local council, in a suburb of 80 per cent Gypsies. Unfortunately, examples of this kind are quite common.

Last year, a Department of Welfare started its performance in a quarter with slum Gypsies, ignoring the fact that the Department of Education of the same administration had already been working there for some time. The latter developed a Compensatory Educational Programme, obtaining quite good results, though they were limited due to the lack of municipal collaboration and support.

Many programmes and public interventions have been initiated without a knowledge of where action was needed. Lack of analysis of the viability of the programmes and social interventions always have negative consequences. Improvisation obstructs the achievements of the proposed objectives, and this, in general, generates apathy and mistrust and the failure of the efforts, dedication and expectations which have been created. Such results have greater effects on the population affected by the programme than on the professionals who intervene in it.

Many social programmes can be seen on paper, on official desks. There are programmes for everything: cultural, health, educational, housing, work, and so forth. I have seen on paper social sensitization campaigns to promote the integration of the Gypsy community – many papers on many desks . . . but where is the concrete evidence of so many programmes on the Gypsy life and population towards which they are said to be directed?

CONCLUSIONS

In this chapter laws of the Social Services have been discussed, and I have mentioned the existence of laws whose purpose is fundamentally to avoid discrimination, and which therefore do not foresee the need for any special service for Gypsies. I totally agree with the principle of normalization of the Social Services and, therefore, of a system of non-segregative access to the collective services of a general character. I believe that the application of this principle to the matter on which I focus, the specific Gypsy culture, should be pursued as well as their present situation. Therefore a program specifically designed for the Gypsy people is needed (not 'Special Services'), in which more and more aspects may be slowly absorbed by the general programmes, so that at the end only the specific aspect of the ethnic difference remains. Due to the situation in which we find ourselves, it is possible that this position (in some cases) has other causes. I could say that to discriminate from the start is as bad as to ignore different and specific situations. I have often found that the different public administrations sometimes ignore the existence of Gypsies in their area or improvise occasional answers to the demands of this population, and to the conflicts derived from the lack of civic coexistence; such improvised answers correspond more to the old-fashioned notions of charitable help, paternalistic or even racist in character, than attitudes favourable to the integration of the Gypsies into the rest of the civil society, with equal rights and obligations like any other group of citizens.

To these evils, often derived from an unfortunate public intervention, there should be added the no less detrimental consequences of the archaic and predominant charity practices which have perpetuated, under new forms, old habits of begging and beneficence. All this has contributed to consolidate attitudes in some Gypsies, who have abusively extrapolated the rights which assist them to enjoy the

Social Welfare Service, given by the administration, and who have not understood that their integration in society also obliges them to adopt responsibilities.

What has fundamentally changed the life of the Gypsies has not been legislation, nor the Social Services given to them, but the evolution of the world and the change produced in the society in which they live. It has been so, I would dare to say, because many social programmes designed for them were made without having in mind their opinion and have been designed from what others think to be best for them. A social change from the outside must not be programmed. Any procedure which does not count on their participation, which does not start taking into account their reality and does not take into account their own options and expectations will always be ineffective, apart from being an imposition and an act of repression.

The complexity of the situation is evidenced when one considers the variability of the Gypsy population. Not only is it a different minority, but it is also heterogeneous. The Gypsies are all just Gypsies to the Gadjes, but amongst themselves there are many differences. All this emphasizes the difficulty of the success and effectiveness in the application of general measures.

The great majority of the Gypsies in Spain live under a marginalized situation, in some cases contending with racism, whose mechanisms should be very well known and taken into consideration when conceiving a programme. A general objective should be proposed for all policies of intervention, the elaboration of a plan, including the necessary steps to reach this objective. Concrete information and the knowledge necessary to establish a realistic and feasible plan is needed, but above all, it is necessary to have the opinion of the Gypsies.

We have seen that many plans are programmed without previous knowledge of the population group to whom they are going to be applied. Sometimes, the intervention of the administration must take place immediately, as some problems cannot wait. The sad thing is that, once the urgency is over, nobody is seriously interested in the subject any more, or in planning the procedure on a long-term basis. An evaluation of the final procedure does not exist either.

When a specific programme is proposed for this population, an adequate theoretical study should be taken into consideration, with information provided mainly by the social, anthropological and historical investigations that have already been undertaken about the subject, which might help us to know and understand Gypsy culture, their social relations, their organizational forms, their historical process and many other aspects of their way of life. It is also worth, before starting any action, at the very beginning, having a first stage of direct contact, with much observation and listening, originating from deep respect for Gypsy life, the ways of which are not the same as ours.

In comparative investigations and studies, performed in Spain (GIEMS, 1976, and elsewhere), it has been shown that the principal factors which prove to be effective in the generation of change inside Gypsy communities are housing and living quarters, work and education. These are main factors on which the administration should act, but taking into consideration the opinion of the Gypsy population, and starting from their point of view, as it is work directed towards the development of this community.

As far as the persons who carry out these programmes are concerned, both professionals and prepared volunteers (I think it is important to note the need for specific preparation), it is essential that they obtain all the available documented information about their work. From this initial information the necessary material can be obtained for the progress and improvement of the designed programme. The collected documentation and the information it contains is of basic importance in order to acquire an adequate knowledge of the Gypsies with whom we work; and it is equally necessary for reflection about the programme and its evaluation in terms of the proposed goals.

Some of these pages might seem somewhat defeatist to those not being used to criticism. However, they reflect the confusion in which these problems are seen, how badly the Gypsies are spoken of, a situation that has existed for centuries in Spain and in other European countries. Fortunately, there are also important achievements, rigorously undertaken and carried out successfully, but there is still much work to be done. The normalization of life as citizens of the same community between men and women from different cultures is very slow and is not exempt from backward steps, tensions and conflicts.

In Spain, during recent years, we have seen important changes, which have given place to different processes in normalization. There is the political process, with the inauguration of the social and democratic state in regard to rights. There is the linguistic process, in which, in spite of difficulties, the normalization of the conditions of the use of local languages (such as Catalan, Basque or Galego) is growing steadily. From the military and religious points of view, the role of the army and the Church are in the process of being modified to suit a pluralistic society such as ours. However, these matters of multi-cultural living together do not seem to grow at the same rate. The outbursts of racism, the perpetuation of the poverty culture amongst these collectives and, in general, the lack of conditions suitable for the development of the Gypsy people and their total integration into society evidence a situation that in no way can be considered as 'normal'.

We believe that the understanding of and respect for the cultural characteristics of the Gypsies can improve the life of all, as well as the fulfilment of the social norms by everybody, which make it possible to live in peace and to maintain equality of rights and responsibilities as citizens. I have had the good fortune to share my life with Gypsies, who wholeheartedly wished to continue to be Gypsies, and who are merely other citizens. With them, I regret so much discrimination and confusion respecting their status and rights. If this chapter helps to focus concern on matters relative to the Gypsies more suitably, and contributes in some way to the better planning of the social interventions affecting them, I shall feel satisfied.

ENDNOTE

I would like to thank Gloria Rubiol for the opportunity she offered me to write this chapter. Because she has worked uninterruptedly in the study of the Social Services I might have hoped that this chapter would have been jointly authored. However, personal conditions and research occupations have made it impossible. My work has been extraordinarily eased by the help of Matilde Barrio, who supplied me with basic documents for the elaboration of the Social Services chapter. From 1967 up to 1973 I worked with Teresa San Roman, first as an informant and later as a field-worker in her research on the Gypsies, enjoying a solid professional and personal relationship. With her, many years ago, I had the opportunity of discovering that my lack of knowledge and gaps in theory, were due to a professional dissatisfaction, which I felt when I worked as a social worker with the Gypsies. I found out that intuition, though fundamental, was not enough. Her orientation was decisive, and with her help I managed to study anthropology in London, and sociology afterwards in Madrid. To find that after all these years our collaboration continues is a great satisfaction, which I cannot omit to mention. Finally, I would like to thank Salvador Carrasco, for his patience and help in completing this chapter, and also Susan Petersen and Silvia Carrasco, for their collaboration with an English translation of this text.

Barcelona, December 1990

REFERENCES

Generalitat de Catalunya (1984) *Mapa de Serveis Socials de Catalunya*, Barcelona: Direccio General de Serveis Socials.

GIEMS (Interdisciplinary Group of Studies of Social Marginalization) (1976) *Gitanos al encuentro de la ciudad: Del chalaneo al peonaje*, Madrid: Edicusa.

Leblon, B. (1987) *Los gitanos de Espana. El precio y el valor de la diferencia*, Barcelona: Gedis, SA.

Ministerio de Asuntos Sociales (1989) *Servicios Sociales. Leyes autonómicas*, Madrid: Ministerio de Asuntos Sociales.

San Roman, T. (1976) *Vecinos gitanos*, Madrid: Akal.

— — (1981) *Realojamiento de la población chabolista gitana*, Ajuntament de Barcelona: Area de Serveis Socials.

— — (1984) *Gitanos de Madrid y Barcelona. Ensayos sobre Aculturación y Etnicidad*, Barcelona: Universidad Autónoma (Bellaterra).

— —(ed.), (1986) *Entre la marginación y el racismo. Reflexiones sobre la vida de los gitanos*, Madrid: Alianza.

San Roman, T. and Garriga, C. (1975) *La imagen paya de los gitanos*, Revista de Trabajo Social No. 60, Barcelona.

Sanchez, M. H. (1977) *Documentación selecta sobre la situación de los gitanos españoles en el siglo XVIII*, Madrid: Editorial Nacional.

7 From exclusion to dependence: Aborigines and the welfare state in Australia

J. C. Altman and W. Sanders

EUROPEAN SETTLEMENT AND ABORIGINAL POLICY, 1788 TO THE 1950s: A REGIME OF EXCLUSION

An indigenous population of hunter-gatherers has inhabited the Australian continent for at least the last 50,000 years. At the time of the first European settlement in Australia in 1788, the indigenous population probably numbered between 250,000 and 750,000 (Smith, 1980; Mulvaney and White, 1987). During the nineteenth century, as European settlement spread, the Aboriginal population was reduced through disease and direct contact to perhaps a quarter of its original number. The indigenous population was, in aggregate terms, rapidly outnumbered by the settler population which by 1850 had reached about 450,000, and by 1900, 3.5 million. By the end of the nineteenth century, then, Aborigines constituted probably 5 per cent or less of the Australian population, though there were still areas in the more sparsely settled northern and central parts of Australia where they predominated.

Australia in the nineteenth century comprised six British colonies, each focused on a coastal port city and each with a gradually expanding rural hinterland. In the course of the century each of these six colonies was granted self-government from Britain and each developed its own policies for dealing with its Aboriginal inhabitants. Though there were some differences in the policy approaches of the colonies, there were also many similarities. Each enacted special bodies of law which set Aborigines apart from the larger population of colonial citizens in a separate legal category. This was done in the name of 'protection', the purpose of which, depending on one's optimism or pessimism, could be variously interpreted as a process of 'smoothing the dying pillow' or of training Aborigines for future full citizenship. 'Reserves' of land were set aside for the purpose of collecting together and supervising groups of Aborigines. Public officials were appointed with titles such as 'Protector of Aborigines'. Through these legal and administrative mechanisms, colonial governments ostensibly developed a high degree of control over the lives of their Aboriginal minorities. However, in reality the day-to-day task of directly supervising and managing all Aborigines within their territories was often beyond the capacity of the government official concerned. Responsibility was often delegated to missionaries and employers of Aboriginal labour, and many Aborigines just slipped through the protection policy net. These latter groups lived an officially unsanctioned existence either on the fringes of European settlement or in the remote hinterland unoccupied by settlers.

After federation of the six colonies into the Commonwealth of Australia in 1901, the new State governments continued to manage their Aboriginal minorities in much the same ways as their colonial predecessors. The exception was South Australia, which in 1911 ceded the remote northern section of its territorial claim to the Commonwealth. This arrangement for the government of the Northern Territory meant that the new Commonwealth government's jurisdiction included a large area of the Australian continent in which Aborigines still outnumbered Europeans and which contained a sizeable proportion of the national Aboriginal population. The Commonwealth, like the nineteenth-century colonies, developed the approach of a separate legal status for Aborigines in its administration of the Northern Territory and similarly set aside reserves of land for their use, supervision and management.

In the early years of the twentieth century, the central rationale of Aboriginal policy in Australia continued to be 'protection'. The Aboriginal population, particularly its 'full-blood' component, was probably still decreasing. However, there was also an increasing recognition that a 'part-Aboriginal' population was emerging which was already significant in southern or 'settled' Australia and was likely to increase further. From the 1930s 'assimilation' became the declared goal of Commonwealth and State government policies at least for these Aborigines, and the emphasis swung more clearly to training for future full citizenship.

By the 1950s, the Aboriginal population was officially estimated to number between 70,000 and 80,000, or about 1 per cent of the total Australian population. The Aboriginal population seemed now, however, to be stabilizing, or perhaps even increasing, and 'assimilation' became the central term of government policy towards *all* Aborigines. Under the new policy, only officially defined in 1961, Aborigines were supposed in time to:

> attain the same manner of living as other Australians and to live as members of a single Australian community enjoying the same rights and privileges, accepting the same responsibilities, observing the same customs and influenced by the same beliefs, hopes and loyalties as other Australians.
>
> (Commonwealth Parliamentary Debates, House of Representatives,
> 20 April 1961: 51)

The mechanism for achieving assimilation was the granting of exemptions to individual Aborigines from the special bodies of State and Territory law. These 'assimilated' Aborigines were then supposed to take their place in the larger body of Australian citizenry, no longer officially categorized as Aborigines and no longer of a separate legal status.

With the shift to assimilation as the declared goal of governments, the term 'welfare' came increasingly to be used as part of the lexicon of Aboriginal policy. Protectors of Aborigines often became welfare officers and protection authorities, welfare authorities. This Aboriginal welfare system was not, however, in any sense part of the modern Australian welfare state. Indeed, those in the Aboriginal welfare system were generally excluded from the provisions of the mainstream Australian welfare system by their separate legal status. The Australian social security legislation, for example, had since its establishment contained explicit provisions disqualifying Aborigines from eligibility for income support payments. Industrial awards, regulating wages and conditions of employment also had exclusionary provisions, as too did laws relating to the electoral franchise. Even the Australian Constitution contained two provisions which specifically excluded Aborigines; the one excluding them from being counted in any reckoning of the numbers of people in the Commonwealth, and the other excluding them from the Commonwealth power to make laws in relation to the people of particular races. Even where there was no clear legislative, regulatory or constitutional basis for Aboriginal exclusion, mainstream functional agencies of government generally claimed that responsibility for Aborigines did not lie with them, but with the special-purpose Aboriginal welfare authorities. After all, why else did these authorities exist?

Breaking down exclusion: a tentative start

The pattern of exclusion of Aborigines from the rights and benefits of the Australian welfare state began to be dismantled in the middle years of this century. One of the first ways in which this was to occur, and one that would assume great importance for the economic status of Aborigines over subsequent years, was in the social security system. During the 1940s, the child endowment (family allowance) payment made for the care of dependent children became payable for all Aboriginal children, except the 'nomadic' (Commonwealth Acts No. 8 of 1941 and No. 5 of 1942). The provisions of the social security legislation relating to the more substantial pension and benefit payments were also amended during the 1940s from wholesale exclusion of Aborigines to a formulation which allowed eligibility to individuals who were either exempt from State or Territory laws 'relating to the control of Aboriginal natives' or whose 'character, standard of intelligence and social development' made it 'reasonable' to grant such eligibility (Act Nos 3 and 19 of 1942 and No. 10 of 1944). The interpretation of these pension and benefit provisions which gained acceptance within the Commonwealth's social security administration at that time was that they allowed eligibility only to those Aborigines who lived away from the reserves administered by the State and Territory Aboriginal welfare authorities. These Aboriginal welfare authorities soon became concerned that the availability of pension and benefit payments off reserves provided an incentive for Aborigines to move away, and from the late 1940s, these authorities, along with others, sought to have pension and benefit eligibility for Aborigines extended (Neville, 1947; Rowley, 1971a: 390). This objective was achieved in 1959, when provisions of the social security legislation were changed throughout to include all Aborigines except the 'nomadic and primitive' (Act No. 57 of 1959). By 1966 even this last qualification was removed from the social security legislation (Act No. 41 of 1966). In a statutory sense at least, Aborigines were now included in the social security system on the same basis as other Australians.

The role of the Aboriginal welfare authorities of the 1950s in supporting the inclusion of Aborigines in the Australian social security system may seem a little surprising. At that time, these authorities kept a close watch over their Aboriginal charges, seldom giving them much money. Why then push for Aboriginal eligibility for social security income payments? The answer lies in the provisions of the social security legislation which allowed payments to be made to third parties on behalf of eligible applicants. These provisions had already been used during the 1940s and 1950s to direct child endowment payments to State and Territory Aboriginal welfare authorities, rather than directly to Aboriginal parents. In the negotiations leading up to the legislative changes of 1959, agreement was reached between the Commonwealth's social security administration and the various State and Territory Aboriginal welfare authorities that these provisions would be similarly applied to pensions and benefits. The Aboriginal welfare authorities would be the recipients of social security payments on behalf of many Aborigines. They would be allowed to retain the greater proportion of the payments for expenditure on the welfare of their charges, having only to pass on a 'pocket money' component to individuals. Direct payment would only be made to individual Aborigines once they had demonstrated their 'ability to handle money wisely' and to 'manage' their 'own affairs' (Commonwealth Parliamentary Debates, House of Representatives, 3 September 1959: 930; Department of Social Security, 1960: 3). After 1959, the Aboriginal welfare authorities stood to gain a considerable Commonwealth contribution to their recurrent budgets through access to the pensions and benefits of their charges. It is little wonder, then, that they were at the forefront of public pressure for the legislative inclusion of Aborigines in the social security system.

During the 1960s, many other aspects of the exclusion of Aboriginal people from Australian legal and administrative institutions began to be tentatively dismantled. In 1965 the Commonwealth electoral franchise was extended to Aborigines of voting age on a voluntary basis. (For other Australians of voting age enrolment to vote had long been compulsory.) A number of industrial awards regulating conditions of employment were also extended to cover Aborigines, the most celebrated being the pastoral (or cattle) industry award extended to Aboriginal people from 1968 (Rowley, 1971b; Stevens, 1974). In 1967, a constitutional amendment referendum was proposed and passed deleting the two exclusionary references to Aborigines from the Australian Constitution. This was of itself a significant achievement, as from Federation to 1967 there had been 26 proposed constitutional amendments put to referenda and this was only the fifth to be passed. Furthermore, Australians gave these amendments the highest 'yes' vote yet recorded, with nearly 91 per cent voting for the change (Crisp, 1970: 40–57).

The success of the 1967 referendum opened up the possibility of the Commonwealth government becoming more directly involved in policy towards Aborigines on a national scale. A new Office of Aboriginal Affairs was established within the Commonwealth government's bureaucratic apparatus, quite separate from its existing Northern Territory Aboriginal welfare administration and with a clearly separate and national role to play. The Office began to make special-purpose grants to the States for expenditure on Aboriginal welfare and economic development and also began to provide some funding for Aboriginal community organizations. 'Assimilation' was discarded as the key term of Aboriginal policy in favour of 'integration', though precisely what difference this signified was somewhat unclear (Schapper, 1970: 59–60). Although these were significant changes, they continued to operate through the established structures and organizations of Aboriginal policy, rather than in any way directly challenging them.

On the social security front, in the 1960s pressure was building up to have pensions, benefits and family allowances paid directly to Aborigines, rather than to their welfare authority, mission or employer custodians (Andrews, 1964). In response to such pressure a directive was issued in 1968 by the federal Minister for Social Security that progress towards direct payments to Aborigines should be hastened. However, with the Department of Social Security's 'field' presence among Aborigines being extremely limited, such a directive was to little avail. Most Aborigines were still dependent on the State and Territory Aboriginal welfare authorities for the majority of their day-to-day needs and had little prospect of receiving their social security entitlements directly. There was in any case still an ambivalence in the larger Australian society over the applicability of social security payments to Aboriginal people, particularly in remote areas. Pensions and family allowances were being paid, but unemployment benefit was still being regarded by the Department of Social Security as inapplicable to Aborigines in remote areas (Sanders, 1985).

From exclusion to inclusion: the 1970s revolution

History will record the 1970s as a decade in which federal government approaches to Australia's Aboriginal minority under-went radical change. The 1971 Census was the first in which Aborigines were to count in 'reckoning the numbers of people of the Commonwealth' and the first that adopted a self-identification test of Aboriginality. Previous census questions on Aboriginality had asked for distinctions by racial proportion (for example, half Aboriginal/

half European, or 'full-blood' Aboriginal) and had come under increasing criticism for their racism, unrealism and inappropriateness. In the 1971 Census, approximately 116,000 people self-identified as Aborigines or Torres Strait Islanders. This was some 14,000 more than had been enumerated in the 1966 Census under the old proportional question, but was still only about 1 per cent of the total Australian population of 12.8 million.

The adoption of a self-identification definition of Aboriginality may not of itself seem a significant development in policy. However, it was indicative of a whole change of philosophy in Aboriginal affairs policy developing at that time. Late in 1972, the Whitlam Labor government was elected to office and the established regime of Aboriginal policy began to be transformed in ways that would make the changes of previous years look tentative indeed. The Whitlam government adopted 'self-determination' as the central term of Aboriginal policy. The new federal government declared that it would restore to Aborigines their lost power to determine their own futures and ways of life (Whitlam, 1973). This was intended to indicate a clear break with past policy philosophy, which was now seen as having determined such choices for Aborigines.

Major institutional changes were also embarked upon in conjunction with the change of policy philosophy. A fully fledged federal Department of Aboriginal Affairs (DAA) was established, combining in the first instance both the relatively new and small Office of Aboriginal Affairs with the Commonwealth's much more long-standing and larger Aboriginal Welfare Branch of the Northern Territory administration. With the help of the new DAA, the Whitlam government also established a National Aboriginal Consultative Council, composed of elected Aborigines from around the country and specifically charged with the task of advising the Commonwealth government on issues of concern to Aboriginal people. A Royal Commission to inquire into mechanisms for the granting of Aboriginal land rights was also established and, although its brief was restricted to the Northern Territory in the first instance (where direct Commonwealth administration would ensure quick implementation), there was also a clear understanding that any proposed mechanism for the Territory could become a model for the rest of Australia.

In as bold an institutional move as any, the Whitlam government also declared its intentions to take over the policy responsibilities and personnel of State Aboriginal welfare authorities and incorporate them into the new DAA. Explaining his government's reasons for this take-over to the Council of Commonwealth and State Ministers for Aboriginal Affairs in 1973, Whitlam argued that the intention was not to establish a new 'omnibus' Department of Aboriginal Affairs, like a super-sized State or Territory Aboriginal welfare authority, but rather to create a new Commonwealth DAA which:

> will instead seek to devolve upon a wide range of Federal, State and local authorities, as well as upon organizations of Aboriginals themselves, responsibility for carrying out the policies decided upon by my Government. These authorities would be responsible for Aboriginals in the same matters and in the same way as they now are functionally responsible for the community generally.
>
> (Whitlam, 1973: 697)

This approach would, if realized, reverse the previous pattern of Aboriginal exclusion from the mainstream institutions of the Australian welfare state. The Commonwealth's Aboriginal affairs administration was to provide some overall policy direction and some supplementary assistance for Aborigines, but it was to do so in conjunction with and in addition to, rather than instead of, mainstream agencies at all levels of Australian government. The DAA was to encourage Aboriginal community organizations to incorporate legally for the conduct of their own affairs and for the provision of many of their own services, thereby creating new relations with such organizations somewhat akin to those with non-government community welfare agencies more generally. All this promised to be a major change from the past regime of Aboriginal exclusion from the Australian welfare state, which had only been tentatively challenged in previous years.

The realization of the Whitlam vision required many battles to be fought on many fronts. The DAA did succeed during the Whitlam years in taking over the State welfare authorities in all States except Queensland, where a conservative State government dominated by rural interests maintained its own State Department of Aboriginal and Islander Advancement (DAIA). A Queensland branch of the new Commonwealth DAA was, however, established in 1975 alongside the State government's department. Legislation for land rights in the Northern Territory also reached an advanced stage of preparation during the Whitlam years, though it had to rely for its enactment on the incoming Fraser government, after the Whitlam government lost office late in 1975.

In relation to other agencies in the Commonwealth's administrative apparatus, such as the Department of Social Security (DSS) and the

Commonwealth Employment Service (CES), which were now supposed to serve Aborigines directly, the DAA was constantly pressuring these agencies to take a more active service delivery role. Disagreements abounded as to just where the responsibility of these functional departments stopped and those of the DAA started. But the DAA was always insistent that the functional agencies were not doing enough, and in time they slowly began to do more. The DSS, for example, initiated a process of appointing special-purpose Aboriginal liaison officers in 1977, and the CES had already begun appointing Aboriginal vocational/employment officers.

In relation to State government agencies, such as housing, health and education departments, the DAA's main weapon of persuasion was increased special-purpose grants, which in most States were quickly accepted and used. However, while these agencies did no more than spend their Commonwealth special-purpose grants on services to Aborigines, and this was generally the case, there was a sense in which they were not fully accepting separate responsibility for their Aboriginal clientele. The problem for the DAA was getting State departments to earmark some of their own financial resources for their Aboriginal clients, rather than just taking Commonwealth money.

Throughout the 1970s, the DAA insisted that other agencies at all levels of government should be doing more for Aborigines, while at the same time building up its own array of Aboriginal assistance programmes. These programmes were defined in functional terms such as housing, health, employment and education. The balance that was to be struck here was always a difficult one. On the one hand, as long as the DAA developed its own programmes and expanded its expenditure, it was easy for other government departments to argue that responsibility for matters relating to Aborigines lay with the DAA. Why else did the DAA's programmes exist, and why else was it encouraging and directly funding Aboriginal community-based organizations such as health services, housing associations, legal services and, in remote areas, general community councils? On the other hand, if the DAA ceased to develop its own programmes, or even withdrew financial support from certain types of activity in Aboriginal communities, would the mainstream functional departments adequately fill the void?

The 1980s: a proliferation of programmes

Despite the many battles which needed to be waged, progress had been made by the early 1980s towards incorporating Aborigines in the Australian welfare state in a way reasonably in line with the Whitlam vision of the early 1970s. The central term of Aboriginal policy had been changed by the Fraser coalition government from the somewhat provocative 'self-determination' to the slightly more restrained 'self-management'. The National Aboriginal Consultative Council, the elected national Aboriginal advisory body, had been abolished and reconstituted as the National Aboriginal Conference in 1977, and the DAA had been effectively split in two with the creation of the Aboriginal Development Commission in 1980. However, the basic thrust of philosophical and institutional change remained intact. In even the remotest areas Aborigines were by the 1980s being treated as eligible for all social security payments, including unemployment benefit (Sanders, 1985; Altman, 1985). Aborigines were also increasingly being provided for through a broad range of special Aboriginal assistance programmes operating across a whole range of Commonwealth and State government departments; some provided services direct to Aborigines and some funded community-based service organizations. The underlying rationale for separate Aboriginal assistance programmes was the extreme disadvantage and special needs of the Aboriginal clientele.

Some indication of the growth in Aboriginal assistance programmes over recent years can be gained from Table 7.1, where the ratio of Commonwealth Aboriginal Affairs Portfolio's expenditure on Aboriginal assistance to total Commonwealth expenditure on Aboriginal assistance is calculated. From accounting for over 80 per cent of such expenditure in the early 1970s, the Aboriginal Affairs Portfolio's share dropped to around 70 per cent by the early 1980s and to around 56 per cent at the time of writing. The change has been brought about by the development of Aborginal assistance programmes in Commonwealth agencies outside the Aboriginal Affairs Portfolio. The largest of these programmes, in terms of expenditure, have been in the areas of employment, education and housing. However, in more recent years Aboriginal assistance programmes have emerged in Commonwealth portfolios as diverse as arts, environment, health, community services and communications (see Table 7.2).

Table 7.3 provides a functional breakdown of the Aboriginal Affairs Portfolio's own programme expenditure. There are probably now over 100 Aboriginal assistance programmes and sub-programmes provided across the range of government departments and at various levels of Australian government. Even listing these

Table 7.1 Commonwealth Aboriginal assistance programmes expenditure (not indexed for inflation)

Financial year	Aboriginal Affairs Portfolio (A) (A$m)	Other C'wealth agencies (B) (A$m)	Total (C) (A$m)	(A) as % of (C)
1970/71	20.3	4.4	24.7	82
1971/72	24.0	5.0	29.0	83
1972/73	44.3	14.1	58.4	76
1973/74	78.3	18.4	96.7	81
1974/75	124.8	34.1	158.9	79
1975/76	138.9	47.2	186.1	75
1976/77	121.0	40.5	161.5	75
1977/78	124.3	49.5	173.8	72
1978/79	132.6	19.0	151.6	87
1979/80	140.8	41.2	182.0	77
1980/81	159.4	60.2	219.6	73
1981/82	168.8	90.0	258.8	65
1982/83	198.0	102.4	300.4	66
1983/84	242.8	153.9	396.7	61
1984/85	281.2	186.0	467.2	60
1985/86	295.1	225.1	520.2	57
1986/87	332.1	240.0	572.1	58
1987/88	377.4	278.8	656.2	58
1988/89	450.0	327.6	777.6	58
1989/90	505.8	394.1	899.9	56

Source: DAA (1987) and various annual reports of the DAA

programmes, let alone describing their mode of operation, would now be a major undertaking.

The expenditure identified in Tables 7.1 to 7.3 on specific Aboriginal assistance programmes does not take into account expenditure on Aborigines through general government programmes where Aboriginality is not identified, and this too is a significant amount. Expenditure through the social security system is clearly by far the most important such item. One recent estimate by the economist Fisk (1985: 79), which draws together diverse sources of data on Aboriginal incomes, estimated that social security payments constituted 47 per cent of all Aboriginal personal income in Australia at the time of the 1976 Census and 54 per cent by the 1981 Census. This increase over the five-year period was probably due to change in the interpretation of Aboriginal eligibility for unemployment benefits and to a decline in Aboriginal employment levels, especially in rural

Table 7.2 Mainstream Commonwealth agency expenditure on Aboriginal assistance programmes

	1988/89 (A$m)	1989/90 (A$m)
Dept of Employment, Education & Training	190.9	210.6
including Aboriginal Study Assistance	74.1	74.6
and Aboriginal employment development	72.7	70.8
Dept of Community Services and Health	111.7	136.7
including public rental housing	70.0	92.4
Dept of Administrative Services	10.2	11.2
Dept of the Arts, Sports, the Environment, Tourism and Territories	5.3	6.2
Dept of Social Security	4.6	1.6
Australian Bicentennial Authority	1.3	0.0
Australian Broadcasting Corp	1.1	1.4
Dept of Transport & Communication	0.7	0.2
Australian Electoral Commission	0.7	0.8
Dept of Primary Industries & Energy	0.3	1.0
Special Broadcasting Service – TV	0.2	n/a
Australian Bureau of Statistics	0.2	0.1
Dept of Attorney-General	0.2	0.3

Source: DAA (1989) and Aboriginal and Torres Strait Island Commission (ATSIC) Budget Branch

areas, owing to structural changes in the Australian economy. This level of Aboriginal dependence on social security payments can be compared to an estimated 14 per cent social security contribution to the personal incomes of the whole Australian population in 1984 (Australian Bureau of Statistics, 1986).

Tables 7.1 to 7.3 also do not identify expenditure on Aborigines at the State level of Australian government, except where it is derived from Commonwealth special-purpose grants. Although probably fairly small in comparison with Commonwealth expenditure, such expenditure does exist and is not entirely insignificant. The New South Wales State government established a land rights system in 1983 under which about A$30 million per annum of State government revenue has recently been spent and the Western Australian government has contributed half of a joint Commonwealth–State A$100 million community improvement programme for

Table 7.3 Aboriginal Affairs Portfolio, expenditure by functional programme area

	1988/89 (A$m)	1989/90 (A$m)
Employment	99.0	133.2
Housing	96.7	80.9
Community infrastructure	69.3	78.0
Health	43.5	44.0
Enterprise	27.9	27.4
Heritage*	25.8	0.6
Legal aid	17.0	19.7
Social support	10.1	11.0
Consultation and research	8.3	7.4
Recreation	6.4	4.9
Broadcasting	4.5	7.6
Training	4.1	8.5
Art and culture	2.4	4.1
Land ownership and administration*	0.0	40.3
Administration	58.7	76.6
Total	473.7	544.2
Revenue received	(23.7)	(38.4)
Net expenditure	450.0	505.8

* In 1988/89 'land ownership and administration' was included with 'heritage' figures.
Sources: DAA (1989) and ATSIC Budget Branch

the period 1986–91. In Queensland, the Division of Aboriginal and Islander Advance of the Department of Family Services and Aboriginal and Islander Affairs spends A$36 million per annum. No doubt there are other State government contributions which we have not identified. In the Northern Territory, in particular, where Aborigines comprise 22 per cent of the total population, it is likely that a significant proportion of the Territory budget is expended on Aboriginal clients.

In the current absence of comprehensive information on overall expenditure on Aboriginal people by all levels of Australian government, one has to estimate. Such estimates require projections of Fisk's data on social security, combined with the figures in Tables 7.1 to 7.3 and some rough estimates of State, Territory and even local government expenditure (other than that already identified in Commonwealth special-purpose grants). It is probable that, all told in 1989/90, in the region of A$1,800 million was spent by Australian governments on Aboriginal people. This is clearly a very significant amount and represents expenditure in the region of A$7,200 per Aborigine. Much of this expenditure is not, of course, received directly by Aborigines, but is instead paid to organizations that provide goods and services to them. Another problem with such statistics is that they do not differentiate between negative funding on police, justice and welfare, and positive funding on, for example, post-primary education (Douglas and Dyall, 1985). Information collected on Aboriginal custody rates by the Royal Commission into Aboriginal Deaths in Custody suggests that Aboriginal people are over-represented in negative funding, while their low economic status (Altman, 1988) suggests that they are under-represented in positive funding.

In parallel with this proliferation of government programmes over recent years there has been a rapid increase in the self-identifying Aboriginal population. By the 1986 Census, the Aboriginal and Torres Strait Islander population had reached 228,000, or 1.4 per cent of the total Australian population of 16 million. It is estimated that the current (1991) Aboriginal population totals about 250,000. The high growth rate of the Aboriginal population (4.5 per cent per annum since 1971), which cannot be entirely explained in demographic terms, has led some to see Aboriginal identification, somewhat cynically, as a matter of convenience. However, it can also be seen as a renewed willingness of people of Aboriginal descent to identify as such, now that Aboriginal affairs policy is moving in a more positive direction.

Dependence and programme fragmentation: causes for concern?

The inclusion of Aborigines in the Australian welfare state has not been without its critics. Criticisms are generally of two types. The first points to the extent of Aboriginal dependence on welfare provisions. The second criticizes the proliferation of programmes now available in terms of fragmentation, duplication, overlap and inefficiency.

For a range of historical, structural and cultural reasons, Aboriginal people have remained largely outside the mainstream Australian economy. This is especially so in regions that are remote from labour markets, where a disproportionate number of Aborigines still live, but it is not restricted to Aborigines in these regions. Many Aborigines have therefore become long-term dependants on social security and other social programmes, which are only intended as short-term palliatives, and are that, for most Australians. This has resulted in concern about Aboriginal welfare dependence, which is by no means new. Indeed, such concern has been evident throughout the period of Aboriginal inclusion in the welfare state, and accounts in part for the rather gradual and sometimes quite contested nature of such inclusion. It also accounts for some specific policy and programme developments over recent years.

One such development is the Community Development Employment Projects (CDEP) scheme, initiated in 1977. This scheme was a direct reaction to the prospect of large-scale unemployment benefit payments in remote Aboriginal communities. Its proponents argued that these payments would be counter-productive in such communities, where much socially useful, if not economically viable, work could be undertaken. The CDEP scheme converts individual unemployment benefit entitlements into a grant to community councils for the purpose of undertaking community works, but only where communities seek such a conversion. Community members are, in effect, employed by their community councils to work for their unemployment benefit entitlements.

The CDEP scheme encountered many difficulties during the early years of its operation (Sanders, 1988). However, the DAA persisted in its support of the scheme and eventually received government backing for its major expansion. In 1987, when the Hawke Labor government announced a major re-working of Aboriginal employment programmes, the two issues which the federal government saw as 'paramount' were 'appalling levels of Aboriginal joblessness' and Aboriginal disillusionment with 'the current situation which does not extend beyond the receipt of a welfare payment for many' (Commonwealth of Australia, 1987: 2). The expansion of the CDEP scheme was a major component of the Aboriginal Employment Development Policy launched in 1987. The scheme now has more than 20,000 Aboriginal participants (including dependants) and accounts for over one-quarter of the Commonwealth Aboriginal Affairs Portfolio's budget. The recent rapid growth of the scheme clearly reflects concerns about Aboriginal welfare dependence, although it is arguable that the scheme itself is still a form of welfare provision.

The second line of criticism of Aboriginal inclusion in the welfare state relating to programme fragmentation includes a number of issues. One issue is the inter-relatedness and ultimate unity of

Aboriginal needs for land, better housing, jobs and so on. Programme interventions, it is argued, need to be co-ordinated and integrated if they are to be effective. A second issue is that programme fragmentation leads to interminable inter-governmental and inter-departmental debates about where responsibilities for servicing Aboriginal people lie. A third issue is that Aboriginal communities find themselves almost incessantly dealing with different government agencies and trying to steer some course through their differing rules and programme requirements. A fourth issue is that fragmentation is responsible for special Aboriginal programme expenditures being used as a substitute for, rather than a supplement to, normal government expenditure.

Though concerns about fragmentation of programmes and Aboriginal dependence on the welfare state are legitimate, they can also be overstated. From an historic perspective they overlook the extent to which it has in fact been inclusion in the fragmented array of welfare state programmes that has made additional resources available to Aborigines in recent years and has in the process underwritten many positive developments towards greater Aboriginal autonomy.

Social security entitlements have been especially important in providing a 'base level' of resources both to individuals and, if used collectively as they often have been, to Aboriginal community groups. This base level of social security income can be quite significant, and has provided Aborigines with a degree of economic independence which they did not enjoy even twenty years ago. Whether all this social security income will be maintained is currently a little uncertain, as from 1991 the federal government plans to abolish unemployment benefits and replace them with Newstart, a new employment and training scheme limited to twelve months' duration. How Newstart will be applied to Aboriginal and non-Aboriginal Australians who reside at remote locations where there are very limited labour market opportunities is a matter which will not be clarified for some time.

Access to social security income has also increased Aboriginal people's room for manoeuvre in relation to the many other organizational arms of the Australian welfare state. A basic income entitlement to fall back on is a potentially important strategic resource for Aborigines attempting to negotiate with the adminis-trators of other programmes intended for their benefit. It should also be noted that the sheer number of such programmes and adminis-trators has similarly increased Aboriginal people's room for manoeuvre. Some well-resourced and effective Aboriginal organizations may be able to obtain from one programme, department or level of government that which they cannot obtain under a slightly different guise from another. However, other Aborigines who lack such ability, but are in greater need, may miss out because they find the fragmented array of programmes intimidating and confusing.

There is no doubt that a large proportion of Aborigines are now dependent on the Australian welfare state, but they are not dependent on any one programme or any one agency, as they were under the exclusionary regime of Aboriginal policy described earlier. Escaping from dependence on the welfare state is a legitimate and important goal both for Aboriginal people and for Aboriginal affairs policy in future years, but just to have attained such dependence from the previous position of exclusion has been a major achievement of the last decades.

Changing patterns of inclusion: recent developments and future prospects

The pattern of Aboriginal inclusion in the Australian welfare state which has developed over recent years is not the only pattern which could exist. The present combination of specific Aboriginal assistance programmes, based on claims of disadvantage and special need, and Aboriginal inclusion in general government programmes is unlikely to be sustained for ever. It may be useful therefore to speculate on just how this pattern of inclusion is currently developing and how it may develop in the future.

In March 1990, the federal Aboriginal Affairs Portfolio was re-organized into an Aboriginal and Torres Strait Islander Commission (ATSIC). Impetus for this re-organization emerged from the disbanding in 1985 of the Commonwealth government's previous structure for elected Aboriginal representation, the National Aboriginal Conference, and reservations about the effectiveness of existing Aboriginal affairs administrative structures, including programme fragmentation and duplication. The model for the new Commission attempted to combine previously separate representational and administrative elements. The Commission is staffed by public servants, but its peak decision-making body consists of twenty Aboriginal Commissioners – seventeen Aboriginal-elected and three ministerially appointed. The Commission has a regional structure of 60 elected regional councils, each of which will play a role in determining the expenditure of Aboriginal assistance money within their region. Under the legislation this role is to apply to some extent not only to Commission expenditure, but also to the Commonwealth, and even State and Territory government, expenditure. This regional structure reflects the attempt to overcome programme fragmentation and lack of co-ordination. However, in reality the role of ATSIC regional councils is likely to be restricted primarily to Commission expenditure, and even within that, it will have to compete with central bureaucratic determination of 'national' priorities. Other federal departments are likely to guard their own abilities to determine their expenditure of Aboriginal assistance moneys, and State government agencies are certain to do so. Although in some ways appearing to strengthen the role of the Aboriginal Affairs Portfolio in Aboriginal assistance expenditure, we suggest that ATSIC will be unable to reverse the trend of the last twenty years towards greater mainstream welfare-state expenditure on Aboriginal assistance and proportionately lower Aboriginal Affairs Portfolio expenditure (see Table 7.1).

A more likely development in future years is, in our judgement, an even greater move towards mainstream provision. Perhaps this will mean a growing use of mainstream government departments to administer the now familiar special Aboriginal assistance programmes and a simultaneous further decline in the role of the programmes and expenditure within the Aboriginal Affairs Portfolio. Perhaps it will mean the disappearance of specific Aboriginal programmes and their incorporation within the general programmes of functionally defined government departments. The Northern Territory, which since 1978 has been granted a form of Territory self-government not unlike that of a State, has already moved in this direction, and some State governments are considering similar moves. Such a development will no doubt be highly emotive and keenly contested, as it could be compared with previous unsuccessful and culturally damaging assimilation policies. Aborigines may claim that their special needs and extreme disadvantage are once again being ignored by governments, if specific Aboriginal assistance programmes begin to disappear.

However, it may also be the case that even greater resources and expertise are available to Aborigines through inclusion in mainstream programmes than will ever be available to them through specific identified programmes. The social security example has supported this view in the past, and may well be emulated in other functional areas of government activity in the future. The likely outcome for Aboriginal community-based organizations, such as community councils, health services, legal services, and so on, is that they will increasingly draw their resources from government programmes directed not just at Aboriginal people, but at the community more generally. A shift to greater mainstream provision for Aborigines may also assist Aboriginal affairs policy-makers in their constant battle to ensure that special Aboriginal programme expenditure is used as a supplement to normal government expenditure rather than as a substitute. An additional argument is that substitution funding will never cease while there are separate budget allocations for Aboriginal people, and that the only means to overcome under-spending on Aboriginal citizens by functional departments is to move towards greater mainstreaming. Another possible advantage of greater mainstreaming is that expenditure on Aboriginal assistance will become less visible. In many depressed rural areas poor non-Aboriginal Australians already feel excluded from the range of programmes available to Aboriginal people. If the current (1991) rural recession deepens and is sustained, the risks of such a backlash will increase.

Despite our judgement that there is likely to be an even greater move to provision for Aboriginal people through mainstream welfare-state programmes and administrative structures, it is unlikely that separate programmes for Aboriginal people will disappear altogether in the foreseeable future. Special programmes may, however, change their present form. ATSIC may move away from programmes and expenditure defined primarily in functional terms (as in Table 7.3) towards programmes defined more in terms of Aboriginal community types and different Aboriginal circumstances. In the 1970s it was difficult for the federal government and the DAA to move in such a direction because of wariness about making distinctions between different Aborigines. So disreputable had the old proportional racial distinctions become, that to see anything other than a single, homogeneous Aboriginal population was unacceptable. Hence the DAA's programmes from 1972 basically mirrored the functional programme divisions of land, education, housing, health and employment and made few, if any, distinctions between Aboriginal circumstances. Over time, a new willingness has developed among Aboriginal affairs policy-makers to recognize the diversity of the circumstances of the Aboriginal population. This diversity does not inhere in the people themselves, as the old proportional distinctions implied, but is a result of differential European settlement in the various regions of Australia.

That differential settlement pattern is evident from Map 7.1. This compares Aboriginal and total populations for each of the States and

Territories of Australia as measured at the 1986 Census of population and housing; the figure also indicates the proportion of Aboriginal people living in major urban centres (with populations greater than 100,000), other urban centres (1,000 to 99,999), rural localities (200 to 999) and other rural areas. The differences are significant, with the Northern Territory standing out as still having a far higher proportion of Aborigines in the total population (22 per cent) and a far higher proportion of its Aboriginal population (69 per cent) living outside urban areas, compared to Australia-wide averages of 1.5 per cent and 34 per cent respectively. At the other extreme are heavily settled southeastern States where Aborigines are much more urbanized and their proportion of the total population much lower. In between come Queensland, Western Australia and South Australia. Each combines a southern or coastal region of fairly dense European settlement, where Aboriginal proportions of the total population and degree of urbanization are much like southeastern regions, and a more remote and sparsely populated hinterland, where Aboriginal proportions of the population and degree of rural residence resemble patterns in the Northern Territory.

During the 1980s, the Commonwealth Aboriginal Affairs Portfolio identified several categories of Aboriginal communities which reflect this differential pattern of settlement. These categories included:

A1 Discrete Aboriginal townships in remote areas often located on Aboriginal land and likely to be responsible for their own municipal-type services.

A2 Outstations and other small groups in remote areas linked to a resource organization in a nearby Aboriginal township or other regional centre.

B1 Aboriginal communities in State or Territory capital cities and major urban areas.

B2 Aboriginal communities whose members are residents of country towns mixed in with a predominantly non-Aboriginal population.

B3 Groups of Aborigines living at an identified location or camp site near or within an urban area and having different arrangements from the town for municipal services, or no such facilities at all.

In recent years the Aboriginal Affairs Portfolio has developed some programmes directed at specific community types such as the Accelerated Community Infrastructure Programme, Town Campers Assistance Programme and the Aboriginal Communities Development Programme. While such programmes are restricted to the general area of community infrastructure, they do attempt to cross strict functional

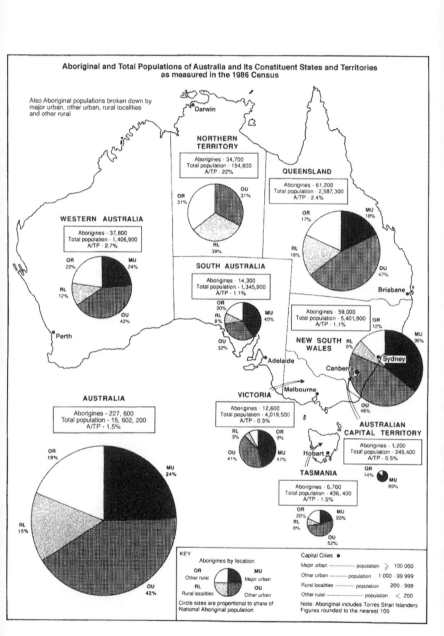

Aboriginal and Total Populations of Australia and its Constituent States and Territories as measured in the 1986 Census

Also Aboriginal populations broken down by major urban, other urban, rural localities and other rural

NORTHERN TERRITORY
Aborigines · 34,700
Total population · 154,800
A/TP · 22%
OR 31% | OU 31% | RL 38%

QUEENSLAND
Aborigines · 61,200
Total population · 2,587,300
A/TP · 2.4%
OR 17% | MU 18% | RL 18% | OU 47%

WESTERN AUSTRALIA
Aborigines · 37,800
Total population · 1,406,900
A/TP · 2.7%
OR 22% | MU 24% | RL 12% | OU 42%

SOUTH AUSTRALIA
Aborigines · 14,300
Total population · 1,345,900
A/TP · 1.1%
OR 20% | MU 40% | RL 8% | OU 32%

NEW SOUTH WALES
Aborigines · 59,000
Total population · 5,401,900
A/TP · 1.1%
OR 12% | RL 6% | MU 36% | OU 46%

AUSTRALIA
Aborigines · 227,600
Total population · 15,602,200
A/TP · 1.5%
OR 19% | MU 24% | RL 15% | OU 42%

VICTORIA
Aborigines · 12,600
Total population · 4,019,500
A/TP · 0.3%
RL 3% | OR 9% | OU 41% | MU 47%

AUSTRALIAN CAPITAL TERRITORY
Aborigines · 1,200
Total population · 249,400
A/TP · 0.5%
OR 14% | MU 86%

TASMANIA
Aborigines · 6,700
Total population · 436,400
A/TP · 1.5%
OR 20% | MU 20% | RL 8% | OU 52%

Darwin, Perth, Adelaide, Melbourne, Hobart, Brisbane, Sydney, Canberra

KEY
Aborigines by location
OR Other rural | MU Major urban
RL Rural localities | OU Other urban
Circle sizes are proportional to share of National Aboriginal population

Capital Cities ●
Major urban ———— population ≥ 100 000
Other urban ———— population 1 000 - 99 999
Rural localities ———— population 200 - 999
Other rural ———— population < 200

Note: Aboriginal includes Torres Strait Islanders
Figures rounded to the nearest 100

Map 7.1 Aboriginal and total populations of Australia and its constituent States and Territories as measured in the 1986 Census

demarcations between various types of services. In other instances functionally defined programmes such as the Aboriginal Employment Development Policy have been differently designed and applied in relation to different community types. All this may be hastened by the decentralization inherent in the establishment of 60 ATSIC regional councils, which are likely to focus strongly on the totality of community needs within their region rather than on the functional programme divisions of the bureaucracy.

Such a restructuring of programme orientation would be a recognition of the fact that extremely varied cultural forms seem highly likely to persist in different parts of Aboriginal Australia, ranging from modern hunter-gatherers in Arnhem Land to groups living in inner-city Sydney or Melbourne. These economic, political and social differences will require policy flexibility and diversity. There is no doubt that many Aboriginal people and their leaders living in communities in more settled Australia want full incorporation into the mainstream economy. Other Aboriginal people, living primarily in remote communities, are seeking to maintain important cultural and economic components of their traditional life-styles, and consequently reject total economic incorporation. There may be a need to develop a better policy balance between the goal of equality between Aboriginal and non-Aboriginal Australians on one hand, and the diverse circumstances and aspirations of the Aboriginal population on the other. Programme structures more clearly focused on different Aboriginal community types may provide a better means to achieve such a policy balance.

Postscript: the retreat of the welfare state, economic restructuring and the reduction of dependence

Throughout the 1980s, expenditure on Aboriginal welfare has increased in real per capita terms, despite the rapid growth of the self-identifying Aboriginal population and inflationary pressures. In Australia, as elsewhere in the developed world, there is now a general retreat of the welfare state. There are already some indications that federal government-forecasted budget outlays on Aboriginal assistance programmes from 1991/92 to 1993/94 may decline in real terms (Commonwealth Parliamentary Debates, House of Representatives, 11 October 1990: 2800), and the welfare state may be less generous in its provisions for Aboriginal people.

A related issue for the 1990s and beyond, is how Aboriginal people can break away from this dependence in times of economic restructuring. The Australian economy as a whole appears to be in relative decline and is struggling to restructure and improve its position in the world economy. Labour markets will be tight, and those, like many Aborigines, with few skills, little work experience and a locational disadvantage will have difficulty finding gainful employment. It is difficult, therefore, to see how the economic situation of Aboriginal people can be improved and their welfare dependence lessened in the immediate future.

REFERENCES

Altman, J. C. (1985) 'Aboriginal Employment in the Informal Sector: The Outstation Case', in D. Wade-Marshall and P. Loveday (eds) *Employment and Unemployment: A Collection of Papers*, Darwin: North Australia Research Unit.

— — (1988) 'Economic Status', in J. Jupp (ed.) *The Australian People: An Encyclopedia of the Nation, Its People and Their Origins*, Sydney: Angus & Robertson.

Andrews, S. (1964) *Social Service Benefits Still Denied to Aborigines*, Location unstated: Council for Aboriginal Rights, Coronation Press.

Australian Bureau of Statistics (1986) *Household Expenditure Survey, 1984, Australia: Summary of Results*, Canberra: Australian Bureau of Statistics.

Commonwealth of Australia (1987) *Aboriginal Employment Development Policy Statement, Policy Paper No. 1*, Canberra: Australian Government Publishing Service.

Crisp, L. F. (1970) *Australian National Government*, Melbourne: Longman Cheshire.

Department of Aboriginal Affairs (1987) *Aboriginal Statistics, 1986*, Canberra: Australian Government Publishing Service.

— — (1989) *Annual Report, 1988/89*, Canberra: Australian Government Publishing Service.

Department of Social Security (1960) 'Social Service Benefits and Aborigines', *Social Services Journal*, 13(1): 3.

Douglas, E. M. K. and Dyall, J. (1985) *Maori Under-development*, Wellington: Maori Economic Development Commission.

Fisk, E. K. (1985) *The Aboriginal Economy in Town and Country*, Sydney: Allen & Unwin.

House of Representatives Standing Committee on Aboriginal Affairs (1990) *Our Future Our Selves: Aboriginal and Torres Strait Islander Community Control, Management and Resources*, Canberra: Australian Government Publishing Service.

Mulvaney, D. J. and White, J. P. (eds) (1987) *Australians to 1788, Australians: A Historical Library*, vol. 1, Broadway, NSW: Fairfax, Syme & Weldon Associates.

Neville, A. O. (1947), *Australia's Coloured Minority: Its Place in the Community*, Sydney: Currawong Publishing Co.

Rowley, C. D. (1971a) *Outcasts in White Australia, Aboriginal Policy and Practice*, vol. 2, Canberra: Australian National University Press.

— — (1971b) *The Remote Aborigines, Aboriginal Policy and Practice*, vol. 3, Canberra: Australian National University Press.

Sanders, W. (1985) 'The Politics of Unemployment Benefits for Aborigines: Some Consequences of Economic Marginalization', in D. Wade-Marshall and P. Loveday (eds) *Employment and Unemployment: A Collection of Papers*, Darwin: North Australia Research Unit.

— — (1988) 'The CDEP Scheme: Bureaucratic Politics, Remote Community Politics and the Development of an Aboriginal Workfare Program', *Politics*, 23(1): 32–47.

Schapper, H. P. (1970) *Aboriginal Advancement to Integration: Conditions and Plans for Western Australia*, Canberra: Australian National University Press.

Smith, L. R. (1980) *The Aboriginal Population of Australia*, Canberra: Australian National University Press.

Stevens, F. (1974) *Aborigines in the Northern Territory Cattle Industry*, Canberra: Australian National University Press.

Whitlam, E. G. (1973) 'Aborigines and Society: Press Statement', *Australian Government Digest*, 1(2): 696–8.

8 Bi-culturalism, social policy and parallel development: the New Zealand/Maori experience

Ian Culpitt

[R]acism has operated in specific ways over the historical development of the welfare state, . . . with a certain consistency which makes the present relationship of 'race' to welfare not simply a post-war, or 'crisis' phenomenon but the emergence, in particularly harsh form, of a nationalism and racism intrinsic in the provision of welfare. . . . The nationalist and often racist assumptions of the welfare state come not only from 'above', but from 'below' too, in the labour and social reformist movements.

(Williams, 1987: 26)

The urgency with which ethnic and, in particular, indigenous ethnic claim rights are argued has been highlighted by successive reviews of separate welfare states (cf. Greenland, 1984; Mishra, 1984; Fleras, 1985; Jayasuriya, 1987; Williams, 1987; Pearson, 1989, 1990). These claim rights have dominated the moral high ground of the social policy debate in western welfare states. Australia, Canada and New Zealand, especially, have had to respond to a striking increase in public rhetoric about the unique welfare claims of their respective indigenous populations (cf. Pearson, 1984; Mullard, 1985). They all have indigenous populations that are economically disadvantaged with significantly greater levels of unemployment. So effective has been the political agitation for the satisfaction of indigenous treaty rights that the spectre of racial conflict has become a prominent feature of the demands for social justice 'as well as the most threatening to social stability in many advanced countries' (George and Wilding, 1985: 133; cf. Tauroa, 1982; Awatere, 1984; Spoonley *et al.*, 1984; Cleave, 1989).

THE POLITICAL DEBATE

The forceful and dramatic articulation of the special cultural and social needs of indigenous people represents the emergence of a unique set of political and moral claims for economic and social entitlement. These claims challenge the fundamental structures of welfare entitlement traditionally based on individual rights. There is little or no statutory provision for entitlements based on tribal or other group affiliations. New Zealand politics and social policy are critically involved in an ethnic resurgence of its Maori population. In this chapter Maori cultural revitalization will be related to the wider international debate about the benefits of privatized or contracted social services to indigenous people. We will need to consider how these policies about the provision of contracted social services shape the welfare debate and offer governments a particular policy instrument to redress economic and social disadvantage. The introduction of these policies provides a politically viable way for governments to respond to the unique claim rights of their indigenous citizens. In order to facilitate this development, a range of agreements will have to be developed with indigenous and ethnic groups about how they might develop some 'form of private agency' that would fulfil the purposes of administrative contracting.

UNIVERSAL WELFARE PROVISION AND ETHNIC PARTICULARISM

Public recognition of the power of the political and welfare claims of differing ethnic groups reflects the shift from an old welfare paradigm based upon religious and political codes of obligation to a new paradigm based upon the legitimacy of claim rights (Morris, 1986; Culpitt, 1992). This paradigm shift in welfare policy, from one based on paternalistic obligation to one which highlights the social legitimacy of welfare rights, has not only created a climate for the recognition of these indigenous claim rights but has also helped to direct and even fashion them. These ethnic welfare claims seek to redress economic inequality by promoting new administrative mechanisms that recognize the principle of group entitlement, which is clearly contrary to the usual pattern of legislated individual entitlement. As Outlaw has argued:

> According to the logic of 'ethnicity' as the paradigm for conceptualizing group differences and fashioning social policy to deal with them, the socially divisive effects of 'ethnic' differences

were to disappear in the social-cultural 'melting-pot' through assimilation, or according to the pluralists, ethnic identity would be mediated by principles of the body politic: all *individuals*, 'without regard to race, creed, color, or national origin', were to win their places in society on the basis of demonstrated achievement (i.e., merit). For both assimilationists and pluralists, *group* characteristics (ethnicity) were to have no play in the determination of merit; their legitimacy was restricted to the private sphere of 'culture'.

(1990: 60)

The old welfare paradigm depended upon established and intricate codes of social obligation. Its social validity depended on the normative power of the church and the state, because both 'institutions' combined to define 'appropriate' social work intervention with indigenous peoples. However, the normative power of the state and the church has been over-ridden and can no longer be sustained. This is particularly relevant to those societies where there was an assumption that ethnic peoples could and ought to be assimilated into the dominant political and social fabric (cf. Jackson, 1987: 5). A new welfare paradigm has emerged, based upon the political imperatives of social rights, which has confronted the implicit assumptions of the old professional welfare paradigm. This new paradigm, which supports the rights of indigenous people to be protected from overt intervention by professional and sometimes paternalistic groups, has exposed the 'hidden hand' behind the benign paternalism of a professional practice that is assimilationist.

The crumbling of this old paradigm, and the emergence of a welfare rights paradigm, followed, in part, from the numerous social challenges that have been thrown at statutory and conferred authority: such an intrinsic part of contemporary ethnic consciousness (cf. Delacampagne, 1990). The emergence of contemporary ethnic consciousness has been spurred by the recognition of these realizable claim rights. The formation of appropriate ethnic social policy involves not only a reconsideration of the basis for entitlement but also the decentralization of a bureaucratic and centrist welfare system and devolution to tribal authorities. In a New Zealand context, this attack on the 'legitimacy' of welfare services provided on the basis of individual entitlement represents an aspect of a general political argument about economic and structural inequalities and how they are perpetuated through institutionally racist administrative policies

(Brosnan and Hill, 1983; Poole, 1985; Trlin and Spoonley, 1987; *Ka Awatea*, 1991).

THE RHETORIC OF 'INSTITUTIONAL RACISM'

Institutional racism is typically defined as the patterning of social rules and laws and the structuring of customs and social practices which systematically produce inequalities in income, employment and access to education which actively disadvantage ethnic and indigenous groups (Jackson, 1987: 11). However, if this concept remains unexamined, and assumes the status of unchallenged 'truth', then this will allow 'policy developments ostensibly attempting to remedy racial inequalities, to remain at the level of rhetoric' (Williams, 1985: 323). The public 'noise' of this rhetoric about institutional racism is significant. It is easy for the white majority to query the legitimacy of these demands because they come couched in such high radical rhetoric reflecting absolute ideological prescription. However, the *Pakeha* (see Glossary, page 274) majority will have to bear the stridency in order to listen for the echoes of where substantive and not the illusions of procedural equality can be found (cf. Jayasuriya, 1987).

The stridency and 'noise' of the debate reinforces the rhetorical use of institutional racism and the belief that there are simple and self-evident solutions denied expression and action because of the destructive power of the 'white majority'. Most claims for the satisfaction of abridged or unfulfilled rights are couched in terms of high rhetoric simply in order to be heard. Negotiating the 'hidden shoals' of such rhetoric will require a rather less defensive reconsideration of the nature of institutional power. Further research is needed to define the scope of racial inequalities and to examine how current welfare policies perpetuate these inequalities (cf. Williams, 1985: 332). Consequently, public and academic discussion of these questions must tread a tortuous path between the traditional safety of detached reflection and analysis and the lure of rhetorical excess. It remains to be seen whether New Zealand is yet willing to hear the substantive claims of its indigenous Maori population or whether these claims will be rejected as 'unacceptable noise' (cf. Trlin and Spoonley, 1987: 209; Vasil, 1988).

Contemporary Maori politics is grounded again in a mood of protest that has steadily grown over the past 25 years (cf. Hohepa, 1978; Awatere, 1984; Fisher, 1984; Greenland, 1984; Walker, 1984, 1987). The main strategic objective of such protest was to attack the 'system' which was seen to be dominated by *Pakeha* policies and organizations (cf. Armstrong, 1987). Together with the whole-hearted rejection of 'mono-cultural' welfare family and child protection policies, this protest coalesced around the demand for the restoration of the rights and resources which it is believed the Treaty of Waitangi guaranteed in 1840 under the second or *Tino Rangatiratanga* clause which guaranteed, in the Maori version, protection of their traditional chieftainship status (cf. Hazlehurst, 1988: 56; *Puao-Te-Ata-Tu*, Ministerial Advisory Committee, 1986; Orange, 1987). The English version of the second clause of the Treaty indicates that the Maori relinquished sovereignty but the Maori version included the words *'Tino rangatiratanga'* which means chieftainship or sovereignty.

IWI DEVELOPMENT AND ISSUES OF CLASS?

Implicit in renewed demands to 'honour the Treaty' are elements of another important discussion about the relationship of class to ethnicity. Not unexpectedly, the political and social implications of this topical argument are crucial to New Zealand social policy (Trlin and Spoonley, 1987: 200). The debate ranges from those who would argue that the impetus for *iwi* development cuts across and transcends class lines to those who would see the ethnic renaissance of *iwi* development as antithetical to the priority of a class-based analysis (cf. Outlaw, 1990, for an excellent international discussion of these issues). While accepting that 'racism is built into the dominant ideology', Green concludes that sexual divisions within society, and the issues relating to the political claims of indigenous ethnic groups, 'have a deeper and structurally more persistent basis in the history and evolution of all societies than do relations of class' (1986: 61; cf. Balibar, 1990). On the other hand, Webster suggests another point of view, and argues that as a consequence:

> of the unchallenged identification of Maori culture with intuitive conceptions of race, language, spirit, or tradition, rather than with the contemporary Maori as working-class participants in a specific history, spokespersons of the Maori renaissance find themselves committed to several contradictions which debilitate or mislead the progressive potential of the movement. The ethnic ideology thus serves the interests of those enforcing the continuity of this specific history rather than the interests of the majority of Maori themselves – whose control over their own means of production, over what they produce, and over their own personal lives

continues to be eroded despite their continual struggle. In this, their history has been no different from the *Pakeha* working class, although their losses have been more recent and remain bitterly fresh in a more remembered history.

(1989: 54–5)

This contention that the class aspects of Maori alienation are being subsumed by the current social resurgence is supported by a range of arguments which suggest that the talents of the Maori elite engaged in the Waitangi Tribunal claims are being deflected from the more pressing issues of unemployment, health, justice, and education (Levine, 1989: 21). These writers would agree that privatization is a smokescreen that obscures the priorities of the working class. The rigid application of a class-based social analysis depends upon the assumption of the thesis of a dominant ideology. The dominance of a *Pakeha* conception of citizenship and welfare entitlement is being substantially undermined by this ethnic Maori renaissance.

There are contradictory aspects to capitalism that are able to be exploited by an ethnic revival focused on social rights. Specifically, that nation-states 'are always caught in the ''contradiction'' between simultaneous tendencies towards universalism and particularism' (Balibar, 1990: 283). Any renewed attempt to argue for the presumed advantages of a universal system of welfare entitlement will have to deal with Ignatieff's reproof that 'the more evident our common needs as a species become, the more brutal becomes the human insistence on the claims of difference' (1984: 130). Capitalism has changed in response to working-class conflict (namely, in the welfare state) and is deeply affected by the struggles of ethnic movements which articulate demands for autonomy and political respect that cannot be totally explained by class-based analysis. Turner concludes his broad discussion of the emergence of citizenship and social rights in other countries by suggesting that because capitalism is based upon respect for certain autonomous 'rights', it 'creates the condition for its own demise and transcendence in that the conditions for socialism grow out of the struggle for genuine rights in capitalism' (1986: 142).

The struggle for ethnic rights represented by the growth of *iwi* development creates the conditions for that 'transcendence' in that the issues in the bi-culturalism debate are not easily subsumed under the analysis of either the left or the right. It is apparent that any analysis of New Zealand's social relations must respond to the fact that the 'reciprocally juxtaposed relationship between Maori and

Pakeha' has become a 'major institutional feature of those social relations' (cf. Green, 1986: 61). It can be argued that the class aspects of Maori disadvantage may have greater leverage expressed within the context of *iwi* development and claims about the moral power of the Treaty. Certainly, the argument that contrasts ethnic relations and the Maori renaissance with politics (see Webster above) does not reflect the substance of Maori scholarship. On the contrary, it argues that the Maori cultural renaissance represents a search to merge politics and culture.

> Metaphorically speaking, ethnicity provides the paradigm within which political actors work, culture provides the raw materials, and ideology the political fare. The 'new' political ideology emerging from this metamorphosis, though largely a secularized version of primordial symbols and beliefs, is one in which the sacred also persists. There is a link made with a redeemed past and these notions of tradition are seen to transcend the conventions of everyday life. The aphorism 'old symbols, new meanings' pithily expresses the phenomenon of going into the future by way of reclaiming the past. The key symbol between past and future in the present context is land.
>
> (Greenland, 1984: 88)

Current proposals for *iwi* development contend that racial inequalities were inextricably built into the society through the existing patterns of welfare services (cf. Puketapu, 1982; Fleras, 1985; Williams, 1987). This impetus towards *iwi* development has coincided with other arguments favouring the devolution and deregulation of centrally administered services as well as with the range of opinion in support of the privatization of welfare services (cf. Lightman, 1987). The philosophy of *Tu Tangata*, adopted by the original Department of Maori Affairs, rejected the power or relevance to the *iwi* of a centrally planned bureaucracy. Where, however, there is reason for caution is in the pattern and structure of the intervening and intermediary bureaucracies that a transition to full *iwi* authority will require. Turner, interestingly, comes to a defence of the bureaucracy. He argues for a reformist stance and contends that, where:

> there is a commitment to providing a service on an egalitarian basis to a mass of the population there will inevitably be an increase in officialdom, bureaucracy and public control. . . .

Equality demands standards, standards require regulation and regulation can be most effectively achieved by bureaucracy.

(1986: 138)

Ironically, but perhaps not surprisingly, it is this bureaucracy which has been seen to be the major social mechanism of an institutionally racist welfare system. The failure of this welfare bureaucracy has led to the arguments for *iwi* development (cf. Maori Advisory Unit, 1985; *Puao-Te-Ata-Tu*, Ministerial Advisory Committee, 1986). Social policy in New Zealand is involved in an important social experiment. Although initially couched in terms of welfare entitlement, the economic claims of New Zealand's indigenous people have broadened to wider issues of social injustice and even political autonomy. The articulation of indigenous claims against the injustices of the dominant *Pakeha* society have increasingly turned towards and been allied with an analysis of the Maori version of the Treaty of Waitangi that emphasizes the inherent sovereignty of the *iwi*. These political arguments frame the debate, so that the *Pakeha* majority can no longer comfortably expect that these claims can be contained within the same welfare structure and enactments. As with Canada, which has enacted separate welfare legislation for their Canadian Indian nations, so too will New Zealand have to face a similar political imperative to recognize the implicit and explicit claims for self-determination. These claims are couched in terms which are explicitly aimed at returning some form of sovereignty to the Maori which, it is argued, was guaranteed by the Treaty (cf. Awatere, 1984).

IWI DEVELOPMENT AND GROUP ENTITLEMENTS FOR WELFARE

The western tradition is one of justice for individuals and not justice for groups. Thurow suggests that there is a fundamental dilemma, in that:

at the same time ours is an age of group consciousness. Economic minorities argue that group parity is a fundamental component of economic justice and that an optimum distribution of income consists of more than an optimum distribution of income across individuals. . . . However it is done – each society is going to have to establish rules as to when it will recognise groups' demands for parity and when it will resist those demands.

(1981: 147–8)

This dilemma is also highlighted by Outlaw (1990: 78), who similarly argues that 'a new historical conjuncture has been reached', because the fundamental issues that surround justice for ethnic people demand a recognition of the central political viability of group citizenship as well as the traditional individual basis for citizenship which was so integral to the welfare state.

The *iwi* are, within their own *kaupapa* (philosophy) and *kawa* (protocol), elitist. Tribal authorities have distinct patterns of authority that reside in the *kaumatua* (elders) (cf. Cleave, 1989). There are contradictions in a policy that attempts to respect the legitimacy of the *iwi* when the general pattern of welfare policy is still universalist and individualistic. The full implication of group entitlement through the *iwi* is yet to be explored. As the debate continues, the loss of the Maori Affairs bureaucracy and its translation into the Iwi Transition Agency may yet reflect the political pessimism of Webster, Levine and others. The full effects of the privatization of former publicly owned utilities and industries upon this question of *iwi* development is unclear. Boston has argued that

> The whole saga over privatisation and the status of Maori land claims is full of ironies. For example, one of the results of the corporatisation program has not merely been the intensification of Maori efforts to secure justice and to retrieve their lands, but also the strengthening of their legislative capacity to achieve such an objective. This is because the Waitangi Tribunal will for the first time have the power to direct, rather than simply recommend, that land be returned to Maori ownership. Without doubt this is a major victory for the Maori community. . . . The other irony is that a reform program based upon the principles of market liberalism, individualism, private ownership and the clear specification of property rights has been derailed, or at least slowed in its tracks, by an ethnic minority with a very different set of values – communalism, collective ownership etc.
>
> (1988: 81)

This attack on the present individualistic pattern of service delivery also reflects, and is influenced by, the emergence of an ethnic underclass that is anti-statist and not just anti-racist. Cleave develops a concept of 'negative sovereignty' to explain the importance of 'a general anti-state mood in the Maori intelligentsia that is comparable . . . to the way existentialists perceived the modern state and the impossibility of [personal] freedom therein' (1989: 27), although Pearson (1989) and Webster (1989) would argue with the proposition that the Maori intelligentsia can be essentially equated with an underclass. Consequently, any assessment of the political nature of racism and ethnic entitlement must reflect these two aspects of claims for sovereignty under Article 2 of the Treaty of Waitangi. It has become fashionable amongst sections of the *Pakeha* media to reject the radicalism of Maori rhetoric and to treat it as if it were solely the fulminations of the disaffected. But it is important to recognize that this rhetoric expresses real grievances that will not be assuaged by policies that blindly reinforce the normative power of the *Pakeha* majority (cf. Walker, 1987).

RETRIBALIZATION

These claim rights are reflected by the 'retribalization' of purpose and demand that respective *iwi* express in their unique claims for entitlement. Consequently, ethnically sensitive social policies that adopt the legitimate and unique welfare claim rights of *iwi* reveal the vacuity of any contemporary social analysis that continues to base social policies upon concepts of universality and common entitlement. The *iwi* are not homogeneous, and will continue to resist welfare policies that do not represent the matrix of social difference that they encapsulate. In New Zealand these claims are inexorably linked to the provisions of the Treaty of Waitangi and specific questions about economic justice and equity of land ownership (cf. McHugh (1988) for a discussion about the legal basis for Maori claims under the Treaty against the crown; cf. Fitzpatrick (1990) for an international discussion about law and racism). Article 2 of the Treaty (*tino rangatiratanga*) establishes the primacy of the *iwi* as elites within a constitutional framework. Such formal recognition does not confirm them as elites, for they assumed this status long before the signing of the Treaty. It would be a mistake for governments, when developing purchase of service contracting approaches to welfare administration, to consider the *iwi* as a 'quasi-agency', or as a local administrator of centrist policy. The pattern of welfare administration and social policy that *iwi* development will require is unique in that *tino rangatiratanga* establishes the principle of *iwi* 'sovereignty'. As we have seen, this is elitist, and an understanding of the implications of this development cannot be subsumed in social analysis that is construed by a corporate managerial ethos or one that reflects socialist or social democratic analysis of the position of the working class.

This political step towards *iwi* development and *iwi* authority has exciting and far-reaching implications that stretch beyond the typical issues of welfare entitlement and the stigmatization of welfare recipients. These questions must now be addressed in terms of the sovereignty claims of the Treaty of Waitangi. Questions of bi-cultural social justice are no longer just about the procedural aspects of the structure and pattern of future welfare entitlement. They cannot be addressed by current patterns of mandated welfare entitlement, because the particular issues of Maori sovereignty involve the fundamental future political structure of New Zealand and how that political power will be exercised. The force of this political challenge provides New Zealand with a unique opportunity to re-examine those justifications for welfare that depended initially upon the legitimacy of individual claim rights.

One of the crucial political and managerial issues that advanced industrial societies confront is deciding whether it should or should not intervene in the market either to protect or to raise group incomes (Thurow, 1981: 148). Bullivant argues that pluralist societies 'may evolve through time, singly or in combination, to exclude those considered ineligible for group or associative rewards' (1984: 107). New Zealand public and social policy has traditionally denied the group, or tribal, claims of the *iwi* and has treated their members as individual units of an homogenous Maori minority. While it might still be argued that there is a Maori consciousness, that 'consciousness' is increasingly considered to be a *Pakeha* construction of a cultural reality that is in fact complex and diverse. The *iwi* have different histories – their *whakapapa* and *waiata* are different – and they cannot be completely subsumed as 'Maori' because they belong to more fundamental tribal groups from which they take their 'essence'. Emergence of the political power of *iwi* coincides with the proliferation of other interest-group claim rights that reflect aspects of the change to a welfare-rights paradigm with a consequent democratization of welfare. For the *iwi* this democratization of welfare and the ascendance of a welfare-rights paradigm has provided a welcome opportunity to reject those welfare policies which are based upon implicit attitudes of assimilation. It can also be argued that this process of retribalization represents the denial of any process of *embourgeoisement*, although there are some writers (cf. Jayasuriya, 1987; Cleave, 1989) who argue that unless that happens ethnic minorities will continue to be marginal to the dominant economic and social process. Cleave also contends that the concept of 'retribalization' must also be applied to the gangs who represent aspects of an ethnic underclass. He states that:

In fact the lumpen proletariat, the ragged underclass that so worried Marx and Engels, is probably better defined in Aotearoa than in most countries. Here it is criminal, dishevelled, bestial and all of the pejoratives ascribed to it by Marx but with the very significant difference that it is organised on a consistent historical basis as an ethno-underclass. Aotearoa is approaching its fourth generation of tattooed gang members. Practices like gang rape are not novelties, they are ritual constants.

(1989: 27)

It might be contended that any claims for the legitimacy of the 'negative sovereignty' of an ethnic underclass, so deliberately opposed to the state, should not merit serious consideration. While the gangs are equally antagonistic to the *mana* – the spiritual essence – of the *iwi*, as well as to the state, their claims for *iwi* status, in effect for a retribalization, will have to be considered. The fact of their existence and endurability across generations challenges both the obvious inequities of the rejected *Pakeha* economic system and the failure of the *iwi* to exercise control. They are not transitional outcast social organizations in the sense that these provide for a rite of passage from rebellion and alienation to more traditional and less lawless social participation. They represent the stolid face of a form of ethnic resistance, a cultural 'no' that gathers strength as the mana of *Te Tiriti O Waitangi* is flouted by legislation in respect of lands and fisheries that represents a *Pakeha* system of resource usage (cf. Awatere, 1984; Greenland, 1984; Walker, 1987). New Zealand as a nation-state 'remains as an enigma to many Maoris' (Levine and Vasil, 1985: 163). Because the dominant *Pakeha* state retains the statutory power to dominate and even suppress Maori political activity, it will inevitably be seen as their collective instrument. New Zealand is little different from other western welfare states which have resisted the political attempts of indigenous people and their demands that 'social justice be applied to *groups* and that ''justice'' be measured by *results* not opportunities' (Outlaw, 1990: 60). However, because it is not regarded as part of the organic offshoot of their own communities – which encapsulate fundamental group values – the New Zealand state, which cannot be 'one people', will have to develop a reasoned and equitable response to the *tino rangatiratanga* clause of the Treaty. In other countries, such as Australia and Canada where there are not such clear legal and social treaty rights, similar claims are asserted for welfare entitlement based upon respect for the primacy of the family or tribe over individual rights.

The force of the moral argument that impels the current political trend towards separate tribal identity and purpose in New Zealand is overwhelming. A parallel pattern of social services would redress some of this cultural imbalance. Without these new welfare structures, and the creation of new economic initiatives for targeted employment, New Zealand is likely to witness increasing inter-cultural conflict (Fisher, 1984: 41). For these reasons there are aspects of purchase of service contracting that offer the *iwi* and the New Zealand government a model for the provision of decentralized welfare services. This model provides the possibility to redress economic and social grievance and establish group entitlement through contracts with the *iwi*. Adoption of purchase of service mechanisms would reinforce the *iwi* rather than perpetuate patterns of 'welfare dependency' that focus on individual entitlement. This would provide a more effective means to recognize distinctive individual or group claims to services.

The practical dilemma for ethnic minorities is that establishing ethnically separate agencies which express the values and social protocols of a minority culture has often resulted in their being regarded as marginal to other dominant systems of welfare. The great danger about accepting the legitimacy of such separate claim rights is that the welfare bureaucracies will resist and are unable, from existing budgets, to meet the fiscal consequences that would result from the substantial satisfaction of such claims. Accepting the political validity of such claim rights also provokes intense discomfort in the general population that still expects that some moral blame and stigma be attached to those who are welfare recipients. Despite the extent of welfare provision, 'welfare' as a social concept has never been able to rise above a subtle pejorative rhetoric that first developed in response to the Elizabethan Poor Laws where it was stated that 'the relief given to the poor be limited and precarious'. For the *iwi* in New Zealand realization of these issues reinforces the importance of the Treaty of Waitangi as a constitutional and legal defence of these welfare-claim rights.

SERVICE CONTRACTING/PRIVATIZATION

Emergence of these claim rights has, interestingly, coincided with the development of proposals for purchase of service contracting. Contracted social services can contribute significant integrated functions when 'regional, ethnic or racial identities are highly salient (perhaps even on a par with national identities) by providing a structure and purpose for such group organizations' (Gronbjerg, 1983: 774; Reid and Gundlach, 1983: 48). The typical patterns of social and political consensus on how to respond to the issues of social and economic inequality are curiously disappearing at precisely the same time as there is a growth in market-driven economic policy which tends to generate a more unequal distribution of income (cf. Thurow: 1981). It is an ironic observation that those sectors of the population that are arguably the most socially marginal and politically disenfranchised are those that have, in New Zealand at least, an opportunity to use the rhetoric of privatization to debate the merits of parallel development and further their own ethnic purpose. This conjunction is further support for the view that previous sustaining metaphors of welfare will not adequately explain options for current ethnic social policy (cf. Outlaw, 1990).

Any conceptualization of social policy that seeks to promote an integrative or systemic response to problems such as unemployment, physical and mental health and criminality can be dismissed as assimilationist. A new synthesis of the debate about ethnically sensitive welfare policy will have to respond to this challenge to recast former individually based national or state patterns of welfare allocation and distribution. The depth of distrust is such that the institutionally racist aspects of existing welfare dispensations will need to be identified and challenged before a structural *rapprochement* can be established. Arguments about 'unity in diversity' disguise the implicit social control in those political assumptions which respects the cultural value of diversity while maintaining control through the statutory welfare bureaucracies.

The welfare state was founded on the criteria of the 'citizenship of shared entitlement' (Ignatieff, 1989), but the metamorphosis of citizenship obligations into welfare rights compels a drastic reconsideration of the traditional arguments for universal entitlement which were based on citizenship rights. Resolving the intrinsic residual dilemmas created by the old welfare dispensation, based on universal entitlement, requires that the legitimate welfare claims of separate ethnic groups be given priority. Neo-conservative welfare policies are grounded in respect for difference and individuality. It is no longer possible to subsume ethnic differences and simply to argue for the superiority of a system of general or universal social services based solely on the yardstick of citizenship. There are more basic cultural patterns of allegiance, affiliation, identity and commonality that challenge traditional justifications for entitlement established solely on the grounds of citizenship.

It is frequently argued that citizenship rights for primordial indigenous groups can only be fully safeguarded through the development of a contracted and private welfare system. It is also argued that the formation of ethnic social services is the only way to preserve a political system that protects the citizenship values of 'mutual, but specific, rights and obligations' (Gronbjerg, 1983: 785). This challenges the usual community-based 'welfare orthodoxies' which have always presumed that the state is the only possible or viable 'guardian' of these citizenship rights and responsibilities. Privately contracted welfare systems have the ability to sustain and augment the essential voluntary nature of the welfare interchange and can preserve group identity and purpose (cf. Gronbjerg, 1983; Reid and Gundlach, 1983; Taylor-Gooby, 1986). Governments can therefore use purchase of service contracting procedures to support the development of intermediary and specific cultural arrangements which can arbitrate the 'otherwise impersonal link between the individual and the state' (Gronbjerg, 1983: 784). A pattern of contracted social services can usefully distribute resources to specific 'hard-to-reach or controversial groups . . . whom government is obligated to serve but where fear or stigma inhibits utilization' (Kramer, 1983: 423).

These issues can no longer be addressed by recourse to the dominant arguments of either the 'old left' or the 'new right' (cf. Goodin, 1988; Outlaw, 1990). Although aspects of resurgent Maori radicalism have inevitably turned to the revolutionary rhetoric of the 'old left', the rhetoric of the 'new right' is also reflected in the corresponding white 'backlash' (cf. Spoonley *et al.*, 1984). At the core of these issues about welfare claim rights and legislative patterns of entitlement are political questions about citizenship. Implicit in the practice of the 'helping professions' is a fundamental assumption that intervention will lead to greater public participation and to a resolution of the factors that have either caused social dislocation or perhaps even political alienation. There are important conceptual difficulties in continuing to advocate ethnic social policies that implicitly or explicitly aim to 'elevate' to fuller citizenship those seen on whatever criteria or basis of need. Intervention to resolve, overcome, banish, diminish, lessen or remove demonstrated need stumbles over the nature of the 'act' itself. Especially in cross-cultural practice, where the professional is from the dominant culture, the client or client-group can be ascribed a 'lesser status' in that greater moral or social power to sanction deviance or non-compliance is accorded to the donor or giver role, even when it is mediated through professional practice.

The old patterns of paternalistic professionalism will no longer work. Neither will the bewildering range of democratized claim rights be able to provide solutions because they do not fundamentally accept any over-arching conceptualization of mutual obligation: only a strident demand. Two differing aspects of this stridency are seen in the relationships of indigenous New Zealanders with the *Pakeha*. The first is what Cleave calls '*hamama Pakeha*' or 'shouting down the *Pakeha*', which reflects aspects of the challenge of the *haka* where the intimidation is in the 'noise' and the confrontation face to face with those defined as enemies (1989: 21). The second, and more significant, is his observation that these strident welfare claim rights, and associated demands for new culturally appropriate administrative processes, reflect a deeper political concern. This is the belief that the 'noise' of these strident claims 'does not so much cry out for recognition as for redefinition' (Cleave, 1989: 70). The debate is not about accommodation nor is it simply a clamour to be 'heard'. Rather, it is about the establishment of a new, culturally affirmative administrative process. The old welfare consensus, while paternalistic, operated on the assumption of the implied obligation required of the donor, the giver or the 'professional altruist'. The tenor of Maori welfare imperatives suggests the importance of redrafting the welfare consensus to reflect a new theory of 'need-reciprocity'; of seeking political and social validation for a new theory of social obligation.

As we have seen, validation of *iwi* claim rights threatens commonplace assumptions about citizenship and the 'rights of the individual'. The practical administrative dilemma is that to assume that a welfare system can be developed that operates at an individual level for *Pakehas* and at a group, ethnically sensitive level, for Maoris ignores the fact that not all Maoris share common values and that *Pakeha* working-class values may be more similar to Maori group consciousness than middle-class *Pakeha* values. While specific aspects of culturally appropriate social policies have especial significance to New Zealand, the relevance of purchase of service contracting mechanisms in promoting the betterment of indigenous peoples in other countries is often alluded to (cf. Gronbjerg, 1982, 1983; McCready, 1986; Taylor-Gooby, 1986). Such mechanisms will provide only the illusion of separate identity unless they are accompanied by levels of financial support that will sustain the partnership and fulfil the provisions of the Treaty of Waitangi. However, any further analysis of these issues must consider how needs assessments can be determined that are not seen to be inherently paternalistic or racist.

SOCIAL RESEARCH: THE MYTH OF OBJECTIVITY

Excessive or culturally insensitive research leads to the kind of 'cultural heart-sickness' expressed by many Maori with respect to most *Pakeha* research findings and methodologies. A commonplace attitude amongst Maoris in New Zealand, as it is in other social-welfare-state countries with indigenous populations, like Canada and Australia, is that empirical research undertaken simply for the sake of knowing is pointless (Poole, 1985; Stokes, 1985; Williams, 1987). This is not to imply that knowledge is pointless, but that research information which does not lead to remedial action is damaging to the *mana* of those studied. The core of this criticism is that the stance of 'detached observer' is not tenable (Rein, 1977). Acknowledging this poses the problem of the legitimacy and status of 'culturally appropriate' research to those in power, because the empirical models may be more efficient politically in gaining access to economic resources.

For Maori, as for other indigenous peoples, their concept of 'knowledge' implies a knowing of the whole and not the parts (Greenland, 1984; New Zealand, 1988). The concept is related to that which builds up the power and the ability of the *iwi* to prosper and not to categorization or division which, it is assumed, leads to destruction of the *mana* of the *iwi*. Typical of such arguments is Stokes (1985), who suggests that there is an increasing awareness in the Maori world that they have been used as 'guinea pigs' for academic research that promotes *Pakeha* 'expertise' about *taonga* which are intrinsic to their *mana*. She further argues that despite the use of Maori researchers, public respect for the research is usually accorded to the *Pakehas* who collate the research. The most common feature of indigenous criticism of empirical research is that it is not sufficiently practical. Similar constraints are voiced about participant observation research, because often the observer takes no responsibility for the 'consequences' of the research which highlights specific problems. No matter what the research method, ethical issues will face researchers who undertake to study the social needs of indigenous people. Some researchers argue that it is imperative that antecedent commitments be given about how social resources will be re-allocated once the needs are uncovered or clarified by the research (Olson, 1980: 126). There is a growing ethnic 'voice' that needs assessments and other forms of research that do not result in effective action are pernicious (Jayasuriya, 1985, 1987). Siegel, for example, goes so far as to suggest that if no prior 'commitment to planning or restructuring programmes in accordance with those needs [is] identified, no useful purpose is served by an assessment effort' (Siegel *et al.*, 1978: 225). As Stokes concludes descriptive research that 'only reinforces that which is already known is also useless. Isolation of issues with no practical advice or guidelines is damaging to the *mana* of the *iwi*' (1985: 3–4).

Consequently, culturally appropriate needs assessments for respective *iwi* will need to review the nature of appropriate social science research and how it should be used so as to respect the *mana* of the *iwi*, and also to consider whether such a focus might restrict effective resource application. There are difficulties in reconciling social policies which respect the *mana* of *iwi* with the current ethos which supports the privatization and contracting of social services. There is an awkward 'fit' between the business concepts of quality assurance, accountability and cost effectiveness and the *mana* of the *iwi*. Analysis of the Treaty of Waitangi, particularly the partnership clause (*Tino rangatiratanga*), suggests no model for the articulation of culturally appropriate forms of needs assessment. This raises a very important series of questions about how the Treaty can be used to support political initiatives for culturally appropriate research and needs assessment. There are therefore clear distinctions to be drawn between what the Treaty actually said and how it is ideologically construed to support current social-policy analysis. The ideological use of the Treaty of Waitangi poses particular problems in New Zealand, but the issue of social policy analysis, construed individually, has wider significance. As the Royal Commission on Social Policy concluded, New Zealand is a long way from the position where 'respect for individual or group privacy, culture or spirituality [is] recognized in the design, implementation and end use of monitoring and assessment' (New Zealand, 1988, vol. 11: 841). Not only must culturally appropriate methods of needs assessment and analysis be established, but the issue will also have to be addressed about the over-research, or over-evaluation of small, community-based schemes in which Maori figure highly.

As has been suggested earlier, specific patterns and policies of social services are determined by the particular forms and processes of needs analysis used to justify policy decisions about welfare allocation and service delivery. These prior patterns of needs analysis and assessment are thought to be the linchpin of structural racism (cf. Puketapu, 1982; Cody, 1988). The concept of structural racism refers to the prevalence of ethnic minorities in health, crime and employment statistics and to the generally mono-cultural patterns of research used to explain these statistical phenomena (cf. Brosnan and Hill, 1983; Cleave, 1989). The existence and political challenge of an ethnic underclass is avoided by treating all of these indices of crime, illhealth and unemployment as individual phenomena (*Ka Awatea*, 1991). When the group aspect of these statistics is highlighted it is usually only reflected negatively (Trlin and Spoonley, 1987: 194); for example, in the media, coverage of gangs or the health of Maori women where the incidence of smoking is reported in depth. The process of stigmatization of welfare recipients, so destructive of individual autonomy and self-respect, are magnified when the stigmatization is directed to a group. When that group is also an ethnic minority it becomes institutional racism (Jackson, 1987: 10–11). The collective shame of the group is imprisoning, and negatively reinforces group solidarity.

CULTURAL NEEDS ASSESSMENT AND INSTITUTIONAL RACISM

Determining needs assessments that accurately reflect the perceptions of ethnic minorities requires the recognition that most of the research or assessment stances that have an implicit or explicit expert orientation run the risk of being rejected as institutionally racist. Threads of institutional racism can also be seen in those political arguments that reject the validity of ethnic culture and want only to discuss ethnicity as 'a concept whose importance must be assessed along with other potentially significant factors'. Gelfand and Fandetti argue that:

> the use of traditional models or paradigms of ethnic cultures is fraught with serious problems [and that] . . . the tendency is to slip into reification of ethnic culture, that is, to attribute an independent or real existence to a mental creation.

> (1986: 542)

Although such arguments are addressed to an American cultural situation, the arguments are representative of the 'dominant ideology' that seeks to explain the complexity of social life as representative of a 'paramount reality' (cf. Spoonley *et al.*, 1984; Webster, 1989). It is important to realize that this analysis is structured in such a way that the forms and patterns of intellectual discourse are determinedly mono-cultural and how they can be institutionally racist. Williams (1987) discusses the same pattern of mono-cultural social theory and its effects upon an independent black analysis. Aspects of contemporary variables such as 'modernization, urbanization and industrialization' which Gelfand and Fandetti use to argue that ethnic culture ought better to be described as ethnicity, and therefore only as a part of class-based sociological analysis, are the context for the rhetoric of institutional racism and not an argument against it. It will be no solution in New Zealand to attempt to undermine the ethnic cultural claims of *iwi* by assuming that they are reifications – by definition only a mental creation!

Understanding the political use of the concept of institutional racism has never been easy for those bureaucrats imbued with service ideals. The contention of an institutionally racist analysis that there are racist assumptions at the core of what was considered a benevolent welfare system challenges one of the most fundamental assumptions of the welfare state that there could be 'unity in diversity'. This denial that racism could be part of the welfare state arose from its intrinsic assumptions, from its commitment to 'empiricism, its idealism, its inherent nationalism, and its belief in the Welfare State as integrative, universalist and redistributive' (Williams, 1987: 7).

Commenting on a Report to the Australian government, entitled *Don't Settle for Less: A Review of Migrant and Multicultural Programmes and Services* (1986), Jayasuriya challenges the Report's implicit policy of cultural pluralism. He argues that cultural pluralism 'is not a respect for difference so much as it is a reworking of the old liberal assumptions about "access and equity" and "equality of opportunity"' (1987: 494). The assimilationist views implicit in cultural pluralism offer no clear grounds on which to establish the legitimacy of cultural and ethnic differences. Jayasuriya saw the attempts to demolish the myth of 'ethnic inequality' and substitute for it the myth of 'liberal equality' as mischievous and pernicious; merely reinforcing an institutionally racist analysis. Given the disproportionately high statistics of Maori incarceration, admission to psychiatric hospitals, unemployment and the proportion of beneficiaries, the fact of ethnic inequality can no longer be rationalized away. Brosnan and Hill's New Zealand research into employment and occupational data confirmed 'that Maoris are more likely to be found in the lower paid occupations within each group'

(1983: 54) The Ministerial Report, *Ka Awatea* (1991), highlights the most stark analysis of Maori disadvantage in relation to absolute levels of Maori unemployment. It states that while 'Maori comprised 8 per cent of the total NZ labour force in 1990, they currently make up 20.5 per cent of all unemployed people (in the March quarter, 1990)' (1991: 30). These figures are worsening as the economic recession bites even deeper. As Jayasuriya has argued (particularly in respect of Australia but with international application):

> there is no doubt that in general on account of the minority status, ethnic groups tend in varying degrees to be stigmatized, oppressed, subject to prejudice and stereotyping and denied or discriminated against in their access to the valued resources in society.
>
> (1987: 490)

There is, therefore, a profound structural inequality in New Zealand in which the disadvantages of institutional racism are allied with the growing barriers of class deprivation. Recent changes in the pattern of New Zealand's welfare state move it away from the principle of universality towards targeted assistance. Within this is enshrined the neo-conservative principle of 'user-pays' which establishes a welfare system within which movement across 'class' lines is increasingly difficult. The principal 'beneficiaries' of this new system are the indigenous Maori population, whose rates of unemployment have skyrocketed! The dominant political ideology and the policy options are heedless of the social costs of this structured pattern of unemployment. This reflects some common aspects with other similar countries. Jayasuriya, for example, states that 'ethnic minorities in Australia suffer the double disadvantage of ethnicity and class deprivations' (1987: 494; see also Outlaw, 1990). Cleave (1989) also discusses how these twin aspects of ethnicity and class deprivation have in fact led to the establishment of a permanent underclass in New Zealand society.

INEQUALITY: PROCEDURAL OR SUBSTANTIVE?

The concept of minority status is crucial to an understanding of economic and social disadvantage and the discriminatory process. Often associated with this concept of minority status is that of social justice. However, instead of dealing with the actual aspects of structural inequality that minority status confers, most western social-service bureaucracies tend to use the concept of justice in a much more limited sense. It is seen as a principle against which the processes and outcomes of practical policies can be evaluated. Defining social justice narrowly in this way establishes and maintains institutionally racist policies. There are, in New Zealand, complex questions about constitutional power that will need to be addressed if the wider questions of social justice and partnership under the Treaty of Waitangi are to be considered. As Cleave argues:

> It is important to be conscious ... that the Crown is one contractual partner and the tribes are the other; the partners are not the Maori on the one hand and the state on the other. There is no constitutional concept of the *Pakeha* as partner. Maori as well as *Pakeha* pay taxes and they pay those taxes to account for state rather than ethnic spending. The Crown, as it has evolved and is evolving has incurred and will continue to incur debt and when the state is asked or required to pay that debt the respective roles of Maori, the Crown the state and the tribes should be clarified. ... This is not to question the validity of the debt but to ensure that ethnic ascription of blame, that is Maori blame of non-Maori or non-Maori of Maori, for the debt does not replace the correct constitutional arguments.

> (1989: 53)

As has been suggested earlier, the Treaty of Waitangi *per se* is not a sufficient guide to understanding the concept of institutional racism. It is those ideologies shaped by the various perceptions of the Treaty of Waitangi that have used the concept of institutional racism as a motif for seeking redress of far more than the constitutional framework of the Treaty of Waitangi envisaged. This is not to deny the urgency of these claims but to suggest that the argument for them cannot solely depend upon constitutional arguments. It is easier, as Jayasuriya (1987) argues, to talk about procedural equality with respect to the distribution of social services rather than resolve the more difficult concept of substantive equality. Procedural equality refers to the process of decision-making rather than the content of those decisions. Procedural equality is essentially a principle of equality of treatment and not one of distribution. Substantive equality considers the issues of distributive justice. The principle of substantive equality contends that, by definition, a rationale must be made for the justification of any inequality of distribution. Equality in the sense of substantive equality can only be understood in terms of an underlying theory of justice.

Existing policies and patterns of needs assessment with respect to the Maori community often follow the line of procedural equality (cf.

Jackson's 1987 survey of the geography of racism for an international discussion of these issues). No adequate attempt has yet been made in New Zealand to deal with the substantive issues of equality, although it can be argued that the proceedings of the Waitangi Tribunal and recent legal action against the crown by tribes has begun to address these issues of substantive equality (cf. Mahuta, 1987). If the concept of procedural equality is linked, in the delivery of social services, with that of universality (which maintains that common human needs require common solutions), a major anomaly is created in the construction of social policy (cf. *Ka Awatea*, 1991). This highlights the endurability of social structures that establish institutional racism. To maintain that 'common human needs require common remedies' is 'somewhat awkward because for a policy based on the tenets of cultural pluralism it provides no justifiable grounds for differentiation on the grounds of cultural and ethnic "differences"' (Jayasuriya, 1987: 494).

If substantive equality is equated with equality of outcome, then claims for a fair share in the rewards of distributive justice find little echo in current New Zealand public policy with respect to the Maori community. Jayasuriya and others would argue that most needs assessments of ethnic minorities follow the metaphor of procedural equality. This is the pre-eminent assumption of liberal social-policy analysis which holds that 'access and equality' and equality of opportunity are the main goals. Because of these 'liberal' assumptions, there is no commitment to address equality of outcomes or to arrive at a different assessment of needs on that basis. Almost ineluctably the liberal mind-set of the Enlightenment, with its claim to universality, comprehensiveness and consistency, can only conceive of those excluded or alienated from this political dispensation as somehow qualitatively different. As Fitzpatrick argues this:

> imperative, this terrifying consistency puts the . . . colonized beyond the liberal equation of universal freedom and equality by rendering them in racist terms as qualitatively different. . . . Racism was, in short, basic to the creation of liberalism and the identity of the European.
>
> (1990: 249)

Although the liberal welfare system in New Zealand has operated humanely to recognize the variableness of individual talent and achievement, there is a reluctance to extend these 'laudable concepts so that they respond more specifically to the problem of inequalities between Maori and *Pakeha*' (Levine and Vasil, 1985: 165). This reluctance to admit the legitimacy of difference is being challenged in New Zealand by pressure for more appropriate political response to the issues highlighted in the Treaty of Waitangi. It will no longer suffice to consider these issues as if they are essentially administrative. A more fundamental debate about patterns of political power has been enjoined which will not be assuaged by revamping a *Pakeha* centrist welfare system. Maori speak often on *marae* about the urgency of their collective assumption that partnership under the Treaty of Waitangi requires a much greater recognition of the rights of Maori autonomy with respect to the delivery of social services. How that claim and right to autonomy will be answered in the future is one of the most crucial current issues facing New Zealand. Particularly because division of opinion between Maori and *Pakeha* with respect to the Treaty of Waitangi, particularly the implications for social services, is great.

SOCIAL-SERVICE DELIVERY: THE 'FAILURE OF PROFESSIONALISM'

Substantive arguments against professionalism are developed in the landmark report, *Puao-Te-Ata-Tu* (Ministerial Advisory Committee, 1986). Social services which are founded primarily upon the assumptions that result from a commitment to individual practice such as casework are regarded by the authors of the *Puao-Te-Ata-Tu* Report as totally antithetical to a Maori perspective, which is based upon tribal, community and family allegiances (cf. Puketapu, 1982; New Zealand Planning Council Document, 1984; Fleras, 1985). The traditional nature of the dominant social services places clients in a weakened position. These services 'are by their nature individualized on the basis of client need and professional judgement' (Martin, 1982: 189). In this respect, the development of social welfare systems as state administered sets of exchanges appear alienating and destructive to people whose culture places the responsibility for caring not on to specific individuals but on to the *whanau* itself. There is thus a great desire to return to a voluntaristic set of assumptions about the nature of social caring which do not allow for these processes of altruism and support to be divorced from the central cultural myths of mutual obligation. Models of need assessment based upon an awareness of the subjectivity (or perhaps the spirituality) of those being studied are likely to be more useful to

Maori communities. Reviewing the fisheries claim of the Muriwhenua before the High Court, Levine argues:

> [the] Maori view of the sea is tinged with reverence for creation
> and the sanctity of nature, feelings of kinship with other life forms,
> and an ethic of reciprocity. . . . These values . . . bound an ethnic
> category and oppose the theme of economic rationality.
>
> (1989: 18)

The embracing and enfolding concepts of '*aroha* and *awhina*' are
intrinsically part of the daily life of the Maori and there is, within
Maoridom, an explicit rejection of professionalism with respect to the
delivery of social services. As the *Puao-Te-Ata-Tu* Report (1986)
discusses, there had always been a profound suspicion among
different *whanau, hapu* and *iwi* that the process of social casework
was an implicit instrument of cultural alienation. The fundamental
individual or dyadic nature of the casework 'exchange' was rejected
in favour of the more integrative patterning of group communication.
The philosophy of *tu tangata*, which the Maori Affairs Department
embraced, challenged the taken-for-granted, centrist assumptions
about the professional delivery of welfare services. It marked the first
substantial attack on the traditional bias towards centralized
bureaucratic welfarism in New Zealand, particularly in respect of
the delivery of social services to the Maori community. These
initiatives have played their part in arousing the development of an
iwi approach to social-service allocation and delivery. The current
policy direction of the New Zealand Maori Affairs Department,
outlined in the recent report *He Tirohanga Rangapu* (1988), is a
further experimental step towards a position where Maori and Pacific
Island communities are directly funded through contracts to groups,
in order to deliver appropriate services and to make relevant and
culturally appropriate needs assessments that respect the different
kawa and *kaupapa* of *iwi*.

TU TANGATA: REDISCOVERY OF ADMINISTRATIVE MANA

A detailed history of this unique administrative experiment is outside
the scope of this study, but a brief survey will highlight its importance
in redressing the paternalism endemic in welfare bureaucracies that
offer services to minority groups (cf. Trlin and Spoonley, 1987: 205–
6; Hazlehurst, 1988: 56). *Tu tangata* forced the community officers to
look to the *iwi* for their working mandate and not to the government.

It was a brave experiment that sought a complete reversal of the usual patterns of bureaucratic legitimacy. As Fleras has written, 'the relationship between the Maori and government . . . has evolved from one based on dependency, paternalism, and control to one grounded on the principles of development, partnership and self determination' (1985: 39). The clients of Maori Affairs, prior to the introduction of *tu tangata*, regarded it as the legitimate arm of other stronger and potentially more socially controlling agencies such as Justice, Police, and Social Welfare. The implication of *tu tangata* was two-fold. On the one hand it was a general catch cry to all Maoridom to 'stand tall', and on the other a specific challenge to the Department's Community Officers to go back to the *marae* of the respective *iwi* to recognize 'the stance of the people'.

> This stance reflected the viewpoint that Maori people did not require 'welfare', which had strong connotations of dependency, but rather preferred to move along a path of self-help, self sufficiency . . . with a strong emphasis on the 'development' ethic. Community development as opposed to individual casework became an important focus.
>
> (New Zealand Planning Council Document, 1984: 34)

The degree of community consultation that this change implied gave fresh impetus to the administrative notions of accountability and transparency. Learning the specific needs requirements of *iwi*, *hapu* and *whanau* meant that the *marae*, and not the bureaucrat's office, became the appropriate focus for dialogue. In essence, this returned some administrative power back to the local community and used the age-old forum of the *marae* for the enunciation of future plans, the disbursement of grant money and the creation of new systems of fiscal accountability. This process became known as the *kokiri* process. *Tu tangata* was an explicit attempt to return management to the people and sought a complete reversal of typical bureaucratic patterns of pyramidal decision-making. Assessment of the success of such wide-ranging social experiments is difficult. *Tu tangata* was not a social experiment in the sense that it could be 'undone'. *Tu tangata* was not just about the structure of Maori welfare administration. Nor was it simply a bureaucratic mechanism for greater community involvement and participation. It was the first enabling step in the ongoing political reappraisal of the relationship between Maori and *Pakeha*. It generated a great deal of troubled debate about the proper meaning of words and phrases such as *Pakeha*, *tangata whenua* and *tauiwi* (cf. Spoonley *et al.*, 1984; Pearson, 1989, 1990).

There is no doubt that *tu tangata* helped to spark the process of *iwi* development. However, the processes of devolution, laudable in principle, can mask cut-backs in the level of direct funding and the necessary support required to maintain these initiatives (cf. Levine and Vasil, 1985: 46). The procedural process of *tu tangata*, as an example of a devolutionary strategy, reveals some of the dilemmas implicit in the current paradigm of welfare rights. The stronger *iwi* have clearly responded to these initiatives. Those *iwi* that have been slower to seize these initiatives are less able to respond in such a climate of devolution. The stronger and more forceful *iwi* will garner more resources than the weaker. There can be no return to the dependency of the former Maori Affairs Department, but it is possible to argue that a 'competitive market' for *iwi* in respect of social welfare entitlement creates a different set of difficulties. Governments can 'legitimately' withdraw from the debate and point to the cultural imperatives of local decision-making. But that devolution of power can hide an abandonment of state responsibility and funding.

Commenting on social policies that have attempted to validate multi-culturalism in Australia, Jayasuriya suggests that emphasis on the particular aspects of cultural differences within a concept of 'unity in diversity' may not create new political or economic challenges to the existing patterns of wealth and power. Enhancing ethnic self-esteem through respect for diversity, while maintaining the normative power of existing political and social bureaucracies, serves to diminish challenges to the entrenched power of the nation-state. Policies that emphasize multi-culturalism and pluralism may just reflect the maintenance of the *status quo* (cf. Bullivant, 1984). Rejecting multi-culturalism for migrants, Jayasuriya comments:

> In other words, the legitimate aspirations of migrants as members of minority groups for a fair share of the resources and social rewards of society at large – the public domain of life – may be impeded by an excessive and exclusive concern with the 'privatised' aspects of social and cultural life.

> (1985: 26)

Arguments about respect for ethnic difference that do not address existing patterns of wealth distribution perpetuate structural inequality. For this reason, the ethnic political debate in New Zealand has been construed as bi-cultural. This sharpens the political agenda which would otherwise be avoided by a pluralist or multi-cultural focus.

PUAO-TE-ATA-TU: THE NEW/OLD TRIBAL 'VOICE'

Puao-Te-Ata-Tu literally means daybreak, or perhaps dawn. The fundamental revision of appropriate ethnic administration that the *Tu Tangata* scheme had set in motion was the precursor to this report. The issue of Maori–*Pakeha* relations was no longer just the preserve of the Department of Maori Affairs. A uniquely rapid reappraisal of all government departments was in train. It is clear that *tu tangata* was not an experiment, but a cultural watershed that coincided with a revision of historical scholarship regarding the Treaty of Waitangi (cf. Orange, 1987). The Advisory Committee that wrote *Puao-Te-Ata-Tu* noted that there are major gaps in the understandings between Maori, Pacific Island and *Pakeha* in this country with respect to the nature of the provision of social services. They wrote that:

> [a major] thrust of this report is the support of positive initiatives to enable Maori people to care for their own, we have concerned ourselves with operating mechanisms. The Committee suggests that the Social Welfare Commission has overall responsibility for the direction of national budgets for institutions, family and community development projects and for diversionary pro-grammes for channelling negative spending into positive invest-ments. The funds released as a result of diversionary policies should be targeted for work, training and cultural activities through tribal authorities.

> (1986: 37)

Commenting on these recommendations, the Report suggests that the government should work through Maori tribal authorities to allocate funds for positive initiatives and outcomes with respect to the *Maatua whangai* programme. The report argues that *iwi* are committed 'to the attainment of socio-economic parity' between Maori and *Pakeha* by the provision of social and economic resources to meet Maori needs on Maori terms (cf. *Puao-Te-Ata-Tu*, Note 139: 36). A recent Maori economic development commission has also recognized that negative funding, or funding that compounds negative outcomes for Maori people – dependency, unemployment, institutionalization and so on – should be redeployed. The *Puao-Te-Ata-Tu* Report also recognized that transfer of funds from negative spending to positive initiatives would, for a time, increase total government expenditure and new programmes would have to be established. But it assumed that double funding would reduce and finally cease, as permanent savings would occur through reductions in admission to institutions and unemployment benefits (*Puao-Te-Ata-Tu*, Note 140: 36–7).

Endorsement was also given to the initiatives of some tribal authorities to undertake entrepreneurial activities such as tourism and small business schemes. The Report argued that such entrepreneurial schemes capitalize on the considerable flair that Maori have for such schemes, and that it is a way of moving away from economic dependency. The Report was careful to suggest that it is 'essential for authorities to invest in urban as well as in rural areas if they are to give the economic leadership for which young Maori people are looking' (*Puao-Te-Ata-Tu*, Note 141: 370. The Report suggested that the Social Welfare Commission would allocate funds to committees – district and institution, in consultation with tribal authorities, having regard to needs and priorities. The committees would be accountable for the operation of the budgets and for monitoring the projects. This is to ensure that initiatives and positive development are soundly based and in the interests of both child and family (*Puao-Te-Ata-Tu*, Note 143: 37).

The substantive orientation of this particular report was that major new funding mechanisms must be found in order that the Maori community rediscover its sense of purpose within the matrix of social services. This resulted in an explicit recommendation – 11 (d) – 'that funds be allocated to Social Welfare District Offices with a high Maori population to provide some remuneration to Maori elders who provide assistance to social welfare staff in dealing with Maori clients' (*Puao-Te-Ata-Tu*, 1986: 41). The tenor of this report reflects some of the aspects of distributive social justice which, as Jayasuriya (1987) outlined, required that an appropriate ethnic social system justify the reasons for the continuation of procedural inequality. As Cody suggests, 'the onus [is] on the department to establish that the iwi could not meet the demands of the people effectively' (1988, IV: 240). Purchase of service contracting offers one possible way in which a new administrative mechanism may be developed to meet this precise range of needs. The nature of such an administrative mechanism will need to be negotiated with each separate *iwi* so that an appropriate social organization could be developed that would represent the welfare rights claims of separate *iwi*.

IWI DEVELOPMENT: TRIBAL INITIATIVES TOWARDS AUTONOMY

As the Royal Commission on Social Policy outlines, *iwi* development, through the devolution of responsibilities for resources to *iwi* authorities, has considerable support from Maori people (New Zealand, 1988, 111(1): 177). It is important to note that consideration of needs assessment with respect to *iwi* authorities is not essentially different from the notion of community-based or consumer-based needs assessment approaches. It is often easy to assume that there is something intrinsically different about *iwi* development which sets it apart from the overall demand by communities for accountability with respect to assessment of needs and the structures of service delivery required.

While questions of *iwi* development and needs assessment have uniquely different features, it is important to note the similarity with other community- and consumer-based initiatives. For instance, how Maori society considers and determines the appropriateness of various policies involves dramatically 'different understandings of the principles of participation, transparency and representativeness' (Royal Commission on Social Policy, 1988, 11: 848). Maori policy-making is a complex matter, with the intersecting demands for feedback and accountability between all the levels of *whanau, hapu, iwi* and even tribal *rununga* requiring a considerable amount of time. To come to an adequate needs assessment of a particular *iwi* requires a detailed understanding of the protocols of that particular *iwi* with respect to the pattern of devolved decision-making. Culturally appropriate needs assessments must reflect the *mana* of the *marae* and the processes of *korero*, and not the application of static and expert research models. Transparency with respect to the way that decisions are made and information transmitted within the context of these particular protocols raises major difficulties for *iwi* at the present time. Urbanization, and the consequent dispersement of *hapu* and *iwi*, have also created major difficulties for the gathering of statistical information in a culturally appropriate way. The particular nature of representativeness within Maori society poses other issues and questions for needs assessments. Being *tangata whenua* gives additional status to certain peoples in particular areas. The representation of needs assessment, based upon simple majority calculations, does not adequately take into account the fact that even if *tangata whenua* are numerically fewer they have claims that the *tangata kainga* (Maori people who have come to reside in a particular district) do not have.

Adequate needs assessments of *iwi* authorities must also recognize the different nature of leadership. There are leaders who are well versed in addressing the contemporary aspects of Maori development, but there is also significance and *mana* of the *kaumatua* group, the leaders and elders upon whom the spirit and integrity of the *iwi* depend. And as the Royal Commission Report indicates (1988, 11: 851), while they would not necessarily be expected to take an active role in all aspects of policy-making, their evaluation and support of a policy is crucial for its effective implementation. Needs assessments, therefore, which do not take account of the attitude and responses of the *kaumatua* group will be flawed.

However, the social welfare exchange, far from being a social mechanism for the creation of citizenship (Weale, 1983), is in New Zealand, particularly with relevance to the Maori and Pacific Island Communities, a mechanism for cultural oppression and destruction. The rejection of state-administered social-welfare systems is almost complete. The provisions of social welfare services, as we have discussed, are seen as hidden forms of institutional racism which are subtle attempts to coerce people into a definition of citizenship that is more appropriate to the dominant culture.

MAATUA WHANGAI: TRIBAL INITIATIVES?

It was argued in the Report of the Administrative Review Committee, 1987, entitled *Performance and Efficiency in the Department of Social Welfare*, that 'social policies and structures used to date have not worked for Maori people', and that:

> the most appropriate vehicle for dealing with these problems was through the development of self-determination in terms of Maori control over social policy resources relating to Maori people. The creation of uniquely Maori solutions to the problems was advocated. Avoidance of dependency in terms of control of resources and service was considered by the *hui* to be very important. It was also recognized that the Maori community themselves need to address some of the causes of the problems they are facing.

(1987: 77)

Establishment of the *Maatua Whangai* programme marked an attempt to deliver social services in a culturally appropriate way and is the first direct effort to give *mana* to tribal authorities. However, as we have seen, the *iwi* are very different, and they therefore confront different issues. No understanding of the problems as well as the successes of the scheme have yet been detailed, and the differing patterns of social-service delivery within *Maatua Whangai* need to be more clearly understood. As the *Puao-Te-Ata-Tu* report outlined, the Maori people initially expected much of the *Maatua Whangai* programme but have, however, been substantially disappointed (1986: 23).

The *Maatua Whangai* programme actively sought to assist *iwi* to restore their tribal networks. However, as Puketapu (1982) outlined, success for Maori involved economic development as well as tribal authority and identity. The actual moneys given to the establishment of such a radically different programme were meagre, and this undermined the programme's *mana*. In part, such initiatives stumble over the problems that the welfare bureaucracy experiences in translating different cultural expectations into existing patterns of welfare entitlement. Arguments in favour of purchase of service contracting already canvassed, which draw their inspiration from market models of effectiveness and efficiency, simply will have no place with respect to the redrafting of purchase of service contracting arrangements with Maori *iwi*.

As the Ministerial Report, *Ka Awatea*, argues:

> From a Maori perspective separation of the policy and operations functions is certainly not in keeping with the holistic image of the Maori. Maori would say that 'it is like having two arms waving in the breeze without a body. Similarly, one leg attached to a tree, and the other to a fence post, each without a body, are good reason for the legs to wither away'.

(1991: 74)

The challenge, managerially and administratively, that such redrafting of social policy requires may well put New Zealand back in the forefront of social-welfare legislation for the future. It is hard to overestimate the importance that these particular mechanisms may be able to demonstrate in relationship, for example, to the Treaty of Waitangi and to the establishment of culturally based services which are sensitive and as free of institutional racism as possible. The unintended consequence of the recent (1984–90) Labour government's privatization strategy has been to highlight the complex problems associated with the ownership of Maori land and the patterns of inter-generational rights and responsibilities. There is the potential for divisive and damaging race relations if the expectations now generated by these policies are not accepted as legitimately part of the political equation. As Boston states, 'astute political management will be required during the next few years to navigate New Zealand successfully through the uncharted waters which lie ahead' (1988: 85). How separate *iwi* are to create or re-organize their tribal authorities into some form of private agency administratively for the sake of purchasing services in order to substantiate programmes such as *Kohanga Reo* and *Maatua Whangai* will need careful consideration. It is vital for New Zealand's race relations that new patterns of service delivery be found.

CULTURALLY SENSITIVE MANAGEMENT: REDEFINITION, NOT RECOGNITION

Developing new and culturally appropriate policy initiatives that may lead towards some resolution of these issues also requires an administrative stance of experimentation and discovery. Development of social policy and consequent legislation is frequently 'bedevilled' by the internal dilemma of bureaucratic management which seeks to 'get it right' at any one point in time and then to impose that normative definition of needs and needs assessment universally across the population. Administrative policy that emphasizes experimentation and discovery is more useful than that which seeks certain answers. What is urgently required is the development of a social policy and welfare analysis which recognizes difference. To accomplish this will require especially a managerial practice that acknowledges difference within the framework of a structural analysis of bi-culturalism. It will be important for managers not to recast these issues and take the easy option of procedural rather than substantive equality (cf. Jayasuriya, 1987). It is respect for people, particularly their cultural self-image and dignity, that is the rationale for contracted welfare schemes which respect these cultural preferences. As Goodin argues, 'policymakers must therefore always give dignity and self-respect precedence over preference and choices in case of conflict' (1982: 246).

Variable definitions of what constitutes a private agency in a cultural context will need to be developed, and new funding mechanisms will need to be created. The *iwi* cannot be construed as a quasi-agency representing the authority of a centrally planned welfare bureaucracy. Contracting with *iwi* can be seen to be part of a practical recognition of sovereignty, and the administrative procedures used to facilitate a contracting approach must recognize the status of the *iwi*. Consideration will need to be given to the specific pattern of systems of monitoring and evaluation that would need to be developed with respect to the culturally appropriate programmes. For example, how would governments therefore deal with single supplier service providers? How would the principle of competition which is intrinsic to the argument for purchase of service contracting be appropriately established with respect to Maori communities?

An important question about policy planning and implementation arises given the use of 'universal' funding criteria. If all grants are equally applied, then there will be no encouragement for local initiative in determining the validity and appropriateness of needs assessment techniques. Such funding criteria do not allow for the development of an argument for selected or targeted funding, nor for a process of experimentation. For example, not all issues of needs assessment can be generalized across respective *iwi*. Consequently, some local variations can be expected and different needs assessments will inevitably be made. A stated objective of differentially seeding moneys to local projects would allow for a mosaic of research that would enhance an overall commitment to a planning and experimental model. The ease with which smaller schemes can be assessed represents a major problem that Maori have in dealing with bureaucratic rationality that concentrates solely on issues of manageability.

The New Zealand Royal Commission on Social Policy Report (1988) highlighted the administrative anomaly in which many of the larger expenditure categories of major social-service departments and agencies were not evaluated while there was an excessive evaluation of the smaller, community-based schemes. This poses particular problems for the auditing and monitoring functioning of government. Many of the *iwi* do not have the range of managerial skills necessary to administer grant or contract money according to established bureaucratic processes. There are common tribal assumptions and group integrative processes that regard money as a resource and means of social solidarity. It will consequently be used according to tribally determined need which will not necessarily accord with the implicit reasons for which it was initially granted. *Pakeha* New Zealand will need to understand the spiritual dimension of 'well-being' and the vital importance of this notion in Maori communities. Most of the typical models of needs assessments and systems of monitoring and evaluation are materialist when they embrace the empiricist tradition. They reflect assumptions that needs are essentially practical and measurable and that they have little to do with values. For example, if the state bureaucracies are to be ethnically responsive, they will need to understand the function of *koha* (the gift of money), and how the rituals that surround it give practical expression to tribal identity. *Koha* is money which is offered to the host tribal group in exchange for hospitality and as an acknowledgement of the tribal *mana*. Totally new models of social-service delivery, administration, monitoring and evaluation will need to be developed. Gronbjerg suggests that private philanthropy with the concept of voluntaristic exchange is:

> especially important in a pluralistic society where ethnicity, region, race and religion provide salient identities. A private welfare system that bases its services on the distinctive needs of existing groups would fill a number of needs. Such a system would maintain group identity and purpose in an otherwise undifferentiated mass. It would provide an intermediary structure for negotiating the otherwise impersonal link between the individual and the state.

(1983: 784)

McCready, substantiating these particular points, has stated that 'it is relatively easy to observe that people often feel most attuned to their own religious and/or cultural backgrounds being reinforced by the social services they receive' (1986: 255). It is possible that purchase of service contracts might provide potentially advantageous mechanisms for the administration of existing cultural programmes, such as *Kohanga Reo* and *Maatua Whangai*. But, as has already been argued, such contracting must go beyond the provision of procedural equality. Contracts with *iwi* can be a mechanism for the redress of the sovereignty issues as well as establishing the basis for group claims for welfare entitlement.

Analysis of the issues surrounding culturally appropriate needs assessment and allocation of resources suggests that the task can never be separated entirely from the process. Using the rhetoric of the Maori the 'head' is not 'talking to the heart'. It is organizationally 'absurd' for managers to resist openly the political imperatives of an analysis of institutional racism and to dismiss the challenge as rhetorical and therefore unacceptable. But there are factors of open compliance and hidden defiance whereby public statements do not represent private action. The 'public face' of the manager who 'recognizes the legitimacy' of ethnic claims may nevertheless give way to the 'private face' of the corporate or organizational bureaucrat who is required to defend the protocols of the organization for efficiency or choice in the allocation of budgetary resources. The nature of the debate is such that any managerial stance which denies the fact of political imperatives avoids the heart of the issue. But managers will also need to consider the practical consequence of hidden defiance that acts at a more complex level to reinforce precisely the racist assumptions that are being challenged. Because of the politically and personally sensitive aspects of these questions, research is necessarily tentative. There are other limits to what policy responses can be made that occur because of limited resources, ambiguity of objectives, internal organizational competition and political will (Minogue, 1983: 73). As Minogue says, 'issues of policy analysis do not lend themselves to neutral, value-free, scientific analysis' (1983: 82–3; cf. Rein and White, 1977). The power of the political process to cut across strategic planning initiatives and impose an 'arbitrary will' can lead to institutional paralysis. Yet discrete analysis of issues and problems can move the responses of senior policy-makers away from opportunism towards experimentation and discovery.

PARALLEL DEVELOPMENT AND SOCIAL-SERVICE DELIVERY: A WAY AHEAD?

In New Zealand, the rhetoric of assimilation was distilled into the catch-cry of *He iwi kotahi tatou* – 'we are one people' – (Hohepa, 1978; cf. Jackson, 1987; Outlaw, 1990). The Maori renaissance has achieved a recognition of difference and separation in the cultural sense, and the assumption of cultural unity has been thoroughly discredited. It will, however, be a source of continuing political difficulty to establish how that separation will be effected both politically and economically. While ethnic cultural loyalties can complement national feelings of trust and identity, they can also threaten them. New Zealand sits uneasily with the challenge of the Maori renaissance and still collectively fears cultural diversity. For the modern nation-state to function effectively and independently, a power structure must exist which compels allegiance to common legal, social and economic norms. The pivotal question, what constitutional and political changes are required in order to give expression to *tino rangatiratanga*, will remain? Bi-culturalism and sovereignty are established as the nodal points for the arguments about substantive justice.

What is at stake in this debate is not accommodation but structural change in order to redress historical and current grievances that have become culturally reified into the political demand for substantive power – which must inevitably mean control of economic resources. There is a developing body of Maori opinion that seeks parallel development within the Department of Social Welfare in relation to resource allocation, service delivery, executive monitoring of programme effectiveness, and needs assessment. This may well require restructuring the Department of Social Welfare into ethnically separate organizations. Senior managers in the Department of Social Welfare will have to respond to the body of Maori opinion which seeks, under Article 2 of the Treaty of Waitangi, greater access to funding resources that would establish parallel and even separate social-service delivery systems. The Maori community is no longer willing to accept 'passively their status as a subjugated minority'. Vasil argues that they:

> are being increasingly politicised and it is only a matter of time before they are roused and mobilised for political action. They no longer have expectations; now they demand the fulfilment of their rights and entitlements. And these are derived by them from their status as the *tangata whenua*, of which they now have an acute consciousness, and the Treaty of Waitangi. To them the Treaty of Waitangi confers on them certain legal rights and their indigenousness a special status.

> (1988: 21)

One important implication of the Treaty of Waitangi is that social services which help to 'define' a community should be understood and mediated by the *iwi* themselves. As has been argued earlier the *iwi* are elites, and acceptance of *iwi* authority is also an acceptance of a separatist and anti-bureaucratic bias. The clear implication in all of this is that New Zealand may well need to devolve the existing welfare bureaucracy into more than one Social Welfare Department. While this is a radical policy direction, it can be argued that it has already been implicitly endorsed through the acceptance of contractual approaches to social-service funding. Yet the public and bureaucratic response to the possibility of ethnically separate welfare-service delivery is confused with pejorative assumptions that this is the first step in political and social apartheid.

However these issues are resolved, autonomy in the determination of *iwi* needs identification, assessment and clarification of appropriate social-service delivery patterns will need to be protected. Greenland has written that the 'tenor of Maori politics is more conducive to a study of mood and metaphor, of cultural values and leadership style, rather than to a conventional study of political thought or institutions' (1984: 88). The importance of the 'spiritual dimension' in Maori decision-making, so alien and troubling to the 'bureaucratic mind', will have to be accepted and respected (cf. Levine, 1989). That will require the development of a flexible and sensitive bureaucracy which respects different patterns and forms of knowledge. This is particularly important because adequate needs assessment of particular *iwi* requires a detailed understanding of the protocols of that *iwi* with respect to the pattern of devolved decision-making. Rejection of the importance of these protocols on the basis of 'bureaucratic rationality' will inevitably reinforce racist assumptions. Despite extremist rhetoric about 'apartheid', some aspects of the implications of parallel development will need to be resolved. Other countries have embarked on this direction. For example, the concept of the parallel administration of religiously and ethnically different social services is part of the practical structure of Canadian social services.

OTHER PATTERNS, MODELS AND POSSIBILITIES

Some aspects of the public debate about the Treaty of Waitangi, and in particular, a more equitable provision of welfare to the *iwi*, regards the issues as essentially unique to New Zealand. While this is in some sense appropriate, it is also useful to place the internal debate in an international context. Ethnic peoples throughout the western world have common perceptions about their particular disadvantages under the pattern of 'benevolent paternalism' typical of most welfare states. Where the ethnic minority is also an indigenous minority there are even greater similarities. Canada, as has been mentioned, has recently enacted legislation that places it in the forefront of countries ready to establish legislation that respects the rights and privileges of ethnic minorities, with special focus on the rights of the indigenous Canadian Indian.

The recent directions of ethnic social policy in Canada can be seen as possible models for New Zealand to evaluate in the search for social policy that is perceived to be culturally appropriate by the Maori ethnic minority. Despite the fact that the Canadian government is concerned to promote a multi-cultural social policy, as New Zealand wrestles with the implications of bi-culturalism it can still look to Canada for an example of how ethnic policies are translated into legislation. In Canada, separate social-service organizations and agencies have been established that respect different ethnic and cultural demands. In Ontario (for example) there are legislatively distinct Catholic Children's Aid Societies, a Jewish Children's Aid Society, Metropolitan Children's Aid Societies and separate agencies for Canadian Indians, all constitutionally empowered to deliver the same social services in uniquely different ways. Each operates with separate administrative and service systems where the identification of needs and service delivery patterns are culturally, indigenously and religiously distinct.

The Canadian government Report *Equality Now: a Report of the Special Committee on Visible Minorities in Canadian Society* (1984), influenced the Canadian government when it established, in 1988, a new Multi-culturalism Act. The Canadian government sought, through this legislation, to recognize and promote multi-culturalism in order to reflect cultural and racial diversity and to establish the principle of ethnic diversity as an intrinsic part of the national character. In clause after clause, the patterns and expectations of diverse ethnic and other cultural groups were considered to be more important than any one single facet of the Canadian character. However, such legislation has all the hallmarks of procedural rather than substantive equality (Jayasuriya, 1987). Despite such criticisms and the realization that most governments have been able to render politically marginal the claims of ethnic peoples, it is this institutionalizing of difference through legislation which is especially important. It provides an example of how the principles of parallel development can be promoted. Canada has been able to articulate and place on to the statute books policies that respect not only the cultural differences of French-speaking Canadians and Canadian Indians but also those of a variety of other smaller ethnic minorities. There appear to be no substantial reasons why New Zealand should not similarly proclaim the same salient principles in arriving at a recognition of the constitutionally different rights of the *tangata whenua*.

ECHOES, ILLUSIONS AND PROMISES

These political and social issues have elements of high drama in that recognition of the essentially bi-racial and bi-cultural character of New Zealand society would require a clear commitment to the parallel development of social services in New Zealand. As such, further steps might be taken towards honouring both the spirit and the principles enshrined in the Treaty of Waitangi. There are confused and troubling echoes, like the rumbling in the Marabar Caves of Forster's *A Passage to India*. The collapse of the paternalistic certainties of the old welfare paradigm echo in the uncertainty with which the state welfare bureaucracies accommodate themselves to the challenge that their policies are racist and that parallel systems of welfare administration are required. There is a troubling 'noise' that echoes more generally in the public relationship of the races and the fact that a powerful ethnic underclass cannot be ignored. The 'noise' echoes in the confrontation and intimidation of those defined as enemies and the stridency of claim rights mirrors beliefs that the 'noise' of these claims 'does not so much cry out for recognition as for redefinition' (Cleave, 1989: 70). The illusions reflect those assumptions that the resolution of these issues can easily be translated into managerial and administrative procedures. The promises to honour the Treaty, however they are understood, are equally fraught.

While purchase of service contracting may be promoted as providing a possibility for the development of culturally appropriate social welfare processes, it is clear that a degree of consultation and the administrative re-working of fiscal transfer arrangements would not be cheap. Arguments that purchase of service contracting can deliver social services at a lower cost simply will not work with respect to the urgent demand facing New Zealand to redraft its social services in a culturally appropriate way for both Maori and Pacific Island communities. This will require the *Pakeha* majority:

> to stop blaming the Maori for most of their problems and treating them as lesser beings who are essentially incorrigible and incapable of becoming partners in a modern and prosperous New Zealand. They have to stop thinking of themselves as the only civilised people and the Maori as only a defeated and subjugated minority. It is time the *Pakeha* accepted the Maori as the *tangata whenua* and accorded them their due dignity and mana.
>
> (Vasil, 1988: 23)

REFERENCES

Armstrong, M. J. (1987) 'Interethnic Conflict in New Zealand', in J. Boucher, D. Landis, and K. A. Clark, *Ethnic Conflict: International Perspectives*, Newbery Park, CA: Sage, 255–78.

Awatere, D. (1984) *Maori Sovereignty*, Auckland: Broadsheet.

Balibar, E. (1990) 'Paradoxes of Universality', in D. T. Goldberg, *Anatomy of Racism*, Minneapolis: University of Minnesota Press, pp. 283–94.

Banton, M. (1983) *Racial and Ethnic Competition*, Cambridge: Cambridge University Press.

Beacroft, L. (1987) 'The Treaty of Waitangi – A Century Ahead', *Aboriginal Law Bulletin*, 28: 6–8.

Boston, J. (1987) 'Transforming New Zealand's Public Sector: Labour's Quest For Improved Efficiency And Accountability', *Public Administration*, 65: 423–42.

— — (1988) 'From Corporatisation to Privatization: Public Sector Reform In New Zealand', *Canberra Bulletin of Public Administration*, 57: 71–86.

Brosnan, P. and Hill, C. (1983) 'Income, Occupation And Ethnic Origin In New Zealand', *New Zealand Economic Papers*, 17: 51–7.

Bullivant, B. M. (1984) *Pluralism: Cultural Maintenance and Evolution*, Clevedon, Avon: Multilingual Matters, 11.

Campbell, M. J. and Armstrong, R. H. R. (1982) 'Providing Community Services for a Minority Group. The Case of the Australian Aboriginal', *Planning and Administration*, 9(2): 47–59.

Chau, K. L. (1989) 'Sociocultural Dissonance among Ethnic Minority Populations', *Social Casework*, 70(4): 224–30.

Cleave, P. (1989) *The Sovereignty Game: Power, Knowledge and Reading the Treaty of Waitangi*, Wellington: Victoria University Press for the Institute of Policy Studies.

Cody, J. (1988) 'Personal Social Services: Implications of the Principles of Social Provision', *The Royal Commission on Social Policy Report*, vol. IV: 233–50.

Culpitt, I. R. (1992) *Welfare and Citizenship: Beyond the Crisis of the Welfare State?* London: Sage.

Delacampagne, C. (1990) 'Racism and the West: From Praxis to Logos', in D. T. Goldberg, *Anatomy of Racism*, Minneapolis: University of Minnesota Press, pp. 83–8.

Evison, H. (1987) 'Maori Claims to the Waitangi Tribunal', *New Zealand Monthly Review*, XXVIII (298): 2–3.

Fitzpatrick, P. (1990) 'Racism and the Innocence of Law', in D. T. Goldberg, *Anatomy of Racism*, Minneapolis: University of Minnesota Press, pp. 247–62.

Fleras, A. (1984) 'From Social Welfare to Community Development: Maori Policy and the Department of Maori Affairs in New Zealand', *Community Development Journal*, 19(1): 32–9.

— — (1985) 'Towards 'Tu Tangata': Historical Developments and Current Trends in Maori Policy and Administration', *Political Science*, 37(1): 18–39.

Gelfand, D. E. and Fandetti, D. V. (1986) 'The Emergent Nature of Ethnicity: Dilemmas in Assessment', *Social Casework*, 67(9): 542–50.

George, V. and Wilding, P. (1985) *Ideology and Social Welfare*, London: Routledge & Kegan Paul.

Goldberg, D. T. (1990) *Anatomy of Racism*, Minneapolis: University of Minnesota Press.

Goodin, R. E. (1982) *Political Theory and Public Policy*, Chicago: University of Chicago Press.

— — (1985a) 'Self-Reliance Versus the Welfare State', *Journal of Social Policy*, 14: 25–47.

— — (1985b) 'Vulnerabilities and Responsibilities: An Ethical Defense of the Welfare State', *The American Political Science Review*, 79(3): 775–87.

— — (1988) *Reasons for Welfare: The Political Theory of the Welfare State*, Princeton, NJ: Princeton University Press.

Green, P. (1986) 'Race and Racism In Aotearoa', *Sites: A Journal for Radical Perspectives on Culture*, 12: 59–62.

Greenland, H. (1984) 'Ethnicity as Ideology: the Critique of Pakeha Society', in P. Spoonley, C. Macpherson, D. Pearson and C. Sedgwick, (eds.) *Tauiwi: Racism and Ethnicity in New Zealand*, Palmerston North: The Dunmore Press, pp. 86–102.

Griffiths, H. (1988) 'Working with People in Marginal Communities', *Social Policy and Administration*, 22(2): 166–77.

Gronbjerg, K. A. (1982) 'Private Welfare in the Welfare State: Recent US Patterns', *Social Service Review*, 56(1): 1–26.

— — (1983) 'Private Welfare: Its Future in the Welfare State', *American Behavioral Scientist*, 26(6): 773–93.

Hazlehurst, K. M. (1988) *Racial Conflict and Resolution in New Zealand*, Canberra, Peace Research Institute: Australian National University Press.

Hodge, J. L. (1990) 'Equality: Beyond Dualism and Oppression', in D. T. Goldberg, *Anatomy of Racism*, Minneapolis: University of Minnesota Press, pp. 89–107.

Hohepa, P. (1978) 'Maori and Pakeha: The One People Myth', in M. King, (ed.) *Te Maori Ora: Aspects of Maoritange*, Wellington: Methuen, pp. 98–111.

Ignatieff, M. (1984) *The Needs of Strangers*, London: Chatto & Windus.

— — (1989) 'Citizenship And Moral Narcissism', *The Political Quarterly*, 60(1): 63–74.

Jackson, P. (1987) 'The Idea of ''Race'' and the Geography of Racism', in P. Jackson, (ed.) *Race and Racism: Essays in Social Geography*, London: Allen & Unwin, pp. 3–21.

Jayasuriya, D. L. (1985) 'Multiculturalism: Fact, Policy and Rhetoric', in M. E. Poole, P. R. Delacey, and B. S. Randhawa, *Australia in Transition: Culture and Life Possibilities*, Sydney: Harcourt Brace Jovanovich, pp. 23–34.

— — (1987) 'Ethnic Minorities and Social Justice in Australian Society', *Australian Journal of Social Issues*, 22(3): 481–97.

Kimmel, M. S. (1987) 'Reconstituting Community: Moral Economy and Community-Based Social Movements in Industrial Nations', *Community Development Journal*, 22(4): 270–80.

Kramer, R. M. (1983) 'Contracting for Human Services: An Organizational Perspective', in R. M. Kramer and H. Specht, (eds) *Readings in Community Organization Practice*, (3rd edn), Englewood, NJ: Prentice-Hall, pp. 421–32.

Levine, H. B. (1989) 'Constructing Treaty Rhetoric . . .,' *Sites: A Journal for Radical Perspectives on Culture*, 18: 17–22.

Levine, S. and Vasil, R. (1985) *Maori Political Perspectives: He Whakaaro Maori Mo Nga Ti Kanga Kawanatanga*, Auckland: Hutchinson.

Lightman, E. S. (1987) 'Welfare ideology, the market and the family', *International Social Work*, 30(4): 309–16.

McCready, D. J. (1986) 'Privatized Social Service Systems: Are there any Justifications?', *Canadian Public Policy*, XII(1): 253–7.

McHugh, P. (1988) 'The Legal Basis for Maori Claims Against the Crown', *Victoria University of Wellington Law Review*, 18(1): 1–20.

Mahuta, B. (1987) 'Te Whenua, Te Iwi', in J. Phillips, *Te Whenua, Te Iwi: The Land and the People*, Wellington: Port Nicholson Press, pp. 82–7.

Martin, E. (1982) 'Consumer Evaluation of Human Services', *Social Policy and Administration*, 20(3): 185–200.

Minogue, M. (1983) 'Theory and Practice in Public Policy and Administration', *Policy and Politics*, 11(1): 63–85.

Mishra, R. (1984) *The Welfare State in Crisis*, Brighton: Harvester Press; New York, St Martin's Press.

Morris, R. (1986) *Rethinking Social Welfare: Why Care for the Stranger?* New York: Longman Paul.

Mulgan, R. (1989) 'Bicultural Democracy – Some Unresolved Problems', *Sites: A Journal for Radical Perspectives on Culture*, 18: 57–60.

Mullard, C. (1985) *Race, Power and Resistance*, London: Routledge & Kegan Paul.

New Zealand (1988) *The Report of the New Zealand Royal Commission on Social Policy*, vols I–V, Wellington: New Zealand Government Printer.

Olson, J. K. (1980) 'Needs Assessment and Program Evaluation In Impacted Communities', in J. Davenport and J. A. Davenport, *The Boom Town: Problems and Promises in the Energy Vortex*, Cheyenne: University of Wyoming Press, pp. 123–38.

Orange, C. (1987) *The Treaty of Waitangi*, Wellington: Allen & Unwin.

Outlaw, L. (1990) 'Toward a Critical Theory of "Race"', in D. T. Goldberg, *Anatomy of Racism*, Minneapolis: University of Minnesota Press, pp. 58–82.

Parkin, A. (1984) 'Ethnic Groups, Social Change and Public Policy in Australia', *Current Affairs Bulletin* Aug.: 15–26.

Pearson, D. G. (1984) 'Two Paths of Colonialism: Class, 'Race', Ethnicity and Migrant Labour in New Zealand', in P. Spoonley, C. Macpherson, D. Pearson and C. Sedgwick, (eds) *Tauiwi: Racism and Ethnicity in New Zealand*, Palmerston North: The Dunmore Press, pp. 203–21.

— — (1989) 'Pakeha Ethnicity: Concept or Conundrum', *Sites: A Journal for Radical Perspectives on Culture*, 18: 61–72.

— — (1990) *A Dream Deferred: the Origins of Ethnic Conflict in New Zealand*, Wellington: Allen & Unwin.

Phillips, J. (1987) *Te Whenua, Te Iwi: The Land and the People*, Wellington: Port Nicholson Press.

Poole, M. E. (1985) 'Australian Multicultural Policy: Future Prospects', in M. E. Poole, P. R. Delacey and B. S. Randhawa, *Australia in Transition: Culture and Life Possibilities*, Sydney: Harcourt Brace Jovanovich, pp. 59–69.

Reid, P. N. and Gundlach, J. H. (1983) 'A Scale for the Measurement of Consumer Satisfaction with Social Services', *Journal of Social Science Research*, 7(1): 37–54.

Rein, M. (1977) 'Social Planning: The Search for Legitimacy', in N. Gilbert and H. Specht, *Planning for Social Welfare: Issues, Models and Tasks*, Englewood Cliffs, NJ: Prentice-Hall.

Rein, M. and S. H. White, (1977) 'Can Policy Research Help Policy?' *The Public Interest*, 49: 119–36.

Royal Commission on Social Policy (1988) 'Public, Private and Voluntary Provision of Social Services in New Zealand', *Discussion Booklet No. 2*.

Siegel, L. M., Attkisson, C. C. and Carson, L. G. (1978) 'Need Identification and Program Planning in the Community Context', in C. C. Attkisson, W. A. Hargreaves, M. J. Horowitz and J. E. Sorenson *Evaluation of Human Service Programs*, New York: Academic Press, pp. 215–52.

Spoonley, P., Macpherson, C., Pearson, D. and Sedgwick, C. (eds) (1984) *Tauiwi: Racism and Ethnicity in New Zealand*, Palmerston North: The Dunmore Press.

Tauroa, H. (1982) *Race Against Time*, Report of the Race Relations Conciliator, Wellington: Human Rights Commission.

Taylor-Gooby, P. (1986) 'Privatisation, Power And the Welfare State', *Sociology*, 20(2): 228–46.

Trlin, A. D. and Spoonley, P. (1987) 'New Zealand', in J. A. Sigler, (ed.) *International Handbook on Race and Race Relations*, New York: Greenwood Press, pp. 191–212.

Turner, B. S. (1986) *Citizenship and Capitalism: the Debate over Reformism*, London: Allen & Unwin.

—— (1988) 'Individualism, Capitalism and the Dominant Culture: A Note on the Debate', *Australia and New Zealand Journal of Sociology*, 24(1): 47–64.

Vasil, R. K. (1988) *Biculturalism: Reconciling Aotaroa with New Zealand*, Wellington: Victoria University of Wellington, Institute of Policy Studies Press.

Walker, R. J. (1984) 'The Genesis of Maori Activism', *Journal of the Polynesian Society*, 93: 267–81.

—— (1987) *Nga Tau Tohetohe: Years of Anger*, Auckland, Penguin Books.

Weale, A. (1983) *Political Theory and Social Policy*, London: Macmillan.

Webster, S. (1989) 'Maori Studies and the Expert Definition of Maori Culture', *Sites: a Journal for Radical Perspectives on Culture*, 18: 35–56.

Williams, F. (1987) 'Racism and the Discipline of Social Policy: A Critique of Welfare Theory', *Critical Social Policy*, 7(2): 4–29.

Williams, J. (1985) 'Redefining Institutional Racism', *Ethnic and Racial Studies*, 8(3): 323–48.

Wilson, E. (1988/89) 'Feedback – Elizabeth Wilson Responds to "Racism and the Discipline of Social Policy" by Fiona Williams, CSP 20', *Critical Social Policy*, 8(3): 113–17.

Unpublished papers

Administrative Review Committee Report (1987) *Performance and Efficiency in the Department of Social Welfare*.

Fisher, R. J. (1984) 'Conflict and Collaboration in Maori–Pakeha Relations', *University of Waikato Occasional Paper, No. 20*.

He Tirohanga Rangapu (1988) Report of the Ministry of Maori Affairs.

Ka Awatea (1991) Report of the Ministerial Planning Group.

Maori Advisory Unit (1985) Report: *He Ara ki te Aomarama* – Department of Social Welfare

Maori Directorate D.S.W. Head Office (1989) Responses to Omnibus Social Welfare Bill.

New Zealand Planning Council Discussion Document (1984).

Puketapu, K. P. (1982) 'Reform From Within', Paper presented to the Institute of Public Management.

Stokes, E. (1985) 'Maori Research and Development', A Discussion Paper for the Social Sciences Committee of the National Research Advisory Council.

Te Urupare Rangapu (1988) Report of the Ministry of Maori Affairs.

Report of the Ministerial Advisory Committee on a Maori Perspective for the Department of Social Welfare. (1986) *Puao-Te-Atu-Tu.*

Thurow, L. C. (1981) 'Equity, Efficiency, Social Justice, and Redistribution', in *The Welfare State in Crisis: An Account of the Conference on Social Policies in the 1980s,* Paris, OECD, pp. 137–50.

Tu Tangata, Stance of the People (1980) Unpublished Report of the Department of Maori Affairs.

GLOSSARY OF MAORI WORDS AND PHRASES

Aotearoa The original Maori name for New Zealand.
Aroha Love.
Awhina To assist.
Haka Ritual dance, often associated with war.
Hamama Shouting or noise.
Hapu Sub-tribe (a group of *whanau*).
Hui A meeting.
Iwi Tribe (a federation of *hapu* who share common ancestry).
Kaumatua Elders.
Kaupapa Topic.
Kawa Protocol.
Koha A gift.
Kokiri To advance.
Korero To talk.
Mana Prestige.
Marae A formalized Maori meeting place.
Matauranga Knowledge.
Muriwhenua One of the *iwi.*
Pakeha Predominantly white inhabitants of New Zealand.
Rununga Council.
Taonga Treasures or precious possessions (This indicates not only tangible objects but also spiritual values.
Tauiwi Visitor.
Tiriti Maori word for treaty.
Waiata Song.
Waitangi Place where treaty was signed.
Whakapapa Genealogy.

Whanau Family, extended family, including grandparents, parents, children, uncles, aunts and cousins. Also means birth.

Whenua The land or umbilical cord and placenta.

He Ara ki te Aomarama The path to daylight (the future).

He iwi kotahi tatou We are one people.

He tirohanga rangapu Policy of partnership.

He Whakaaro Maori mo nga Tikanga Kawanatanga Maori opinion on government rule.

Hui Taumata National tribal gathering.

Ka Awatea Daylight.

Kohanga Reo A language 'nest'.

Maatua whangai Adoptive parent (in the Maori sense).

Ngati porou One of the *iwi*.

Nga tau tohetohe Years of dispute.

Puao-Te-Ata-Tu Daybreak or dawn.

Tangata kainga Maori resident in an area which is not *tangata whenua*.

Tangata whenua People of the land. When a child is born the umbilical cord is buried in an ancestral place, thus forever tying Maori to their tribal lands.

Te urupare rangapu Partnership responses.

Tino rangatiratanga Sovereignty.

Tu tangata To stand tall.

9 Social welfare of indigenous peoples in Zimbabwe

Saliwe M. Kawewe

The basic principles and programmes of a particular social-welfare system reflect the social, political, economic and cultural environment in which it exists. Thus, the social-welfare system of any country reflects the predominant values of that society (Trattner, 1985; Dixon, 1989; Prigmore and Atherton, 1990). David Gil, who assumes an egalitarian approach, reinforces this point by stating that choices about social-welfare policy are also shaped by cultural elites who are recruited from the more privileged and powerful strata of society. Thus, beliefs, values, ideologies, customs and traditions reflected in social-welfare policy are based on the preference and tastes of the most powerful in society. In looking at the social welfare system in Zimbabwe, Gil's analysis is correct, as will be shown in this chapter.

There are many people in modern society who are critical of social welfare. However, societies 'accept the principle that society ought to provide resources against problematic social situations, downturns in the economic cycle, health crises, and unfavourable living conditions' (Prigmore and Atherton, 1990: 8). Thus, societal responsibility for social welfare is compatible with contemporary styles as an important aspect of a civilized world.

Human beings have varying needs, but the basic ones are the need for growth and the need for security. In order to lead functional and more fulfilling lives, emotional, physical, cognitive, social and spiritual aspects of the basic needs have to be met. Generally, these human needs are met through personal initiative and resources or by family and friends. But when human needs cannot be met within the mutual social networks, societal mechanisms have to be available (Johnson and Schwartz, 1988). The degree to which such social welfare mechanisms are provided varies in terms of government social services and private, voluntary ones.

There are many definitions of social welfare. In this discussion, 'social welfare refers to societally organized activities aimed at maintaining or improving human well-being' (Johnson, 1990: 13). This definition encompasses programmes and measures operated by social work, health, education, public safety and recreation professionals. Further, the definition includes both formally and informally organized services in government and voluntary settings. In looking at social welfare in Zimbabwe, we are primarily concerned with programmes that combat poverty by alleviating and/or preventing it through income redistribution or social compensation as a social-security measure. Poverty in Zimbabwe is insular as it affects the majority of the population in this Third World country as opposed to case poverty, where only a few, scattered poor people would be affected.

Figure 9.1 shows a comparative diagrammatic presentation of First World and Third World social stratification. The poor consist of the working class, peasants and the landless, the jobless and the destitute. Programmes and activities provided by the social-welfare system to provide social security to the citizenry are referred to as social services. The concept of social services as used here is derived from conceptions by Adeyeri (1984), Zald (1965), the United Nations Department of Economic and Social Affairs (1971), Pumphrey (1971) and Johnson (1990). Social services are viewed as: (1) methods used to help people who are unable to provide for themselves; (2) methods used to control social deviance; and (3) methods used to help individuals, groups and communities improve their social functioning by improving the standard of living and providing recreation. These services are generally provided through social insurance and public assistance programmes at the government level, and through voluntary acts of service at private levels. The use of the concept of income maintenance in Zimbabwe has been avoided, as 70 per cent of the population lives in rural areas where there is no income to maintain, and, likewise, the same is true of a sizeable number of urban dwellers, as reflected in the socio-economic structure in Figure 9.2. Further, because of limited resources and an inheritance of the colonial system, social-welfare programmes are mostly residual, piecemeal, and highly selective to the extent that the majority of the population that would otherwise be eligible to receive assistance do not. Zimbabwe does not have social-welfare programmes that prevent people from becoming poor when they lose an income even in urban areas, because most people who earn an income are poor, and public assistance is allocated on a scale that is less than prior wages. Public

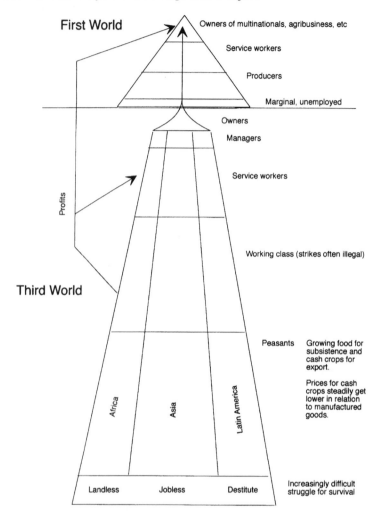

Figure 9.1 Social profiles of the First and Third Worlds
Source: A. Hope and S. Trimmel (eds) (1989) *Training for Transformation: a Handbook for Community Workers*, adapted from Chris Hodzi's illustration

assistance, sometimes referred to as public welfare, is called 'social-welfare assistance' in Zimbabwe. These types of programmes, unlike insurance or 'entitlement' programmes, are not based on work-related contributions or trust funds. Eligibility for public-assistance benefits is based on a means test for proving destitution.

An understanding of the current social-welfare programmes for

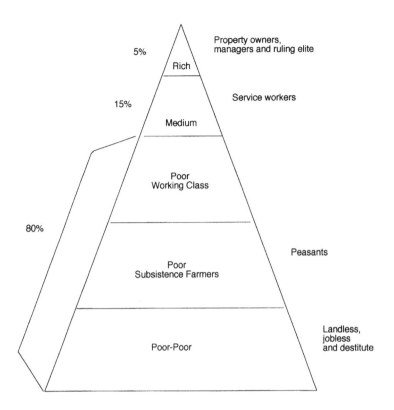

%=Percentage of the Population

Figure 9.2 Pyramid showing percentage of rich and poor

indigenous populations is better understood when placed in a historical perspective, which will enlighten us on what happened in the past, since the past shapes the present and the present is the past for the future. Understanding the present, based on the past, may shed light on how to negotiate the path to the future.

Social welfare for indigenous populations in Zimbabwe will be assessed on the basis of the degree of government (traditional, colonial and Zimbabwean) involvement in providing integrated and comprehensive social services covering the following programmes and client groups: (1) education; (2) health; (3) housing; (4) workers' compensation; (5) unemployment insurance; (6) old-age retirement benefits; (7) family and children's services; (8) disability and survivors' benefits; (9) refugees; (10) rural versus urban focus; (11) responsiveness to human needs.

DEMOGRAPHIC INFORMATION

Zimbabwe is named after some highly sophisticated ruins which were built by the Shona-speaking people in the eleventh century. These ruins mark a great Shona kingdom that flourished in the region now covered by Zimbabwe and Mozambique – the Empire of Monomotapa. Although weakened by internal forces, conflict with the Portuguese and later the Ndebele from the Zulu Empire in South Africa, this Shona kingdom finally collapsed in the 1890s with the coming of the European colonizers. The most recent ruins were built in the fifteenth century. They are a symbol of Shona pride, and hence Zimbabwe replaced the colonial name Rhodesia, so called after Cecil John Rhodes.

Zimbabwe's population is about 11 million people. It comprises 150,873 square miles and has a literacy rate of 30 per cent. The population of 5–19 years in schools is 37 per cent.

The Shona people comprise 80 per cent of the population; the Ndebele comprise about 15 per cent; and the European descendants constitute 5 per cent of the population. The Matabeleland region experiences the most cyclic droughts. Some indigenous people have alleged it is a curse from the ancestral spirits for their historical intrusion of Zimbabwe, causing bloodshed and Chief Lobengula's concession, which led to the colonization of Zimbabwe. There are no obvious differences in physical appearance between them, as they belong to the Bantu group. Both the Shona and Ndebele share similar traditional customs, except that the Ndebele make click sounds when they speak. Both groups believe in ancestral honourship, paying dowry for wives married, the practice of polygamy, belief in one God, and celebrations at birth, marriage and death. Both emphasize high respect for older people. Both resented colonialism, though they were arch enemies. At present, both tribal groupings are becoming modernized, while still clinging to their heritage. The Shona people are the majority in the ruling party.

HISTORICAL CONSIDERATIONS: TRADITIONAL ARRANGEMENTS

The origin of mutual aid as a reflection for a concern for humankind can be traced as far back as the origin of the human species. The historical and cultural situation of the indigenous population in Zimbabwe cannot be understood without considering their inherent hospitality towards humanity. When ancient people discovered the use of tools, they opted for more permanent settlements, as opposed to wandering through hunting and food-gathering. In Zimbabwe, before foreign intrusion, the Shona-speaking people had developed agricultural communities with their own complex civilization. The Zimbabwe ruins, built around the thirteenth century, are a hallmark of that civilization. The core institution was the family. In traditional society, every individual belonged to this primary group. The family consisted of extended family members. They usually involved a man accepted as the family head, who settled marriage, divorce and legal disputes, and was responsible to the kraal head. The family head had the responsibility of handling social and domestic problems as well as land allotment and the spiritual welfare of the family. Then came the kraal headman, who had similar responsibilities to those of the family head, except at a higher level, and he was in charge of affairs relating to many families within a geographic area. He was answerable to the village headman above him. The village head commanded great authority and spiritual powers. He was appointed by the Chief, and at times tribal spiritual mediums were consulted for succession. He had great judicial and spiritual powers, and handled serious cases within the same line of responsibilities as the kraal head. He was also responsible to the Chief for the social well-being and conduct of people in his jurisdiction. The Chief had the overall authority in a tribe, was elected to office through spiritual prophecy and was the ultimate court of appeal (Cormack, 1983).

The coming of the Ndebele-speaking people, descendants of Tshaka the Zulu, did not disrupt this traditional structure drastically. These newcomers developed a similar traditional structure, though they lived by raiding and looting. Some of the Shona-speaking people were conveniently located in the southern part of Zimbabwe. From these Shona they got all the cattle they could place their hands on, killed all the men and women they could lay their spears on, and abducted all the beautiful girls and handsome boys they cast their eyes on. These raids became less frequent as the then peace-loving Shona became more sophisticated in territorial defence, making it more difficult for the Ndebele to benefit from warfare. However, there was general animosity between the Ndebele and the Shona people before the European intrusion in Zimbabwe.

Within each tribe, there were effective political, economic and socio-cultural mechanisms to ensure social security for the residents on the basis of the mores of each tribe. Social welfare was provided for everyone from the cradle and, therefore, was institutionalized to the grave. Education was transmitted informally through the social networks. Age was directly related to high status, and role performance on the part of the elderly was associated with wisdom. Elderly people were taken care of by the kinship group and died with dignity, as they were considered closer to God as they grew older and, therefore, were a blessing to have. People with mental health problems received mutual support from family and community. There was no housing problem, as it was a communal responsibility to build as many huts as were needed. They also lived in equilibrium with their environment.

People used natural materials for building – soil, water, grass and bark. In traditional society, children belonged to everyone in the community. Because the tribes were patrilineal and patrilocal, in cases of divorce, which were rare, the children stayed with the community where they were born, consisting of the patrilineal extended family members. Because everyone knew everyone else in the community, child welfare and social control of deviant behaviour was effectively handled communally. In the case of disability or death, the kin provided the safety net. There were no workers' compensation or unemployment insurance programmes. Traditional society was typically agrarian. Land was owned communally, and the headman or chief was only a custodian. The society was responsible to the needs of every person within the context of the society's mores.

FOREIGN INTRUSION

The early Europeans who came to Zimbabwe were Portuguese traders in the 1830s and missionaries in the 1850s. The missionaries settled in the southwestern part of Zimbabwe (Matabeleland) inhabited by the Ndebele-speaking people. They were followed by the 'pioneers' and colonists led by Cecil John Rhodes, who tricked a Ndebele Chief, Lobengula, into signing the Rudd Concession in 1888 which was used in 1890 to declare Zimbabwe (a larger area than Matabeleland) a colony of the British South Africa Company (BSAC) administration. The 1890 settlers went to settle in the Shona-speaking people's region

(Mashonaland). They settled in Harare, the most fertile area, with beautiful scenery and weather. This European settlement disregarded African land rights. In 1894, the Colonial Lands Commission set aside small patches of semi-arid land for the exclusive occupation of Africans and designated the rest of the fertile land for colonial use. In 1930, the Land Apportionment Act was passed as an effort to resolve the land issue. With this Act, 45 million acres, comprising 71 per cent of the country's grade one arable land, was owned by the Europeans, while 45 million acres, almost half of which is poor farming land, was allocated to the indigenous population, which comprised 95 per cent of the population, resulting in 7.3 acres per individual African and 162 acres per individual European settler.

The missionaries were motivated by the religious desire to spread Christianity. They established the first schools in order to teach Christianity by enabling the natives to read the Bible. The precondition for missionary education was joining the church. These early missionaries supported many 'assumptions, attitudes, and policies of the colonial government' (Mungazi, 1989: 15). They strengthened the colonial paradigm and forgot the real purpose of education and the values of Christianity. Christianity was used to pacify the indigenous people. Later, these sectarian organizations became the first providers of social-welfare services for indigenous people in the form of recreation, health and education services.

In their altruistic efforts, both sectarian and non-sectarian voluntary organizations put persistent pressure on the colonists to cater to the social-welfare needs of the indigenous people. The colonial government's initial reaction was systematically to alienate these liberal organizations. The little provision undertaken for welfare services by non-sectarian voluntary organizations, like African Welfare Societies, which formed a federation in 1936, were often led by Europeans. Owing to their persistence, these voluntary organizations became more effective in gaining support and in co-ordinating efforts with local governments in order to improve indigenous people's conditions of living.

Thus, during the early colonial period, education, health, mental health, housing, and children's and adults' services were provided through voluntary acts of service, especially in urban centres. In rural areas, other than sporadic missionary activity, the traditional safety net continued to provide social security to the inhabitants (Kaseke, 1988; Cormack, 1983).

COLONIAL GOVERNMENT

When the European colonists came to Zimbabwe in 1888, they came under the pretext of visiting. Once granted visitation rights by the illiterate Chief Lobengula, they used trickery, by making him write an 'X' to authorize the visits (Rudd Concession). This was later interpreted by the Europeans as a legal concession to own Zimbabwe. In 1890 they settled, as they were attracted by prospects of mineral wealth, as gold deposits could be seen along river banks, and in addition there was ivory, fertile soil and beautiful weather. These colonists unilaterally established locales which eventually mushroomed into urban centres. The colonial government imposed itself on the indigenous society and quickly established a relationship of rider and horse by making the indigenous people hewers of wood and haulers of water for the Europeans. The indigenous people were deprived of all their human rights. Despite earlier tribal conflicts, the Shona and Ndebele united in the first Chimurenga War of resistance, which was waged in 1896 to resist colonial rule. They were defeated by the more sophisticated weaponry used by the Europeans. The Africans were driven to semi-arid land, while the settlers shared the rich, fertile land amongst themselves and established commercial farms. The traditional African hospitality to strangers had led to their being cheated and subjugated into servitude. The Africans showed further resistance to European rule by refusing to work for them. However, the colonial government soon imposed various taxes, like hut tax and poll tax, which indirectly forced the Africans to seek cash by selling their labour. Further, they drew a cheap labour force from indigenous populations of neighbouring British colonies (aliens). Thus, the young, male, indigenous people were to provide labour for the commercial farms, mines and urban centres owned by the capitalist-minded colonists. The women, children and elderly were mostly found in rural areas. Legally, the urban areas were designated European, but the Africans could stay there temporarily by obtaining passes authorizing them to be in the city working or looking for employment. Later, the law was changed in order to accommodate Africans in the cities' African townships, but the pass laws continued until independence.

Initially, there were no social services for the Africans because their urban residence was considered to be of a transient nature, but this turned out to be a myth. The colonial government held another myth: that the indigenous people lived more cheaply, and that they deserved this quality of life. This myth was based on the superiority complex the Europeans had regarding the indigenous tradition. It was expected that their needs would be met within the peasant rural kinship structure (Gargett, 1973; Hampson and Kaseke, 1987; Cormack, 1983). The fragmented social-welfare schemes like old-age pensions, public assistance and occupational pensions were developed only for Europeans (Kaseke, 1988). The colonial government gave little attention to the needs of the indigenous people in either urban or rural areas until after the Second World War. As a result of urban population growth in the 1940s, and the impact of that war, the social conditions and social needs of the African townships overwhelmed the voluntary charitable efforts, due to limited resources. The deteriorating social conditions forced the local authorities and the government to assume legal responsibility for the African urban population whose needs for welfare services were increasing. The rural needs for indigenous populations were systematically neglected.

During this period, the local governments promoted entertainment through recreation in urban areas. Beer halls were emphasized, as it was believed that if the Africans became exhausted by using their excess energy in recreation and intoxication, they would be less political. The main purpose of this activity was to redirect them from socio-economic conditions and make them passive, in order to avoid political confrontation that might result from social and psychological frustration. Although no resources were directed to any other area of human need, alcoholism was promoted, and paternalism was evident in the provision of social services, inhibiting meaningful progress. Expansions in the 1950s included the formation of women's clubs and youth clubs. In the 1960s, local authorities added library and handicraft centres. Some of the predominant factors (Cormack, 1983) which influenced the types of welfare services and amenities given to the indigenous people were: (1) prevailing ideologies that indigenous people were inferior by virtue of their dark skin; (2) lack of know-how on the part of government welfare personnel; (3) limited financial resources allocated to various local governments; (4) misguided beliefs that the African urban population was transient in nature, as their permanent and rightful place was on the semi-arid rural Tribal Trust Lands; and (5) the misconceived level of sophistication and changing needs of the indigenous people.

The colonial government delegated the responsibility for the welfare and management of the urban areas to European-controlled municipalities (local governments). They used proceeds from beer sales in the African beer halls to fund the services. Despite being trustees of the government, the local authorities maintained autonomy in managing indigenous people's affairs. Most local authorities reflected colonial interests which they represented. They showed no interest in or perception of issues reflecting African concerns. Therefore, there was not a comprehensive and explicitly formulated or described social-welfare policy for Africans. This general tendency of neglect in social-welfare services and underdeveloped social policy was typical of all indigenous urban areas in the country with the exception of Bulawayo, which had the best social-welfare system of all the urban areas at that time. Each local government had autonomy in operating indigenous affairs. It appears the Bulawayo authorities were more progressive in their philosophy towards the Africans there. Further, historically Zimbabwe was colonized because the Ndebele Chief signed the concession. It is possible that the colonial authorities might have accorded preferential treatment to this tribe which erroneously endorsed the colonization of the country. The major beneficiaries of social services were the European inhabitants who lived in separate neighbourhoods because of racial discrimination, and the disenfranchisement and deliberate exploitation of the indigenous people (Hampson and Kaseke, 1987; Kaseke, 1988; Kawewe, 1986).

In order to assess the responsiveness to human needs of the colonial social-welfare services for indigenous populations, we will review selected programmes and client groups.

Education

Educationally, there was a partnership between the government and the missionaries until 1949, when the Native Education Department assumed responsibility for most educational services in the African townships. In smaller urban centres and rural areas, the local community retained educational responsibility based on profits from beer sales and voluntary philanthropic efforts. Although primary and secondary school education was universal for Europeans, it was not universal for the indigenous people due to discriminatory colonial policies. Many indigenous children and adults remained uneducated, especially in the rural areas.

Those who received an education were supposed to be efficient menial workers. Education facilities were organized on a 'bottle-necking' system and, therefore, these workers mostly had elementary school education. Historically, elementary schools were established before high schools. When high schools appeared on the scene, they were few and scattered. Entrance to high school was very competitive, allowing only a limited few to be catered for. The same principle applied for entrance to the only university in the country, and entrance to technical training schools.

Health and mental health

The first health services were established in the African townships because of a phobia on the part of Europeans that disease would spread from the African to the European sections of the cities. Initially, urban indigenous people were forced to take medical screening examinations as they could not be trusted voluntarily to seek modern cures to disease. In addition, some local authorities established isolation hospitals for people with communicable diseases like tuberculosis. Indigenous people with mental health problems were imprisoned or institutionalized. They were treated harshly.

The central government encouraged local governments to utilize self-help in operating health services. Local governments established maternity centres and primary medical care services like out-patient treatment, family planning clinics and post-natal clinics. The government had responsibility for larger general hospitals' curative and preventive services, medical education, training and research. Indigenous medical services were financed from treatment charges, local beer profits and government grants. Many indigenous people were either too far from health centres or could not afford the cost of health care.

The majority of the indigenous populations, in both urban and rural areas, resorted to traditional healing methods by the use of herbs, spiritual mediums, and witch doctors. Indigenous healers have always been consulted for medical, social, economic and political problems. They charge a fee for their services to non-family members. Some learn to become healers, but the majority inherit the skill from their ancestors. The healers claim they can cast spells, cleanse away bad luck, and explain the cause of hardship and illness. The clients are given instructions on how to perform rituals, and use roots and herbs. The types of healers range from family-based to regionally recognized ones. Such a belief system has continued to this day.

Housing and living space

No single authority was responsible for the provision of housing. The situation was exacerbated by the unco-ordinated, scattered, poor building by the government, local authorities and statutory bodies like the Rhodesia Railways. The colonial government lacked interest in the social and environmental conditions in the African areas of residence in both urban and rural areas (Cormack, 1983). The local authorities in urban areas controlled both indigenous townships and European suburbs, because, according to land distribution based on the Land Apportionment Act, all urban areas were legally European land. The indigenous townships evolved as latent functions of colonialism. The colonial authorities had to be as economical as possible in building and operating the African townships since income for housing programmes was derived from housing rents, service charges, and the sale of water and/or electricity. Therefore, housing standards differed, reflecting prosperous centres for Europeans and depressed locations for Africans. The basic principle was that the quality of housing and services were not to exceed the community inhabitants' ability to pay rent for them. Thus, if the local wage level was low, the township standards were equally low.

The indigenous residential areas, both urban and rural, were usually located far from commercial and industrial centres of a town or city. Access to such centres was usually by roads which were relatively better maintained in the urban areas than those in rural areas and those linking rural areas to urban ones. Earlier houses were designed for single men, and had poor ventilation and sanitation and limited privacy. By building small houses for urban workers, the colonial government made it difficult for working men to bring their families to live with them in urban areas. Most African housing lacked electricity, and almost all the houses had corrugated asbestos roofing. Due to urbanization, industrialization, colonial policies, and poverty in rural areas, most people migrated to the cities in search of a better life. The urban areas became overcrowded, and housing shortages became one of the major problems confronting the colonial government. Indigenous people crowded into the single- or two-room houses which initially had been designed for single males.

The rural indigenous people maintained their traditional huts with few modern housing structures. Most rural areas had no sanitation, and people squatted in the bushes, water supply was inadequate, and the environment was destroyed by overcrowding, overgrazing and limited agricultural land. The Colonial Land Apportionment Act controlled the amount of land allocated to indigenous people. The already semi-arid Tribal Trust Land (indigenous reservations) had lost most of its fertility because of overcrowding and lacked enough land to engage in crop rotation. Cow manure was scarce because the number of cattle owned by the Africans was controlled.

Workers' compensation

If indigenous workers were injured on the job, they were usually blamed for negligence and carelessness. The colonial government had no policy governing compensation for work-related injuries or losses for the indigenous people. Any benefits were at the discretion of the employer, and if covered, the employee paid medical costs and was expected to return to his rural home if permanently disabled. Most of the Africans worked in mines and other dangerous industries and contracted occupational diseases.

Unemployment and unemployment insurance

Unemployment and underemployment were serious problems that affected virtually all indigenous people. There were no minimum wage policies. The government ignored the unemployed and sent them to rural areas, or even imprisoned them for being in the European zone without a job. Those in urban areas had to register with the employment exchange before being considered for public assistance. There was a sense of helplessness, hopelessness and frustration with the colonial system. No unemployment insurance was available to the African people. Rural Africans relied on kinship and tradition.

Old-age and retirement benefits

Occupational pensions were not government-controlled and were at the discretion of the employer. Government employees were covered. Indigenous retirees and the elderly were expected to return to the rural areas, as they were considered no longer useful to European employers. Both rural and urban elderly were catered for by the extended family system. Local authorities operated some old-age homes, which were mostly occupied by elderly aliens from neighbouring countries who had sustained the colonial economy by providing a source of cheap labour and doing the dirty work that indigenous people would not do.

Children's and family services

During the early colonial period rural children and families suffered from the separation of fathers/husbands who had to work in urban areas. Most rural families and children depended on family and the community for meeting human needs. Those in urban areas were catered for by voluntary organizations.

In the latter part of the colonial era, the sparse contribution of central government on welfare to African areas was basically of a remedial or residual nature. The most popular methods of service delivery were social group-work in recreation and family casework. Casework in marital counselling was usually ineffective because of the lack of incorporation of traditional mores involved in settling marital disputes by the social-work practitioners. Social-welfare services to families – like probation, child protection, counselling and public assistance in extreme situations of destitution – were mostly provided by local governments and voluntary associations.

Local government social-welfare services for the Africans usually entailed the provision of an outlet for physical energy in the form of recreational services and sports. Such services included boxing, the provision of beer, dancing, sewing and knitting and cinema for both adults and youths (Gargett, 1973). Those families and children who were extremely destitute received tangible services like food rations; children's school fees and housing rent were paid for them.

Government public assistance was given grudgingly to the Africans in both cash and kind, and was based on a very low standard-of-living scale. An example can be found in public assistance allocations for children just before Zimbabwean independence in 1980. An indigenous urban child was allocated less than Z$2 for monthly maintenance, while a European urban child received about Z$35. The colonial government did not acknowledge that nutritional needs for a black child were biologically similar to those of a white child, despite differences in the shade of skin.

The provision of child welfare services was based on a match of funding between central government and local authorities into what were mostly privately operated institutions for children. There were rare cases of indigenous adoptions. Foster-care services for non-relative placements were usually based on inappropriate assessments of indigenous traditional family practices, or resulted from alcoholism, alleged prostitution, insanity and abandonment. Child welfare services were based on judgementalism, and inhumane and punitive practices in cases of juvenile delinquency. Child welfare services reflected the predominant colonial values of racial discrimination against black people regardless of age.

Disability and survivors' benefits

No institutions for the disabled were provided by the central government until the latter part of the colonial period. Survivors and disabled were usually taken care of by voluntary associations, some by local governments and indigenous rural communities. For those Africans disabled at work, benefits for them and their families were at the discretion of the employer, as there was no comprehensive national disability and survivors Act covering Africans. People without relatives applied for public assistance. The mentally disabled were institutionalized at the only mental hospital for indigenous people in Bulawayo or were drugged at major hospitals.

Refugees

There were no programmes for refugees. Illegal immigrants were usually given meagre public assistance in institutions pending deportation. Rural dwellers who were displaced from their homes during the war were mostly catered for by their urban relatives or voluntary local and international organizations.

Rural versus urban forces

Most services provided were in urban areas. Rural areas were seen by the colonial government as a type of indigenous social security or safety net. The rural areas were virtually neglected.

Responsiveness to human needs

The colonial government's social welfare services were based on mythical assumptions held by European colonists regarding the indigenous people's human condition. Services were inappropriate, inhumane, irrelevant and insensitive, and often not available to Africans. In urban areas, in particular, services were given punitively and grudgingly and indigenous residence was viewed as temporary. When the government provided social services for the indigenous people on a massive scale, it was to safeguard the Europeans, as in the case of compulsory health screenings. The indigenous people were believed to be inferior and deserving of living conditions at poverty level. It was held that the indigenous population had inferior levels of human needs. Colonial oppression and racial superiority and the belief that indigenous people belonged in rural areas, were reflected in the harsh social-welfare system.

EGALITARIAN STRUGGLES FOR CHANGE

Colonialism sowed the seed for its own destruction. By conquering and humiliating the indigenous people of Zimbabwe, it aroused in them the need to be free. The desire to be free was further nurtured by the above reflection of a foreign-imposed economic, political and socio-cultural system, based on exploitation and racial discrimination, and reflecting the dominance of the metropolitan sector, and a system of dependent capitalism (Gifford and Louis, 1988). The central issue was that of land, which had religious and economic significance to the Africans and was owned communally. The colonists viewed land as a commodity that could be individually owned and sold. The systematic practice of driving indigenous people to infertile land, apparent in colonial systems throughout the world, also intensified the need for freedom and justice. The indigenous people mobilized themselves and formed organizations designed after 'civilized' western standards of democracy in order to gain their freedom and access to land use. They also utilized all the peaceful traditional methods at their disposal, like consulting the spirit mediums, in their efforts to gain equal rights. The colonial government ruthlessly suppressed all their peaceful efforts by banning political organizations, sentencing influential indigenous leaders to death, administering brutal emotional, cognitive and physical abuse by means of electrical torture, including maimings and castrations; imposing life imprisonment sentences; and harassing and violating the privacy of relatives of suspects.

Under such circumstances, the indigenous people opted for the second Chimurenga War of 1966, which was based on a mixture of Shona and socialist ideology. This was initially waged by the Shona-based ZANU (Zimbabwe African National Union) which had formed a government in exile. A Ndebele-based ZAPU (Zimbabwe African People's Union), which is the older of the two, also established a government in exile and joined the armed struggle motivated by socialist principles as well. Although these governments-in-exile were stationed in independent front-line states like Zambia and Tanzania, they truly functioned like governments. They provided social-welfare services to men, women and children within their memberships. The social-welfare services were in the form of consciousness-raising based on egalitarian principles, provision of food, clothing, shelter, education and military training, and medical services based on availability of donations and membership contributions. They appear to have been viable social-welfare institutions which were responsive to the needs of the exiled indigenous populations. If certain individuals failed to receive social-welfare benefits, usually it was due to depleted supplies, or the interrupted flow of supplies caused by the constant incursion by the colonial army's 'hot pursuits' into the refugee camps, which were often mistaken for guerrilla camps. When freedom fighter camps were attacked, casualties were not as severe as in the refugee camps which were occupied by old women, children, nursing mothers, old men and the disabled or sick. The concepts of equality, justice, freedom, self-determination, self-help, hard work, co-operation and resourcefulness were instilled in the political membership as important aspects in pursuing independence for Zimbabwe.

Within Zimbabwe, new methods of mobilizing the masses were developed within the context of a hostile environment. Here churches played an important role in providing what appeared to be a 'passive' leadership for organizing large numbers of 'passive' indigenous people. Later, an organization with a leadership of this nature, the ANC-Zimbabwe, turned out to be a highly viable political group which opposed the colonial government openly. ZANU and ZAPU continued to operate in the country illegally and underground. Social-welfare services for the freedom fighters were basically supplied by the indigenous rural population. During the war, the rural indigenous people were attacked and harassed by military personnel who claimed to be from the colonial army, while others claimed to be freedom fighters.

Various atrocities were committed against indigenous people during the war. Brutality in the form of murders, massacres, and deprivation was intended to instil fear in the peasants (Jokonya, 1980). As a result of this, many indigenous rural dwellers escaped to the already overcrowded cities and neighbouring countries, where they either joined the freedom fighters or went to the refugee camps. Emotional counselling was not readily available for the refugees and survivors of victims of war during this struggle for survival. During the war, 80 per cent of the country was in the war zone (Jokonya, 1980). The number of people in need of social services overwhelmed the colonial government, which had always neglected African needs.

Because of the success of the indigenous war of liberation and pressure by the international community and as the war was destroying the colonial economy, the colonial government agreed to a peaceful negotiation for Zimbabwean independence.

ZIMBABWE

At independence in 1980, Zimbabwe was faced with a large number of homeless people who had been displaced, or whose homes had been destroyed, during the war. Moreover, the war had caused the destruction of the rural infrastructure, further government neglect of the rural areas, and worsened urban indigenous poverty due to overcrowding, unemployment and lack of adequate government social services. There were masses of people living in railway and bus stations and sleeping on open ground throughout Zimbabwean cities. Apart from aid from voluntary organizations, these people were not eligible to receive aid from the colonial government because of the residence requirement. It is against this background that we will attempt to review the social-welfare programmes of Zimbabwe. Particular emphasis will be placed on how egalitarian principles of the worth and dignity and equality of each human being are implemented through the type of programmes and the methods of service delivery. Further, issues of resources like land will be revisited. Comparisons will be made with the previous discriminatory and insensitive social-welfare system.

Social-welfare services in Zimbabwe are provided on the basis of a partnership between the government and the voluntary associations, as during the colonial period. This style is also typical of most modern societies. The Zimbabwean social-welfare system has both residual and institutional types of services delivered through social-insurance and public-assistance programmes.

Social insurance is mandated by the National Social Security Authority, set up in 1989. It spells out by whom, what, when and where contributions are drawn. Social-insurance programmes are designed to maintain a minimum income to employees whose earning power is reduced or disrupted through forces beyond the employees' control. Social insurance is based on contributions to a particular private scheme and covers such catastrophes as unemployment, sickness and work-related disability, and is available to survivors. Contributions to social-insurance programmes come from the matching of employer and employee funds. Benefits are viewed as a right rather than a privilege, because social-insurance recipients feel that they are withdrawing from their contributions. Thus, there is no stigmatization of recipients. Zimbabwe has made great progress in abolishing racial discrimination in the provision and delivery of the social-insurance and public-assistance programmes. The creation of the National Social Security Authority was a progressive move towards monitoring and consolidating workers' compensation, pensions and retirement schemes, which had been discretionary and operated by private companies and employers.

When public assistance for indigenous populations was introduced during the late colonial period, it was handled by the Department of Native Affairs, and in 1965 it was transferred to the Department of Social Welfare. During that time, assistance was generally given to the disabled, to the elderly who had no kin, to children, and to the sick only after it had been proved that they had no family, and, therefore, could not be sent to the rural areas (Kaseke, 1982). Since the present government adopted the structure of the colonial civil service, the name 'Department of Social Welfare' still stands.

In 1988, the Social Welfare Assistance Act was enacted. Public assistance is non-contributory, and is intended to aid destitute persons whose deprivation is due to old age, sickness, blindness, unemployment, death of the breadwinner, or to disasters such as drought or political disturbances. Assistance is usually given both in cash and in kind. All public assistance is financed through the general revenue which is determined by an annual vote to the Ministry of Labour, Manpower Planning and Social Welfare. Allocation is made on the basis of estimated expenditures submitted by the Department of Social Welfare. Public assistance is of a residual nature based on the Elizabethan Poor Laws. There is a means test to determine eligibility for the 'deserving' poor to be given aid. Such a criterion entails proof of destitution, citizenship or lawful residence, evidence of job-seeking, and lack of care by relatives. Wealthy relatives are investigated and encouraged to help their kin so that the applicant may be denied public assistance (Social Welfare Assistance Act, Government of Zimbabwe 1988).

These criteria are a legacy of the colonial past. There is little doubt that kinship ties, which are as strong in urban areas as in rural areas, are significant. However, it is inconceivable to expect people who are poor to share anything when they have nothing. For those applicants whose needs are considered more effectively served in rural areas, or for aliens, they are provided with relocation or repatriation assistance.

People considered of questionable character, such as those with a criminal record, suspected prostitutes, and those who give up searching for jobs are viewed as 'non-deserving' and 'lazy', and are denied assistance. For those who have a previous work record, cash benefits are determined by giving 50 per cent of previous monthly earnings. Thus, those who earned more would get more cash allowances (Riddell Commission, 1980; Hampson and Kaseke, 1987;

Kaseke, 1988). Since Europeans had a long history of higher salaries on the eve of Zimbabwean independence, they are likely to have higher benefits than the average indigenous recipients. Further, since most Europeans do not have rural villages to go to and have different cultural values from those of the indigenous people, the screening process for eligibility is tilted against the indigenous people in favour of the Europeans. Further, those indigenous people who earn more will, like Europeans, belong to the category of those eligible to receive benefits, resulting in indigenous people receiving the least public assistance. The social insurance and public assistance Acts are unco-ordinated and place an unrealistic and overwhelming responsibility on the rural areas for social security.

Despite the discrepancies, Zimbabwe, like other Third World countries, has limited resources, and those who receive public assistance are usually considered the privileged of the poor (Kaseke, 1988). Public assistance is given grudgingly and in a punitive way. This stringent and dehumanizing approach to public assistance is considered to be a deterrent to the promotion of perpetual dependence on the social-welfare system. It is also considered to be an approach which gives people an incentive to go to the rural areas where they could be productive and live by subsistence agriculture. Conditions of living are generally no better in rural areas than in urban areas. Sending individuals back to the rural areas implies 'blaming the victim', which is a serious violation of the principle of freedom of choice and was initially a practice implemented by the colonial government. The approach to public assistance is so rigorous and degrading to the applicants that, in addition to office visits, home visits are made to see if there are valuable possessions which could be sold by the applicant to earn a living rather than receive public assistance. Here the principles of self-determination, self-worth and human dignity are undermined. Let us now assess the various social welfare programmes and the degree of government involvement.

Education

One of the sectors in which the Zimbabwean government has had tremendous success is in the area of education. Education ranks high on its list of priorities, and free universal primary school education is mandated by law as a right. The new government had to reconstruct schools destroyed during the war and build new ones, embark on an accelerated teacher-training programme, and eliminate all discriminatory barriers by opening elementary and high school education to all Zimbabweans. This approach allowed people whose education had been interrupted by the war or by racism to return to mainstream education. Nominal fees are paid at government high schools, compared to those at private ones. The government views education as a social-security programme that increases employment opportunities for participants and participation in social insurance and decreases potentiality for the need for public assistance. Thus, the education programme prevents unemployment due to lack of skill and also ameliorates the position of those who are qualified to work. However, the programme's effectiveness can be enhanced if the country employs everyone who is qualified to work and capable of it. Many students hold government educational grants in high school, at various technical colleges and at the University of Zimbabwe. There are a number of educational programmes aimed at consciousness-raising to (1) counteract the damage caused to the human mind by years of colonial subjugation, and (2) deal with scars left by the protracted war of liberation.

Many constraints have hindered the realization of the government's educational goals and aspirations. The most obvious ones are the shortage of teachers and schools; long distances to be travelled by students to schools without adequate public transportation; and scarcity of financial resources, making it impossible to provide secondary education and vocational training for all who can benefit from them. The rural areas are the most affected by these constraints.

Health and mental health

Health services are financed from general taxation. The Ministry of Health has a number of preventive and treatment programmes in both rural and urban areas. However, the distance from health-care services is a major problem, especially for rural populations. Although health care is free for those earning less than Z$150 per month, the quality of care has suffered from lack of medicines in government pharmacies, and private pharmacies are extremely expensive and unaffordable to ordinary people because prescription medicines cost an average of Z$50 each. People who earn over Z$150 a month pay for health care on a sliding scale. The local government clinics and mission health centres inherited from the colonial past charge fees for services as government subsidies are not enough to cover their health-care costs. Government expenditures on health care are about 1.4 per cent of its GDP. The large hospitals in the main urban areas cater to severe cases which require more advanced services than those in township and rural settings. Life expectancy is about 56 years, which is typical of Third World countries.

Private medical services are provided through insurance plans, and these have tax-free employer-employee contributions. Major insurance companies have complied with the government's request for a cut-rate insurance plan from 1986. Under this plan participants pay Z$15.20 per month and the employer contributes the other half (Hampson and Kaseke, 1987). A social insurance time-limited health-care programme pays for covered wage earners on sick and maternity leave on full pay for six months, and half pay thereafter, operated under the Workers' Compensation scheme now administered under the National Social Security Authority Act. The various isolation facilities for people with contagious diseases have continued to operate, and the government provides immunization services.

Mental health is also covered by the Ministry of Health, which has established psychiatric units that are attached to major hospitals. These deal with patients who are mentally handicapped. AIDS has been the greatest incapacitating disease under the auspices of the Ministry of Health. Lack of statistics, as well as of a cure, poor education on prevention, limited financial resources and international negative stereotyping have contributed to defensiveness on the part of African governments with regard to reporting the disease and seeking aid. These factors have allowed the AIDS epidemic to spread beyond recognition. Although health care is based on universal coverage to people below a certain income, there is an obvious gap between the urban and rural health services. This disparity also exists between the indigenous and European health services, because those who can afford to pay for hospital care and medication receive better-quality service. Most indigenous people cannot reach the health-care services due to lack of free transportation for those without an income, in both the urban and rural areas. A voluntary association has been created to co-ordinate various traditional healers and to maintain ethical standards for practitioners. This association has attempted to integrate traditional healing with modern medicine. The traditional healers are easily accessible, relatively inexpensive, and use non-scientific methods, which sometimes work. Roots and herbs are used to cure certain illnesses. Although diseases like AIDS have no known cure, traditional beliefs are used to explain any illness.

Housing and living space

Since the elimination of racial discrimination, in urban areas, upper and middle-class indigenous people share residential areas with Europeans. This was introduced under the new political and socio-economic order brought about by independence.

Cormack (1983) indicates that indigenous townships, which were initially established by local governments during the colonial period, have the following characteristics. First, there are blocks of single rooms designed for single people, but usually occupied by families. Second, there are two-room, semi-detached houses with external cooking facilities. Third, three- or four-room semi-detached houses have been built, of varied designs and different construction qualities. These constitute the greater proportion of indigenous housing. Most of the buildings have external bathrooms. Fourth, there is hostel-type housing, sometimes of multi-storey blocks in which up to four persons share a room, and use communal washrooms, cooking and toilet facilities.

The following problems are noted with regard to these buildings: (1) they are small; (2) they are not tall and, because they do not have high ceilings, they become too hot for most of the year and too cold in winter; (3) they have rough interiors, making wall cleaning difficult; (4) lack of electrical supplies for lighting and cooking causes the indigenous occupants to seek other sources of fuel and lighting, in order to avoid smoke damage and discoloration of the interior and of furniture – besides which the fuel used is a health hazard; (5) there are serious sewage problems with townships in smaller urban areas and in the mines; (6) the buildings are generally roofed with corrugated asbestos, which is known to cause cancer and, therefore, is a health hazard.

Some of these houses have been upgraded by the new government, which has had them fitted with interior and exterior private water supplies and solar heating systems. Larger urban areas do not generally experience sewage problems.

The local government urban housing is designed similarly to colonial housing schemes. In rural areas, the government has sponsored resettlement schemes for people displaced during the war, indigenous people from overcrowded Communal Lands which used to be Tribal Trust Lands, and for demobilized ex-combatants. These rural reserves have not changed drastically. They are characterized by traditional mud, poles and grass-thatched huts with a few, scattered modern houses. Sanitation and drinking water are serious problems in rural areas. Most communal lands have become unhealthy living environments due to lack of vegetation to filter the air and provide supplies for building traditional housing. Limited land and financial resources and the reluctance of some to leave the land where their ancestors were buried has created further problems in living space, through overcrowding. Mobility is limited due to poor rural roads and lack of transportation.

Workers' compensation

Social insurance service for the sick employee is called Workers' Compensation, and is now amalgamated into the National Social Security Schemes. It covers self-employed people whose maximum monthly earning is about Z$1,333. This excludes a large number of minimum wage earners like domestics, agricultural labourers, mine workers and those in the underground economic sector. Despite this discrepancy, this scheme is by far the largest social insurance programme among the national social security schemes in Zimbabwe. It is compulsory for qualified employers and employees to participate in the scheme. The scheme pays pension allowances during temporary disability. Lump sum payments, and medical rehabilitation expenses, are paid to employees or dependants on injury or death incurred while working. There is a wage ceiling per annum for each member, and about 900,000 people are covered by this programme (Hampson and Kaseke, 1987). Table 9.1 shows income and expenditures for the period 1983–84.

Rehabilitative services for those with work-related injuries are covered in the form of out-patient care, physical therapy and retraining in alternative skills and trades appropriate to the participant's abilities. In 1984 alone, there were 13,700 injuries and 213 deaths reported to the scheme. However, statistics on actual recipients of benefits for the same period are unknown.

Unemployment insurance

Schemes under the National Social Security Authority Act provide unemployment insurance for covered employees. When employment is lost, a participant gets a lump sum for what he contributed but not what the employer contributed, as the basis for eligibility is working with the same employer until retirement. A notable weakness of the scheme is that employers have indirectly forced employees who are close to retirement to leave employment prematurely, without

Table 9.1 Worker's Compensation Insurance Fund; income and income expenditure

Income	1983 (Z$)	Per cent	1984 (Z$)	Per cent
Contributions	12,604,376	(76.2)	5,550,123	(54.2)
Additional penalty payments	141,138	(0.8)	1,646	(*)
Investment	3,743,732	(22.7)	4,644,007	(45.4)
Miscellaneous	50,724	(0.3)	40,870	(0.4)
Total	16,539,970	(100.0)	10,236,646	(100.0)
Expenditure				
Pensions and allowances	5,707,883	(70.8)	6,621,959	(75.4)
Medical aid expenses	744,339	(9.2)	312,043	(3.6)
Lump sum benefit	1,357,567	(16.8)	1,514,042	(17.3)
Rehabilitation expenses	256,161	(3.2)	330,570	(3.7)
	8,065,950	(100.0)	8,778,614	(100.0)
Surplus	8,474,020		1,458,035	

* Less than .00001
Note: At the time of writing, details of the various schemes under the National Security Act of 1989 were not available.

Source: Hampson and Kaseke, 1987: 287

retirement or unemployment benefits. People who lose employment without having contributed enough into their occupational pensions are expected to apply for public assistance while seeking further employment.

Old age and retirement

The elderly indigenous population has been increasing rapidly and represents approximately 13 per cent of the total indigenous population. In terms of gender, 75 per cent of elderly men and 83 per cent of elderly women live in rural areas. Public assistance is available to a limited few urban elderly. They constitute the largest number of applicants for public assistance.

The elderly can be classified into three groups. The first group consists of labourers for the commercial farming and mining sectors. They usually have neither tenure nor social insurance benefits and migrated to the country during the colonial times. The second group consists of urban elderly, which is the largest population receiving public assistance among the elderly. A small number of urban elderly live on meagre pension benefits, and these have a history of work in towns as menial labourers and have usually migrated from neighbouring countries. The third group consists of the peasant subsistence farmers in the rural areas. These suffer the most, because the present social welfare system was inherited from the colonial government which held misconceptions and myths, regarding indigenous traditions to be inherently inferior. In the rural areas, mutual aid through the extended family network is limited due to the fact that these support networks are barely surviving themselves because of poverty. It might appear that family members neglect them, but the respect rendered traditionally to the elderly is still strong and they receive satisfactory emotional, spiritual and social support, but not enough of their physical needs (like food and health requirements) are adequately met.

In urban areas, a number of the elderly tend to make ends meet through the underground economic sector, which acts as a safety net during this period of need. They engage in various self-help activities like ethnically based mutual aid and burial societies, handcrafts, poultry-raising, selling illegally brewed beer and traditional healing. The informal economic activities provide an income to those below the poverty line.

Social services for the elderly comprise private nursing homes funded through a match of government, state lotteries and private contributions. These institutions are generally operated like almshouses and occupied by the foreign elderly. Repatriation efforts are usually fruitless, as many have lost meaningful ties with their kin. Most current indigenous elderly are not covered by old-age pensions because of prior colonial discriminatory practices which expected the elderly to retire to the rural areas, and left it at the discretion of employers to cover Africans, who usually received inferior benefits. The colonial old-age pensions were eliminated when Zimbabwe became independent, and, therefore, destitute elderly people have only the public assistance option which does not guarantee assistance to every destitute elderly person.

Many occupational pensions that cover indigenous people mushroomed after independence and were included in the Authority Act of 1989. None of the current elderly would benefit from these schemes since the law is not retroactive. Public assistance covers burial costs for destitute persons.

Children's and family services

The Zimbabwean government legally protects children in need of care and their families, under Chapter 33 of the Children's Protection and Adoption Act 1979 and the Maintenance Act (Chapter 35), which provide for the creation of juvenile courts, and the protection, welfare and supervision of minors. The 1979 Act provides guidelines for adequate standards for operating children's institutions and delineates criteria for determining child abuse and neglect. When family destitution contributes to child neglect or abuse, the Department of Social Welfare approves public assistance for the family in order to keep the children in the home. The level of cash assistance is minimal, and covers up to six children. In addition, rent, fuel allowances and education supplies are provided upon the basis of need. In some cases, relative and non-relative foster care is sought. Abandoned babies and war orphans have been placed in foster care and adoptive homes. The Department of Social Welfare usually collaborates with the juvenile judiciary system and the local government in providing child protective services. The local government provides youth programmes as part of their welfare services in urban areas. There are also government-sponsored youth employment and skills training programmes.

Zimbabwe is one of the sub-Saharan African countries that has severe problems in youth employment and skills training (Kasambira, 1987). The voluntary sector operates the children's homes and is subsidized by the government. The department provides for the educational needs of children and youth under its care. Those families that become needy as a result of a breadwinner who is eligible for a social insurance programme are assisted in applying for survivors' benefits under the National Social Security Authority Act which covers pension and compensation schemes.

In rural areas, most children are expected to work in the fields and herd domestic animals when out of school. Social services for children are inadequate and there is a lack of a community consensus on what constitutes child neglect and abuse. Some traditional rural practices could be considered as neglectful and abusive in the modern sense.

Social security for the needy, neglected and abused families with children depends on public assistance in both urban and rural areas. A major weakness of the programme is that benefits are inadequate to meet basic human needs, and, therefore, they do not help recipients to become self-reliant. Even though there is a statute governing public assistance, implementation depends on the officer's ability to read and interpret it within heavy work-loads and high expectations. There is so much discretionary power on the officer's part which is checked only by ethical standards of responsibility. Further, implementation is made difficult by the legal language used in the Acts, making it difficult to interpret. Public assistance approval is not a one-time procedure. Recipients have to be reviewed frequently in order to check change of status.

Although Zimbabwe is a food exporter, malnutrition is a serious problem for the children. About 25 per cent of urban children and 39 to 42 per cent of rural children are affected. The Ministry of Health has embarked on preventive and curative measures through food supplementation, nutrition training, and immunization against childhood diseases. Well-baby clinics are also provided by nongovernment health services.

Although the law protects children and their families, heavy reliance on public assistance as a safety net has kept many recipients in poverty and many needy families unprotected. There are no family allowances, but there is a tax abatement of Z$500 per child, up to a maximum of six children, for families earning an income. There is no social security support for non-taxpaying families.

Disability and survivors' benefits

People who are physically disabled are usually institutionalized if they lack family support or if their disability can only be handled in a hospital setting for appropriate rehabilitation. Mainstreaming and de-institutionalization are emphasized. There are more than 300,000 disabled people in Zimbabwe, and only 29 per cent of them have access to rehabilitation services. About 20,000 of these were disabled during the Liberation War (Nyathi, 1986). Most services tend to be urban-based, and efforts are being made to decentralize them to rural areas. Voluntary agencies like Jairos Jiri Association provide most services for disabled people, in the form of rehabilitation. In rural areas, visiting multi-professional teams are utilized through a mobile service to screen, treat and refer those in need of services.

Two Acts govern disability: the National Social Security Act 1989, and the War Victims Compensation Act 1980, both administered by the Ministry of Labour, Manpower Planning and Social Welfare. The war victims programme is non-contributory and is state-funded. It covers war victims and surviving dependants through government intervention in the form of cash compensation, rehabilitation, vocational training and medical services to provide some social insurance to war victims and ex-combatants. Compensation is based on the degree of disablement. The compensation rates are between 50 and 90 per cent of before-injury earnings.

The National Social Security Authority Act embodies schemes for disabled and dependants that were covered by the Workers' Compensation Act, Chapter 196. Benefits are paid on the basis of the degree of disability and previous earnings. Eligibility is based on the employer's participation in the scheme. Widows and up to five children are covered. The widow receives two-thirds of the worker's pension and 24 months' pension benefits upon remarriage. Disabled people not covered by the two Acts are considered for public assistance (under the Social Welfare Assistance Act), or covered by voluntary organizations.

The two programmes have limitations, as beneficiaries receive less than the usual disabled or deceased person's income. Problems could exist in determining previous income for war victims if they were unemployed or lived in rural areas. A large number of agricultural and domestic workers will not be covered.

Refugees

At independence, the Zimbabwean government was faced with a large number of displaced indigenous people and refugees returning from exile. These had fled from the rural areas. The rural infrastructure had almost been destroyed causing rural and urban poverty to escalate. Also, because the war was concluded by means of peaceful negotiations in Geneva, the new government had to inherit the colonial army and combine it with all the combatants from the nationalist liberation movements. The government embarked on a demobilization programme to reduce the size of the army. Large numbers of ex-combatants were given lump sums so that they could live a civilian life. Those whose rural homes had been destroyed were assigned to resettlement schemes through the government's national reconstruction and rehabilitation projects. Many indigenous people were happy to be free, and co-operated with the government in planning, construction and farming, and engaged in several kinds of co-operative and employment activities (Mandishona, 1987). In general, ex-combatants shared their plans and ideas on how they could be helped, although a sizeable number ended up applying for public assistance as their lump sum had been spent. The Department of Social Welfare, which had the responsibility for rehabilitation, was usually generous to ex-combatants. Assistance with building materials and transportation to rural areas was provided.

Other refugee groups comprise Mozambican and South African political refugees who were settled in refugee camps. The Department of Social Welfare administers the refugee programme, which is funded by the government and other voluntary organizations. These refugees are desperate, and usually work illegally for less than the minimum wage.

Although rural reconstruction, rehabilitation and refugee camps are soundly planned, progress has often been hindered by limited resources in the form of money and land, as former colonial landowners have been reluctant to sell their land to the government. Some of the resettlement schemes have been adversely affected by poor management and the use of inappropriate technology. Those resettlement schemes that have been successful are experiencing land shortages, because their adult children have no agricultural land (Staff writer, 1990).

Rural versus urban focus

There has always been a gap between the rural and urban areas in the provision of social services. The Zimbabwean government has been attempting to redress this imbalance by decentralizing services and creating new ones. During the 1983–84 drought, for example, the cost of public assistance escalated to Z\$42 million, and about 2.1 million rural people received drought relief from the government through the Department of Social Welfare. During the 1980–84 period, Z\$66 million was granted to ex-combatants in the demobilization programme which also utilized rural resettlement schemes on limited government or donated land. Because of the government rural reconstruction projects, many indigenous rural populations have benefited in the areas of education, health, housing, services for the elderly, families and children, women, the disabled and refugees.

One of the most serious rural problems is that of land shortage, creating intolerable problems of living space. Most of the land was owned by a privileged few during the colonial period, and the situaion has not changed fourteen years after independence.

In urban areas, the elimination of racial discrimination in residential areas has opened opportunities to many. Urban areas have more and better-quality services, and freedom of mobility, rural poverty, natural population growth, and the hope for a better future in the cities have increased rural–urban migration, but this has led to overcrowding, unemployment, underemployment and greater poverty. These tendencies have overwhelmed Zimbabwe, a newly independent, Third World country with limited resources.

The rural areas are lacking in employment and youth programmes and those in existence are scattered, and tend to be church-operated or organized by the ruling party's youth wing. The new social-welfare Acts tend to cater to urban dwellers, and most expenditures on social-welfare services are in urban areas. The indigenous rural population has no social security protection from the government other than access to public assistance services which are not easily attainable.

Responsiveness to human needs

Zimbabwe's social security scheme is based on the newly created National Social Security Authority and the Social Welfare Assistance Acts. It appears that the needy and unemployed are not protected by any safety net. Agricultural workers comprise 20 per cent, while the other 50 per cent are rural subsistence farmers lacking skills and opportunities to join the labour force. Slightly over 70 per cent of the indigenous population live in rural areas. The social security programme excludes those people who are generally considered needy due to poor nutrition, ill-health, sanitary conditions, lack of educational facilities, poverty-level income, lack of tenure and weak kinship networks. Then there are over 10 per cent unemployed in urban areas. The future of such people is bleak unless more fertile land and projects generating rural employment and eligible for participation in the present social security scheme are created. The Zimbabwean social welfare system reflects limited responsiveness to the needs of the indigenous population. Those covered are a small percentage of those who would benefit from coverage. Public assistance, which should be an option for everyone excluded from the social insurance system, is only available to the privileged few.

CONCLUSION

The history of Africa and elsewhere has shown that the inability of the current social-welfare system to live up to expectations and promises, and the persistent inability of the political and socio-economic process to respond to concrete community preferences, redistribute resources efficiently and fairly, and redress inequalities can cause frustrations which could explode in destructive ways. In fact, it is these frustrations which led to the War of Liberation.

There are legitimate problems facing the government, like debt deficits and a dearth of foreign exchange, but to the ordinary person these problems are remote, especially when there are indigenous elites who own land that they do not utilize and live in luxury like the former European oppressors. Even if the government has limited resources to sustain a comprehensive social-security scheme, to throw the majority of the indigenous people 'to the wolves' leaves a great deal to be desired. Those who are most needy are not catered for, and even the recipients of public assistance are stratified on the basis of prior earnings. It may have been necessary to inherit a colonial structure, but to continue without major reformation of the social-welfare system may serve a self-defeating purpose.

Suggestions

Limited resources are often cited as an obstacle to a comprehensive, government-funded and -administered social-security programme, but it is debatable whether this is so. A comprehensive and pragmatic social-welfare system is needed. It is the government's responsibility to provide social security to all citizens, under the national motto, 'Unity, Freedom and Work', and demands that any civilized society protect its citizens. Further, the socialist ideals held by the government are not in contradiction with civilized standards. The concept of 'deserving' and 'non-deserving' poor is colonial and outdated.

The resources could come from within Zimbabwe by means of government efforts. The government, through democratic processes, could redistribute the current land owned by Europeans and the indigenous elite by imposing high property taxes and limiting the amount of land per person, as well as by monitoring and recovering land not in use. Further, the government could consolidate the civil-service bureaucracies and positions that go with it, and lower salaries for particular highly paid figureheads. Also, the government could enforce rural social welfare and social development without regard to immediate monetary returns, and focus on developing and monitoring work habits, practices and use of appropriate technology that would eventually lead to agricultural surplus on a massive scale. Kaseke makes the point clearly by suggesting:

> A unique administrative framework could be set up to enable the rural population to participate in a contributory social security. The success of such an approach depends on linking it to a strategy of

rural development geared towards increasing the productivity of the poor.

(1988: 5)

Finally, the government could evolve a social-insurance system that covers people in both regular employment and self-employment by reaching out to mine workers, agricultural workers, domestic workers and those engaged in underground economic activity. Covering such people could generate more money into the trust funds. Rewards and incentives based on gender could be eliminated to avoid economic discrimination against women.

Even if the old-age pension was racially discriminatory, the government could have made it non-discriminatory rather than eradicating it entirely. The majority of sufferers are indigenous people since the Europeans usually have social security by virtue of their historical position of economic power which originated during the colonial period. To expect the social-welfare system for indigenous people to be loosely organized is to expect lower quality of life for them, which would seriously undermine their dignity, freedom, unity and work potential.

REFERENCES

Adeyeri, C. L. K. (1984) 'Social Services in Nigeria', in C. Guzette, A. J. Katz and R. A. English (eds) *Education for Social Work Practice: Selected International Models*, New York: Council on Social Work Education for the International Association of Schools of Social Work, pp. 71–9.

Bender, L. D., Leone, B. and Rohr, R. (eds) (1988) *Problems of Africa: Opposing Viewpoints*, St Paul, MN: Greenhaven Press.

Cormack, I. R. N. (1983) *Towards Self-reliance: Urban Social Development in Zimbabwe*, Gweru: Mambo Press.

Cramer, J. (1945) 'Memorandum on Social Security in Relation to the Needs of the Native Population', *NADA*, 22: 56–60.

Devittie, T. D. (1976) *The Underdevelopment of Social Welfare Services for Urban Africans in Rhodesia, 1923–1953*, Harare: University of Rhodesia.

Dixon, J. (ed.) (1987) *Social Welfare in Africa*, London: Croom Helm.

Dixon, J. and Scheurell, R. (1987) 'Social Security in Australia and the United States: A Comparison of Value Premises and Practices', *Journal of International and Comparative Social Welfare*, III(1–2): 1–13.

— — (1989) 'Social Security Traditions and Their Global Content', in Brij Mohan (ed.) *Glimpses of International and Comparative Social Welfare*, Canberra: International Fellowship for Social and Economic Development, Inc., pp. 109–39.

Federation of African Welfare Societies (1950) *African Welfare in Southern Rhodesia*, Bulawayo: Philport and Collins, Ltd.

Gargett, E. S. (1973) 'The Changing Pattern of Urban African Welfare

Services', A paper presented to the Rhodesian Provincial Division of IANA., pp. 1–5 (unpublished, in National Archives of Zimbabwe).

— — (1977a), with comments by M. Ndubiwa, 'Social Administration in a Changing Society: Issues in Development', Seminar Series, reporting No. 9, Harare: Centre for Applied Social Sciences, University of Zimbabwe.

— — (1977b), *The Administration of Transition: African Urban Settlement in Rhodesia*, Gweru: Mambo Press.

Gifford, P. and Louis, R. (1988) *Decolonization and African Independence*, New Haven, CT: Yale University Press.

Gil, G. D. (1989) 'Social Sciences, Human Survival, Development and Liberation', in Brij Mohan (ed.) *Glimpses of International and Comparative Social Welfare*, Canberra: International Fellowship for Social and Economic Development, Inc., pp.176–89.

Ginsberg, H. L. (1989) 'What the United States Can Learn About Social Welfare from Third World Nations', in Brij Mohan (ed.) *Glimpses of International and Comparative Social Welfare*, Canberra: International Fellowship for Social and Economic Development, Inc. pp. 161–8.

Government of Zimbabwe (1980) *War Victims Compensation Act, 1980*, Harare: Government Printer.

— — (1988) *Social Welfare Assistance Act, 1988*, Harare: Government Printer.

— — (1989) *Social Security Authority Act, 1989*, Harare: Government Printer.

Hampson, J. and Kaseke, E. (1987) 'Zimbabwe: The Welfare System Environment', in John Dixon (ed.) *Social Welfare in Africa*, London: Croom Helm.

Henson, P. (1990) 'Racism in Zimbabwe: There is a Lot of it About', *MOTO*, No. 91, 14, Gweru: Mambo Press.

Hope, A. and Timmel, S. (1989) *Training for Transformation: A Handbook for Community Workers*, 1, 2, and 3, illustrated by Chris Hodzi, Gweru: Mambo Press.

Jackson, J. and Mupedziswa, R. (1988) 'Disability and Rehabilitation', *Journal of Social Development in Africa*, 3(1): 21–30.

Johnson, H. W. (1990) *The Social Services: An Introduction*, 3rd edn, Itasca, IL: Peacock Publishers, Inc.

Johnson, L. C. and Schwartz, C. L. (1988) *Social Welfare: A Response to Human Need*, Boston: Allyn & Bacon, Inc.

Jokonya, T. J. B. (1980) 'The Effects of the War on the Rural Population of Zimbabwe', *Journal of Southern African Affairs*, 5(2): 133–47.

Kachingwe, E. (1981) 'Services for Urban Africans in Zimbabwe: The Role of Social Work Education in the Distribution of Services', Dissertation, Ann Arbor, MI: University Microfilm International.

Kasambira, P. E. (1987) 'Youth Skills Training', *Journal of Social Development in Africa*, 2(2): 35–48.

Kaseke, E. (1982) 'Social Assistance in Developing Countries: The Case of Zimbabwe', Unpublished MSc dissertation, London School of Economics and Political Science.

— — (1988) 'Social Security in Zimbabwe', *Journal of Social Development in Africa*, 3(1): 5–19.

Kawewe, S. M. (1986) 'Planning for Education for Social Development in

Zimbabwe: An Assessment of Zimbabwe's Students and Lecturers Concerning Their Perception of the University's Curriculum in Terms of Providing Skills Necessary to Carry Out National Reconstruction Tasks', *Dissertation Abstracts International*, 47, 315A, University Microfilms No. DA8604388.

— — (1990) 'Reality is Reality', *Moto*, Gweru: Mambo Press, No. 91, p. 9.

Mandishona, G. M. (1987) 'Population and Development Indicators', *Journal of Social Development in Africa*, 2(2): 69–77.

Mohan, B. (ed.) (1989) *Glimpses of International and Comparative Social Welfare*, Canberra: International Fellowship for Social and Economic Development, Inc., pp. 1–2, 169–75.

Mungazi, D. A. (1989) *The Struggle for Social Change in Southern Africa: Visions of Liberty*, New York: Crane Russak.

Nyathi, L. (1986) 'The Disabled and Social Development in Zimbabwe', *Journal of Social Development in Africa*, 1(1): 61–5.

Patel, D. (1988) Some Issues of 'Urbanization and Development in Zimbabwe', *Journal of Social Development in Africa*, 3(2): 17–31.

Prigmore, S. C. and Atherton, R. C. (1990) *Social Welfare Policy: Analysis and Formulation*, 2nd edn, Lexington, MA: D. C. Heath & Co.

Pumphrey, R. (1971) 'Social Welfare History', in Robert Morris (ed.) *Encyclopedia of Social Work*, 16th edn, New York: National Association of Social Workers, p. 44.

Republic of Zimbabwe (1988) *First Five-Year National Development Plan 1986–1990*, II, Harare: Government Printer.

Rhodesia Council of Social Services (1962–74) *Handbook of Social Services in Rhodesia*, Salisbury: Author.

Rhodesia Government (1971) *The State Service (Disability Benefits Act)*, Chapter 274, Harare: Government Printer.

Riddell Commission (1980) *Report of the Commission of Inquiry into Homes, Prices and Conditions of Service*, Harare: Government Printer.

Rodgers, R. H. (1988) *Beyond Welfare: New Approaches to the Problem of Poverty in America*, Armonk, NY: M. E. Sharpe, Inc.

Southern Rhodesian Council of Social Services (1964) *Record of the Social Services*, Salisbury: Author.

Staff writer (1990) 'Reality is Reality', *Moto*, (Aug.), No. 91, p. 9 Gweru: Mambo Press.

Trattner, W. I. (1985) *From Poor Law to Welfare State*, 2nd edn, New York: The Free Press.

UN Department of Economic and Social Affairs (1971) *Training for Social Welfare, Fifth International Survey: New Approaches in Meeting Manpower Needs*, New York: United Nations, pp. 3–4.

Zald, M. D. (1965) *Social Welfare Institutions: A Sociological Reader*, New York: John Wiley & Sons, pp. 1–3.

Zimbabwe-Rhodesia Government (1979) *Children's Protection and Adoption Act, Chapter 33*, Salisbury: Government Printer.

Zimbabwe School of Social Work and Christian Care (1979) 'A Report on Physically Incapacitated War Victims', Unpublished, Harare: National Archives of Zimbabwe.

10 The impact of the social-welfare system on the Temne ethnic group of Sierra Leone

Alfred A. Jarrett

HISTORICAL OVERVIEW AND SUB-ETHNIC BREAKDOWN OF THE TEMNE

The primary thrust of this chapter is an examination of how the western social-welfare system and other social-welfare-related institutions (that is, education, religion and health) have impacted upon the positive growth and development of the traditional social-welfare practices of the Temne indigenous population. This chapter will: (1) present an historical overview and sub-ethnic breakdown of the Temne; (2) discuss impacts of other ethnic groups on the Temne institutions such as the institutionalization of the Temne culture and traditional social-welfare systems; (3) examine the impact of the non-traditional social-welfare system on the Temne; and (4) discuss intervention strategies necessary for a systemic relationship with other social institutions and indigenous groups.

Sierra Leone is a former British colony in West Africa, which obtained its independence in 1961. It is approximately 72,330 square kilometres in size, with a population of 4 million. This country is located on the west coastal plains of the rich tropical rainforests of West Africa. With its fascinating history, it currently contains fourteen ethnic groups. Four of these can be singled out as the leading groups in the nation: the Temne, the Mende, the Limba, and the Creoles. These four population groups play key roles in the political, educational, economic and manpower development of the nation. However, this chapter will only focus on the Temne group and the impact that the western social-welfare system in Sierra Leone has had upon them and their traditional social-welfare system.

The Temne ethnic group is comprised of four sub-ethnic groups: (1) the Bullom, (2) the Wallah, (3) the Konika, and (4) the Mabanta Temne. The Bullom Temne are settled along the western coastline of

Sierra Leone. Their chief occupations are fishing, gardening and petty trading. The Wallah Temne can be found along the tributaries of the Great and Little Scearcies, the Rokel and the Freetown rivers, and farming is their chief occupation. The Konika Temne ethnic group live (outside the boundaries of the western areas of Sierra Leone) in Waterloo, Hastings, and Tarssor Island. The chief occupations of this group are hunting and farming. The Mabanta Temne are to be found in the interior, northern and northeastern parts of Sierra Leone. The primary occupation of this group is farming.

The presence of these Temne groups in Sierra Leone is the result of a long and varied history and the occurrence of political, economic, religious, social, cultural and traditional events. Multiple assumptions were made about how the Temne came to settle in Sierra Leone. This, it is assumed, started during the sixteenth century, as they migrated into the northern and western corridors of Sierra Leone from Senegal and other countries. The rationale for the migration into Sierra Leone is not quite clear due to the high dependency on oral history. It was only recently that Sierra Leone historians started to develop methods of historical research to document the complex migration movements of the Temne in the past (*Background to Sierra Leone*, 1990). The documentation of Temne activities has uncovered an interesting historical profile that warrants restating.

First, the migratory movement of the Temne was influenced by the activities of the great empires and wars of Africa. The empires established their political hegemony by invading territories and other empires, forcing them to be loyal to their systems of government. Part of the historical literature states that the Temne group was one of those displaced by wars and forced to relocate along the West African coastal plain. According to Langley (1938), the Temnes may have migrated and settled in Sierra Leone thousands of years ago, as the expansion of the African empires from the interior aimed to secure the virgin forest of the mountains and the seas of West Africa. During the migration, the Temne encountered the hostility of several other ethnic groups, such as the Bambara, Mandinka, Manika, Fula, Baza, Ualoka, Limba, Koranka, Kono, Mende, Sherbro and Vai. The invasion and attacks on the Temne by these groups took about three or four generations, which reflects the vanguard of an enormous array of looters from these groups who had already swept much of the coast to the southeast of West Africa. These invaders came into Sierra Leone between 1540 and 1550, and subjugated the Temne by at least 1562 (Wylie, 1977). The constant attacks of these groups forced the Temne to migrate further into West Africa.

The Temne were also attacked by the Krim and Logo ethnic groups as they travelled across Senegal, Guinea, Gambia, Liberia and the Côte d'Ivoire, and these groups tried to prevent the Temne from settling. Eventually, the hostility engendered by these ethnic wars stopped, and the land was divided roughly at a line extending inland from the Sierra Leone estuary, leaving the Temne under the direct administration of the ethnic groups that invaded them. The invaders divided the Temne into kingdoms (Wylie, 1977). These constant attacks helped the Temne to work together for the preservation of their culture and community.

Historical evidence shows that the Temne may have been one of the ethnic groups that succeeded in promoting the expansion of the African empires, especially the Ghana Empire (Langley, 1938). Though Langley did not amplify on his conviction that the Temne participated in the expansion of these empires, there is evidence to infer that they may have engaged in warlike activities. The British or colonial administration asked the ethnic groups in Sierra Leone to pay taxes in order to finance the new protectorate. This was rightly interpreted in Temne customary law as implying that actual ownership of their houses had passed to the British (*Background to Sierra Leone*, 1990). Other groups such as the Mende, Loko and Susu, were also in defiance of British taxation policies. These ethnic groups joined Bai Bureh's group with the aim of eradicating European influence from the country. The Temne's refusal to pay the tax resulted in the Hut-Tax War (*Background to Sierra Leone*, 1990), which was fought for several months.

It can only be inferred – as the historical literature has failed to state specifically – how the Temne reached the soils of Sierra Leone. Thus, it is unlikely for contemporary historians to identify events of the past, and the specific time frame the Temne migrated to and settled in Sierra Leone, because the historical data are inconclusive. Inference can be made, however, that: (1) the Temne were not indigenous to Sierra Leone; (2) they migrated from the northern African countries; (3) they were affected by tribal wars and invaded by hostile groups on the migratory routes; and (4) they assimilated cultures, values, political ideologies, and norms of other groups along the migratory route towards West Africa.

CONTEMPORARY TEMNE

The Temne of today have followed in the footsteps of their ancestors, and aim to be politically and economically competitive in Sierra

Leone society. Further, like their ancestors, they still respect the traditional culture, having strong family beliefs, developing and practising the mutual aid concept, traditional social-welfare systems, and a strong community. As such, the Temne have emerged to become a very popular group and to contribute to the national growth and development of Sierra Leone. Moreover, their population has greatly increased, to the point that they have wide influence on political, economic, educational, social and cultural issues in Sierra Leone.

Vernon DorJaha, an American anthropologist, documents that the migratory and settlement patterns of the Temne are still in effect today. Vernon DorJaha specifically states that:

> There can be no question that the Temnes were entrenched on the peninsula of Freetown and islands and creeks of the estuary of 'Sierra Leone River' by the Sixteenth Century, if not before. To the north, the Temne then stretched as far as the Isles de Los and Muaui-Susu territory, according to Duarte Pachecs Pereira (1506–1508); while to the south it seems likely from the writing of Valentin Fernandes (1506–1510), that at least some of the Temnes still settled in Sherbro Island.
>
> (Langley, 1938)

(Sherbro Island is one of the major islands of Sierra Leone.) The Temne also inhabit the northern part of Waterloo and extend as far north as Kambia in the Port Loko district. To the east of the Kambia line the Temne embrace the Yonni, Kholifa, Bankolenken and Konika chiefdoms. A segment of the Temne are between the Loko and the Limba to the north of Kambia, while other sets of Temne are settling in the Koya chiefdom corridor. The Temne currently inhabit most of the western area and northern provincial corridors of Sierra Leone (Kup, 1961; Langley, 1938; Wylie, 1977; Jackson, 1977).

As the Temne settled, they began to practise agriculture and to own land. They developed territorial units under the leadership of the Council of Elders, which ruled as a government by the people for the people. The Council is comprised of: (1) the chief elders, who have a knowledge of past and present community events, and educate the masses about traditional practices, and act as advisers to the chief; and (2) the paramount chief, who is the leader of the unit chiefdom and who exists as a role model. Under the chiefdom are centralized units, organized corporate activities of various kin groups (predominantly village-based), with a centralized structure headed by leaders who preside over the representatives of the local lineages sitting in the Council of Government. The complex interaction between officials who depend upon the chief for their positions and authority lineages gradually emerged as an effective means of maintaining a basic political equilibrium amongst a highly heterogenous population.

The Council of Government is mandated with the responsibility of keeping the peace and promoting the growth and development of the community. Laws regulating the ownership of property and inheritance is one of the primary functions of the Council of Government. The Temne laws regulating the ownership of property and inheritance are divided into two classes: (1) real property, and (2) personal and movable property. Real property consists of land and houses. Land initially belonged to the chief and the traditional government. At present the chief and the traditional government are not the owners of the land; they have merely overlordship over the land, but have no right to dispossess any landowner of his land. Currently, all land in the Temne community is in reality held by some family, however remote that land may be from a township. However, the chief holds certain properties (such as a farm and a house) by virtue of his being a chief (Langley, 1938). Real property such as land may be loaned at a fixed yearly rate payable in money, rice or kind. When the land is pawned, usually to a wealthy individual, it becomes the property of the loaner in a few years provided the landowner has no need of the land (Langley, 1938), or cannot repay the loan. According to Langley (1938), real property that is transferred from father to son or adopted son follows the rule applicable to real property. Sometimes the real property is composed of domestic slaves. Upon the death of the slave owner the domestic slaves are bequeathed to his eldest brother, who then has charge of the family.

IMPACTS OF THE OTHER ETHNIC GROUPS ON THE TEMNE

Several ethnic groups influenced the supra-system of the Temne. However, the impact of the Mende and Creoles have more bearing on the Temne institution than the other ethnic groups.

The Mende

This group invaded and conquered the Temne during their migration from the Fouta D'Jallon mountains in Guinea, West Africa (Wylie, 1977), who further states that the vanguard of an army of looters who already swept much of the coast to the southeast, invaded Sierra Leone in 1540 and 1550, and subjugated the Temne by at least 1562.

During the Mende invasion, warriors like the Vai, Kono and K'kru tribal groups were recruited into their army to fight the Temne (Wylie, 1977). However, Wylie's allegation that the Mende invaded the Temne was disputed by Little (1967), who reports that the Temne were originally a fighting legion engaged in war activities with others. Little (1967) further states that the conflict between the Mende and Temne started when 'the Temne consolidated themselves in the area north and north-west of the Mende land and in the face of opposition from the Mende' (Little, 1967). Based on these accounts, it is apparent that both the Temne and the Mende were warlike. However, the Temne were conquered and placed under the administration of the Mende authorities. Thus, the Mende administration was able to impose their traditional political organization on the Temne, and 'rapidly enhanced their authority over the conquered [Temne] through diplomatic marriages' (Wylie, 1977).

To get the Temne to adopt Mende administration and customary rules, the Mende destroyed much of the Temne culture, including their artistic skills, and converted their names to Mende names, changed their customary practices, and forced them to adopt their culture and customary norms. Today, great similarities exist between the Temne and Mende cultures, customs and practices.

Contemporary similarities between the Mende and the Temne are: (1) their Islamic and African religious beliefs; and (2) their wish to coexist and thrive in an atmosphere of mutual respect and tolerance (Jarrett, 1990; *Background to Sierra Leone*, 1990).

Creoles

The Creoles have had a great influence on the Temne in Sierra Leone. The name 'Creole' is utilized to refer to the descendants of settlers and liberated slaves from the British colonies. To others, they were African ex-slaves who had involuntarily adapted their culture and habits to reflect those of the west, and who believe that their ways of living were superior to other ethnic groups in Sierra Leone. The arrival of the Creoles in Freetown, the capital of Sierra Leone, between 1787 and 1870, dramatically changed the cultural and traditional social institutions of the nation, and quantitatively added another to the thirteen ethnic groups, making them fourteen groups. The ethnocentric and egocentric attitudes of the Creoles, compounded by the British government's favouritism towards them, are the factors responsible for their drive to convert the Temne to Creolism. Until 1961, when Sierra Leone became independent from Britain, the Creoles were the leaders in education and politics, holding key positions in the Sierra Leonean administrative institutions. Accordingly, they were able to establish policies across the social systems that affected the traditional system of the Temne. For instance, Temne were converted to Christianity, and their traditional names were changed to western names. Further, marriages and legal matters were settled in the eastern and European customary ways. In fact, Temne customary marriages and settlement of legal matters were at times not acceptable in the colonial and neo-colonial courts of law. Likewise, some technology, and the knowledge base (such as school curricula), were disguised and institutionalized to reflect western and European customary practices with the Creoles collaborating with their colonial masters.

The foreign technologies imposed upon the Temne by the Creoles were detrimental to Temne customs and to the functioning of other traditional social systems, such as education, health, agriculture, politics, because their technologies were not institutionalized by the present government.

INSTITUTIONALIZATION OF TEMNE CULTURE AND THE TRADITIONAL SOCIAL-WELFARE SYSTEM

Although it would not be possible here to define the many influences on Temne culture, in this section an attempt will be made to describe some of its salient features as it affects the traditional welfare system.

Language

The Temne language claimed affiliations with several other tribal languages, such as Creoles, Gola, Mende, Susu, French and English. The adoption of the various languages was due to Temne interaction with many ethnic groups during their migration from the Fouta D'Jallon mountains of Upper Guinea to the eastern plains of West Africa and the arrival of the Creoles (ex-slaves from England) in Freetown, Sierra Leone. The integration of the Temne language with other ethnic languages makes it hard to place linguistically. Langley (1938) states that the Temne language is hard to track, inferring that it is allied with the Hamitic and Bantu languages and cultures. McCulloch (1950) also states that the Temne language was composed of Susu, Yalunka, Sherbro, Kono and Koranki languages and cultures. Thus it is seen that many ethnic and other cultural influences influenced the Temne language.

Accordingly, the composition of their language helps the current Temne to maintain pride in their ethnic tradition of the past, in such customary practices as marriage, worship, education, healing and the mourning process. These traditional practices reflect the language and culture through which the diverse standards of the group's heritage are woven into a single whole (*Background to Sierra Leone*, 1990).

Mutual aid

Jarrett (1991) conceptualizes mutual aid as a survival strategy adopted by the hunting society at the start of group consciousness and cohesiveness. Further, mutual aid is the volunteering of self and expertise towards peace and stability of the society as a whole. The essential thrusts of this concept are to promote the stability of the extended family, and to facilitate the community's growth and development. The Temne group deeply believed in the custom and practice of mutual aid. It was particularly important to them because in Sierra Leone most Temne shared a low socio-economic status (Jarrett, 1991). This common circumstance gave rise to the realization that their individual survival was inextricably linked with each other, thus, their collective efforts would enhance greater individual benefit. Jarrett's observations of the Sierra Leoneans illustrate that the pivotal point of ethnic, community growth and development is centred on mutual aid practices and the traditional social-welfare system.

The family and the traditional social-welfare system

The Temne traditional social-welfare system is institutionalised. The strongest focuses of this social-welfare system are the family, the management of services to those in need in the community, and enforcement of rituals, customary roles and practices.

With all the changes which westernization brings to Sierra Leone, the close network of the Temne extended family and management of resources remains a constant source of stability and security in the tribe's customs and ritual practices. From conception to old age, the Temne person can rely on the support of his family and community throughout the vicissitudes of life. The Temne clan allows its members to participate in and benefit from a system of social welfare which is real, immediate and caring and which renders the western social-welfare system unimportant. It is unlikely that a child will need the care of an orphanage, or an old person a geriatric home, or that a divorce will be granted without the practice of traditional customs. In the Temne clan, the family acts as its own social agent and provider (*Background to Sierra Leone*, 1990).

The Temne family is the unit of social, economic and agricultural life. Every member participating in the growth of the family and community has specific tasks and responsibilities in improving the village. For instance, the elderly retain a place in society, and are valued for their wisdom and experience. Likewise, the Temne family unit can be viewed as a microcosm; it is an inter-dependent network in which each member has an assured place with a fair and equitable balance of rights and duties. For example, a talented youth can rely on the help of his family and community in obtaining special training or education, while the untalented youth is not abandoned but encouraged by the family and community to grow (*Background to Sierra Leone*, 1990).

Thus, the inference can be made that the primary functions of the family are education, healing and enforcement of traditional and customary values and laws.

Education

Temne children are expected to develop a knowledge base in the following areas: marriage, occupational techniques and unique roles, parenting, customs, laws and practices. The parenting of a child is a group or community activity. The biological and non-biological parents and relatives in the community collaborate in the upbringing of the children from conception to marriage. During the physical and mental growth of the child, both the female and male extended family members help to expose the child to the roles and activities of manhood and womanhood. To a greater or lesser extent, boys are exposed to these job functions:

- family,
- hunting,
- blacksmith,
- religious and traditional practices,
- healing, and
- fishing.

Girls are trained to become:

- homemakers,
- farmers,
- gardeners, and
- petty traders.

Healing

The Temne have in place a mutual-aid health system that addresses the health problems of the community. The chief priests and healers provide their services to the needy amongst the population as their contribution to progress and stability. The healers are committed to training young adults in the arts of healing, so that the community can be served on a continuous basis. The method of payment is mostly a barter system or free of charge for minor illnesses.

Enforcement of traditional custom, values and laws

The family is responsible for the enforcement of norms, values, rituals, customs and practices. For instance, marriage is a serious event. The elders and the community teach or orientate those concerned with understanding how to engage in marriage, its seriousness and relationship to the stability of the family and community. Marriages do not occur without the presence of godparents. The functions of the godparents are to orientate, supervise, monitor, co-ordinate, evaluate and correct dysfunctions or deviant behaviours occurring in the marriage, and to promote peace amongst couples. The godparents are sanctioned by the traditional court system and the community to ensure the marriage relationship works. Thus, their authority in the marriage supersedes that of the extended family members and the court.

The Temne system of marriage has some similarities to Islamic customary marriage. The Temne and Islamic groups stress the religious and moral commitment to marriage, and the promotion of a homogeneous community (Jarrett, 1990).

IMPACTS OF THE NON-TRADITIONAL SOCIAL-WELFARE SYSTEM ON THE TEMNE

To describe the impact that the non-traditional social-welfare system has had upon the Temne, it is necessary briefly to set out its structure and functions. The Ministry of Social Welfare and Community Development (MSWCD) currently collaborates with other macro and micro social institutions, including international social agencies, to provide the following services to its targeted populations and communities: (1) informal and formal education; (2) community development and health care; (3) case management; (4) children and family social services; (5) prisons; (6) recreational services; and (7) housing services. To implement appropriately these services, the MSWCD has sanctioned three primary departments: (1) the Department of Social Services (DSS), which mostly operates in the capital, Freetown and other towns; (2) Community Development (CD); and (3) Prison, Sports and Recreation (PSR), which operates nationally.

The core functions of the MSWCD are: (1) to establish a solid social foundation for the CD and DSS national programmes; (2) to build a professional social-welfare institution that helps to combat social problems through intervention, prevention, treatment, rehabilitation and remedial measures; (3) to promote, encourage and develop recreation and sports activities; (4) to improve and expand institutions and services dealing with criminal activities, gerontological services, family and women's issues; (5) to upgrade nutritional and health programmes; (6) to establish facilities for the training of social practitioners who are to be capable of social policy formation, programme design, administration and direct practice and evaluation; and (7) to provide and manage needed services and facilities not mentioned above to tribal groups and communities.

The above-stated objectives in theory appear to be beneficial to the welfare of individuals and ethnic groups in Sierra Leone. Unfortunately, the Sierra Leone MSWCD does not help enrich traditional practices and traditional social-welfare systems of the indigenous groups, especially the Temne. The unresponsiveness of the MSWCD can be a result of: (1) the adoption of a western social-welfare system; (2) its residual social-welfare practices, and (3) the centralized implementation of the social delivery systems adopted by MSWCD.

The above three problem areas are of great consequence in undermining traditional social welfare of the Temne in Sierra Leone. Other factors which have undermined the traditional social-welfare system of the Temne include: (1) education and social-welfare practices; (2) religious social-welfare practices; and (3) medical and medical social-work practices.

Education and social-welfare practices

The transfer of western education and social-work practices helped to disrupt the traditional educational/social practices of the Temne. According to Wiley and Wiley (1974), colonial education and social-work practices helped to destroy the indigenous practices of the Temne. First, the colonial educators and social-work practitioners did not permit indigenous ethnic languages, prayers and cultural practices in the regular schools and social-work training centres. In fact, Temne children of school age were inculcated to think that traditional cultural practices would not be academically and economically rewarding or valuable to them when entering the job market. Second, western educators and social-work practitioners failed to promote the traditional culture of the Temne and other indigenous groups. Rather, they manipulated the Temne to believe in and adopt western social-welfare practices in place of the traditional social-welfare customs. Learning and accepting the western social-welfare practices, especially in a predominantly traditional African cultural environment, is detrimental to the Temne traditional social education, because the primary importance in the Temne culture and social-welfare system is that it belongs to African indigenous history and education. In learning and practising western social welfare, the Temne ethnic group is unable to place its cultural relevance in a framework of its own traditional social welfare and practices. Consequently, for the western social-work practitioner and educator, persuading the Temne group to practise the western social welfare system has been a constant losing battle, since the traditional family is antagonistic to it. For the Temne, the implementation of western social welfare in place of the traditional social-welfare system, especially in the indigenous community, has been viewed as colonial encroachment into the Temne family, culture and traditional and social-support systems (Jarrett, 1991).

Religious social-welfare practices

The eastern religious social-welfare practices are detrimental to the Temne and other indigenous groups in Sierra Leone. One of the greatest strengths of the Temne and other indigenous groups is its moral and religious background, which is linked to Muslim and traditional religious practices. The Muslim and traditional religious practices believed in polygamous and traditional marriages and naming of children with African names.

The most depressing act of religious social-welfare practices is the conversion of the Temne to Christianity. Christianity for the Temne comes with price-tags. The first price-tag is manipulating the converted Temne and families to deviate from their traditional religious practices and socialization processes. The second is the changing of traditional Temne names to predominantly western and middle-eastern names. Third, the converted Temne must get married either in a western court of law or church, or in a combination of both. Fourth, converted Temne are expected not to respect or comply with the Temne traditional marriage customs, especially in the event of separation, or divorce or death. Under colonial and neo-colonial governments, marital disputes by converted Temne are settled in a western court of law. According to Jarrett (1991) and Mazuri (1986), in the event of a polygamous marriage those women who are married according to western custom are viewed as the legitimate wives and the lawful owners of the husband's property in the event of a divorce or death. Fifth, the religious social-welfare practices favour the concept of the nuclear family over that of the extended family. The converted Temne finds himself in a state of confusion, practising a custom that is foreign to him in a society predominantly of extended families. In the extended family society, nuclear family culture and practices are viewed as evil and antagonistic to the extended family culture and practices. Thus, sometimes the converted Temne finds himself isolated or resented by the dominant culture. At times the converted Temne perceives the extended family as inferior and refuses to conform to its practices.

Medical and medical social-work practices

The implementation of western medicine and medical social work (WMSW) in predominantly Temne indigenous communities has not been successful and has proved to be detrimental to traditional Temne health practices. Some of the multiple impacts of WMSW are addressed. First, the Temne and other indigenous ethnic groups utilize traditional medicine in the healing process. The Temne primarily use plants and traditional psychic medicine in this process.

The primary factors promoting the traditional healers' movement are as follows. First, the traditional Temne government supports and sanctions the use of plant and psychic medicine as a valuable service to the people. Second, the collaboration of traditional Temne healers with other ethnic groups is encouraged, with the establishment of botanical gardens, and the identification of new plants and spiritual techniques that will enhance the healing process; and last, the traditional healers do consult western medicine in the healing process (Ministry of Health, 1990). Western medical professionals and the Sierra Leone health policy-makers have not made an effort to integrate traditional health techniques into the health curriculum to be used in the healing process.

Further, the Sierra Leone health and social-welfare professionals failed to invite, incorporate and develop a liaison with the Temne and other indigenous psychic and traditional healers in the provision of health care and medical research, though this approach has been proved to be effective in Ghana and Nigeria. The Ghana Ministry of Health helped in establishing the Centre for Scientific Research into Plant Medicine (CSRPM). The primary objectives of the CSRPM are to integrate African psychic and traditional healers into medical practices, collaborate in the collection, publication and the dissemination of the research results and other useful technical information. The CSRPM is jointly working with traditional healers in the national hospitals and clinics of Ghana and Nigeria.

The reluctance of medical and social-work professionals to integrate and utilize Temne traditional medicine in the healing process has a major disadvantage. There is a neglect on the part of the government to realize that traditional healing constitutes the only source of medical care for the majority of the Temne and indigenous Sierra Leoneans; especially when about 75 per cent of the indigenous population lives in traditionally rural areas (Ministry of Health, 1990). In fact, the development of the health and social delivery systems in Sierra Leone which excludes the improvement of traditional medicine and healing practice cannot, by any stretch of the imagination, be considered adequate (Ministry of Health, 1990; Jarrett, 1989).

Since traditional medicine and healing practices are not yet recognized by the medical and social-welfare professionals in Sierra Leone, inferences can be made that the health-services system is inadequate and detrimental to the Temne traditional psychic and healing system.

SUMMARY AND CONCLUSION

The literature indicates that the Temne migrated from the Fouta D'Jallon mountains of Guinea, West Africa, and were attacked by warlike groups. In addition, historical evidence indicated that the Temne were also warlike, and invaded and displaced other ethnic groups along their migratory route, and during settlement in Sierra Leone. During the initial phase of Temne settlement, the Mende invaded them and influenced their culture, customs and administrative practices.

The western social-welfare system, because of its residual concept of a centralized service-delivery approach, and because of lack of acceptance of the traditional social-welfare and customary practices, has been detrimental to overall Temne growth and development. Education, religion and western practice and medical social work are factors also identified as having a severe impact on the traditional social institutions of the Temne.

At this juncture, the inference can be made that the Temne have experienced multiple problems in Sierra Leone. Thus, it is imperative for scholars to explore avenues of change which will enhance overall positive growth and development for the Temne, and systematic intervention directed towards the rejuvenation of their ethnic identity and their traditional social-welfare system is needed.

First, political institutions must help the Temne rediscover their traditional political practices by discouraging the importation of foreign technologies that are detrimental to their traditional growth and development. Jarrett (1991) states that the political leaders of Sierra Leone must assist the indigenous groups (including the Temne) in disregarding the myth that they can only attain positive growth and development status by adopting foreign political, educational, health, legal, economic and family ideologies. Further, the political system should mandate an education system in which curriculum designers integrate the Temne language and those of other indigenous groups into the school curriculum. In addition, educators must be mandated to teach students in indigenous languages. Such a practice will do away with the myth that English is the only language of instruction, communication and tool of commerce in Sierra Leone (Jarrett, 1989).

Second, the traditional social-welfare systems of the Temne should be rejuvenated. The rationale for their rejuvenation is that the Ministry of Social Welfare in Sierra Leone is not meeting the social-welfare needs of the Temne. Further, the present social-welfare system is in opposition to the traditional social-welfare practices of the Temne. Thus, the government should help the Temne ethnic group promote its traditional social-welfare practices. In addition, Temne customary marriage practices should be sanctioned by the western court of law in Sierra Leone. More or less, the practice of distributive justice, which, at present, accepts and permits all ethnic practices as equal, should be honoured. Not only Christian marriages should be legally accepted in the court of law, but traditional marriages as well, and in making legal decisions about death, divorce and child-support issues. Furthermore, the Temne should look at the transfer of western religious and welfare practices or morals – such as the naming of children, marriages and other religious practices – for inspiration, never for imitation.

Third, the Temne and other indigenous groups healed the sick before the arrival of western health technology. The success of traditional health practices has been remarkable, and thus must be encouraged and promoted by the government, the Temne and other ethnic groups. There should be a collaborative effort in conducting and promoting the traditional healing practices (1) by establishing and decentralizing plant medicine and psychic technology research centres; (2) by liaison with indigenous traditional health practitioners in the collaboration, publication and dissemination of traditional health and western knowledge; (3) by establishing, where necessary, botanical gardens for medical plants, and performing such other functions as the research institutions may be assigned; and (4) by western health practitioners in Sierra Leonean hospitals and clinics allowing the utilization of traditional health medicine and psychic healing practices.

Fourth, since national economic growth and development in Sierra Leone depends on indigenous groups, emphasis should be focused on the economic promotion of ethnic groups. The Temne should, in collaboration with the government and other indigenous groups, formulate, design and establish new resources and uses for economic input. The Temne should collaborate in the promotion of indigenous market systems for accepting and distributing goods (Rubin and Weinstein, 1974). New opportunities for economic input could arise by the mobilization of new sectors, re-orientating economic activity from a local to a national socio-economic market, and by economic education and marketing.

These opportunities could play a vital role in the development of economic growth by involving all indigenous groups in the nation-building process (Rubin and Weinstein, 1974). Moreover, the Temne must develop specialization in the application and development of traditional technologies and the expansion of domestic and foreign trade which will make it possible to integrate a wide range of traditional and foreign resources. Indigenous groups, including the Temne, must be encouraged to produce traditional technology in excess of local consumer demand for the purpose of investment and growth. Currently, they tend to consume virtually all that they produce. Such an antiquated practice helps to diminish the economic growth potential. Consequently, the lack of economic growth potentials systematically affects the growth of the traditional social-welfare system.

Fifth, the cultural and psychological components should be viewed as vital to a progressive Temne ethnic group. According to Jarrett (1991), the understanding of cultural and psychological sensitivity practice is of fundamental importance, for in the last analysis it is on the cultural and psychological perceptions of an ethnic group that everything depends. The Temne must utilize the mutual aid system and extended family practices as agents to promote their cultural and psychological status. In situations where the Temne have to use the cultural and psychological technologies of foreign nations and other indigenous groups, they must modify such technologies to reflect their cultural and psychological practices (Jarrett, 1991).

Finally, the Temne and the government must realize that a systemic approach to addressing the impact of multiple issues on the Temne and their traditional social-welfare system can be simultaneously creative and destructive by providing new opportunities and prospects at a high price, but at the same time creating social and cultural displacement (Jarrett, 1991). Thus, it is imperative that the Temne adopt a three-dimensional conceptual approach to develop a productive culture, concentrating on: (1) environment, (2) organization and (3) institutions.

First, the environment in which the Temne live must be classified as an aspect of culture that has to be permanently reproduced, maintained and managed. The standard of living that is advocated is one that has new meaning – a combination of traditional and western cultural relevance. Further, the cultural tradition must be transmitted from one generation to the next and still maintain the traditional culture of the ancestors.

Second, the organization of the Temne culture and traditional system must be re-analysed, and suggestions for redevelopment made (Malinowski, 1969). Malinowski suggests that for cultural organization to have purpose, or reach any end, '[the Temnes] have to organise . . . Organisation implies a very definite scheme of structure, the main factors of which [are] applicable to all organised groups' (1969: 39).

Finally, the institutionalization of Temne culture is essential in order to perpetuate growth and development nationally. Thus, Temne should restructure the traditional cultural norms and values from which all their social institutions operate. In the institutionalization of culture the Temne must operate on the fact that the environment, which is neither more nor less than culture itself, has to be permanently reproduced, maintained and managed (Malinowski, 1969).

The institutionalization of Temne culture must be included in the macro, meso, and micro policy formation, planning, implementation and evaluation. Further, the Temne and government authorities should encourage educators to instil cultural literacy in all national institutions, by designing and implementing a national core curriculum (Hirsch, 1987).

The suggested intervention strategies are not exhaustive. However, the need to rehabilitate the cultural and traditional systems of the Temne and other indigenous groups in Sierra Leone will definitely contribute to the national growth and development of Sierra Leone.

REFERENCES

Background to Sierra Leone (1990) Freetown: President, State House.

Hirsch, E. D. Jr, (1987) *Cultural Literacy: What Every American Needs to Know*, Boston: Houghton Mifflin.

Jackson, M. (1977) *The Kuranko Dimensions of Social Reality in a West African Society*, New York: St Martin's Press.

Jarrett, A. A. (1984) 'A Curriculum Design for a National School of Social Work in Sierra Leone, West Africa', Ann Arbor, MI: *Dissertation Abstracts International*.

— — (1989) 'Implications of Transferring Social Technology to Developing Nations and Correct Strategies', *Journal of International and Comparative Social Welfare*, 5.

— — (1990) 'The Encroachment of Rural–Urban Migration in Sierra Leone: A Social Perspective', *International Social Work*, 28(1).

— — (1991) 'The Under-development of Africa: Colonialism, Neo-colonialism and Socialism', Manuscript will be published by University Press of America, Lankam, Maryland.

Kup, A. P. (1961) *A History of Sierra Leone 1400–1787*, Cambridge: Cambridge University Press.

Langley, E. R. (1938) 'The Temne: Their Life, Land, and Ways', *Sierra Leone Studies, XVII*.

Little, K. (1967) *The Mende of Sierra Leone: A West African People in Transition*, London: Routledge & Kegan Paul.

McCulloch, M. (1950) *Western Africa Part II: Peoples of Sierra Leone*, London: International Institute.

Malinowski, B. (1969) *A Scientific Theory of Culture and Other Essays*, London: Oxford University Press.

Mazuri, A. A. (1986) *The Africans: A Triple Heritage*, Boston: Little, Brown & Co.

Ministry of Health (1990) *Plant Medicine*, Ghana: Research Institute of Plant Medicine.

Rubin, L. and Weinstein, B. (1974) *Introduction to African Politics: A Continental Approach*, New York: Praeger.

Ulin, R. C. (1988) *Understanding Cultures: Perspective in Anthropology and Social Theory*, Austin, TX: University of Texas Press.

Wiley, M. and Wiley, D. (1974) *The Third World: Africa*, El Monte, CA: Pendulum.

Wylie, K. C. (1977) *The Political Kingdoms of the Temne: Temne Government in Sierra Leone 1825–1910*. London: Africana Publishing Co.

Name index

Subject index

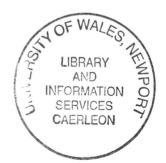
OF WALES
LIBRARY
AND
INFORMATION
SERVICES
CAERLEON

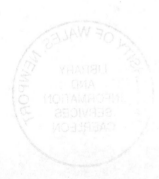